Nursing: Advanced Practice

Nursing: Advanced Practice

Editor: Selina Douglas

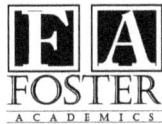

FA
FOSTER
ACADEMICS

www.fosteracademics.com

www.fosteracademics.com

FA
FOSTER
ACADEMICS

Cataloging-in-Publication Data

Nursing : advanced practice / edited by Selina Douglas.
    p. cm.
Includes bibliographical references and index.
ISBN 978-1-64646-148-6
1. Nursing. 2. Nursing--Practice. 3. Care of the sick. I. Douglas, Selina.
RT86.7 .N87 2022
610.73--dc23

Foster Academics,
118-35 Queens Blvd., Suite 400,
Forest Hills, NY 11375, USA

ISBN 978-1-64646-148-6 (Hardback)

Contents

Preface

The main aim of this book is to educate learners and enhance their research focus by presenting diverse topics covering this vast field. This is an advanced book which compiles significant studies by distinguished experts in the area of analysis. This book addresses successive solutions to the challenges arising in the area of application, along with it; the book provides scope for future developments.

Nursing is a health care professional sector concerned with the care of individuals, families, and communities so that they can achieve, recover and maintain quality of life and optimal health. It aims to ensure care for all patients and maintain their credentials, code of ethics, standards, and competencies. Some of the primary branches of nursing are cardiac nursing, perioperative nursing, orthopedic nursing, obstetrical nursing, palliative care, etc. Nursing has the widest range of all healthcare professions. It is divided depending on the needs of the person being nursed. The major populations in nursing are adult-gerontology, paediatrics, neonatal, informatics. This book provides comprehensive insights into the field of nursing. It traces the progress of this field and highlights some of its key concepts and applications. This book is an essential guide for both academicians and those who wish to pursue this discipline further.

It was a great honour to edit this book, though there were challenges, as it involved a lot of communication and networking between me and the editorial team. However, the end result was this all-inclusive book covering diverse themes in the field.

Finally, it is important to acknowledge the efforts of the contributors for their excellent chapters, through which a wide variety of issues have been addressed. I would also like to thank my colleagues for their valuable feedback during the making of this book.

Editor

Practice nurse involvement in primary care depression management

Jodi Gray[1*], Hossein Haji Ali Afzali[1], Justin Beilby[2], Christine Holton[3], David Banham[4] and Jonathan Karnon[1]

Abstract

Background: Most evidence on the effect of collaborative care for depression is derived in the selective environment of randomised controlled trials. In collaborative care, practice nurses may act as case managers. The Primary Care Services Improvement Project (PCSIP) aimed to assess the cost-effectiveness of alternative models of practice nurse involvement in a real world Australian setting. Previous analyses have demonstrated the value of high level practice nurse involvement in the management of diabetes and obesity. This paper reports on their value in the management of depression.

Methods: General practices were assigned to a low or high model of care based on observed levels of practice nurse involvement in clinical-based activities for the management of depression (i.e. percentage of depression patients seen, percentage of consultation time spent on clinical-based activities). Linked, routinely collected data was used to determine patient level depression outcomes (proportion of depression-free days) and health service usage costs. Standardised depression assessment tools were not routinely used, therefore a classification framework to determine the patient's depressive state was developed using proxy measures (e.g. symptoms, medications, referrals, hospitalisations and suicide attempts). Regression analyses of costs and depression outcomes were conducted, using propensity weighting to control for potential confounders.

Results: Capacity to determine depressive state using the classification framework was dependent upon the level of detail provided in medical records. While antidepressant medication prescriptions were a strong indicator of depressive state, they could not be relied upon as the sole measure. Propensity score weighted analyses of total depression-related costs and depression outcomes, found that the high level model of care cost more (95% CI: -$314.76 to $584) and resulted in 5% less depression-free days (95% CI: -0.15 to 0.05), compared to the low level model. However, this result was highly uncertain, as shown by the confidence intervals.

Conclusions: Classification of patients' depressive state was feasible, but time consuming, using the classification framework proposed. Further validation of the framework is required. Unlike the analyses of diabetes and obesity management, no significant differences in the proportion of depression-free days or health service costs were found between the alternative levels of practice nurse involvement.

Keywords: Depression, Practice nurse, Primary care, Collaborative care, Cost-effectiveness, RAC-E analysis

* Correspondence: jodi.gray@adelaide.edu.au
[1]Discipline of Public Health, The University of Adelaide, Adelaide, South Australia
Full list of author information is available at the end of the article

Background

Globally, depression is the most common mental health disorder with a point prevalence between four and ten percent [1]. Depression has been identified as a health priority area in many countries, including Australia. It is estimated that 11.6% of Australians have experienced a depressive episode at some point in their life [2] and depression costs the Australian economy AU$14.9 billion per year [3]. Depression is the second most frequently managed chronic problem in Australian general practice [4].

Multiple systematic reviews and meta-analyses have found that collaborative care for depression is effective [5-7], and cost-effective [8,9]. Collaborative care involves a team based approach, where team members include the primary care physician (GP), a case manager (often a practice nurse) and a mental health specialist (e.g. psychiatrist, psychologist). The case manager's role includes the systematic identification, management and follow-up of depressed patients. Adequate mental health training for the case manager was found to be a key determinant of effectiveness. The Australian Government offers financial incentives for general practices to employ practice nurses and to expand and enhance their role within the practice [10]. A practice nurse is a qualified nurse employed by a general practice to provide nursing management under the supervision of a general practitioner. The number of practice nurses in Australia increased from 3,255 in 2003–04 to 10,085 in 2009–10, with 58% of practices employing a practice nurse [11]. In 2009–10, Government practice nurse incentives totalled AU$55.3 million [12]. To date, studies of the Australian practice nurse workforce have been mainly descriptive, with little focus on models of practice or determining impact on health outcomes [13].

In Australia, the TrueBlue randomised control trial is the main study of practice nurse management of depression [14-16]. It examined clinical outcomes (e.g. reduction in depression score) associated with practice nurse led collaborative care for the management of moderate to severe depression comorbid with type 2 diabetes or coronary heart disease. The intervention comprised intensive training, supporting materials, access to a local facilitator, and monthly peer-support teleconferences. While both the intervention and control groups demonstrated a significant reduction in depression intensity after six months, the reduction was significantly larger in the intervention group.

As with the TrueBlue study, internationally, much of the evidence on the effectiveness of nurse involvement in collaborative care has been gathered via RCTs [5-7]. However, limitations exist, particularly when evaluating health care interventions with complex treatment pathways that are best represented as models of care. Questions remain about the external validity of RCTs conducted under highly controlled conditions with carefully selected patient populations [17]. Compared to RCTs, observational studies can offer greater external validity, and determine the effectiveness of interventions as applied in a real world setting.

Risk adjusted cost-effectiveness (RAC-E) is a method of analysis for identifying important differences in routinely provided services. RAC-E analysis has previously been applied to hospital services [18]. The Primary Care Services Improvement Project (PCSIP) was a retrospective observational study, which used RAC-E methods to assign general practices to models of care based on observed differences in practice nurse activity in the provision of clinical-based services. Three case studies were conducted [19,20], with this paper reporting on the depression case study.

RAC-E analysis uses routinely collected data to identify patient characteristics, and to track health outcomes and health care costs. Standardised assessment tools for depression are not consistently used within general practice or recorded in routine data. While previous studies have used proxy measures, such as antidepressant prescriptions, there is no clearly defined methodology to determine depressive state in the absence of standardised assessment tools or diagnostic interview [21-23]. As an illustrative case study of a RAC-E analysis, the PCSIP aimed to evaluate whether, from the perspective of the health-care system, a high level model of practice nurse involvement in the management of depression in primary care was more cost-effective than a low level model of practice nurse involvement. A secondary aim was to develop and test the feasibility of a depression state classification framework for use with routinely collected, general practice data. This paper describes the methodology developed to classify the depression status of patients, and reports the within trial cost-effectiveness findings of the RAC-E analysis.

Methods

Practice recruitment and classification of model of care

The recruitment of general practices and patients has been described in detail elsewhere [24]. Practices were recruited from within the Adelaide Northern Division of General Practice (ANDGP), which is located in the northern suburbs of metropolitan Adelaide, South Australia. All 66 practices in the ANDGP were contacted. Ten practices with practice nurses agreed to participate in the PCSIP.

Practice nurses within the participating practices were surveyed to determine their level of involvement in clinical-based activities in the management of depression (e.g. patient education, self-management advice, monitoring of treatment adherence). Level of involvement was determined based on two questions within the survey: (1) What is your best estimate of the percentage of patients with

DEPRESSION that are seen by you [i.e. the practice nurse] in your practice? (2) In an average consultation with a DE-PRESSED patient, what percentage of time do you spend providing education and self-management advice, monitoring clinical progress, and assessing and enhancing treatment adherence? Where the average response of the practice nurses within a practice was greater than 50% on both these questions, the practice was considered to show a high level of practice nurse involvement and assigned to the high level model of care. If high level criteria were not met, the practice was assigned to the low level model of care.

To identify any further differences between the models of care, the following were also analysed: responses to other questions in the practice nurse survey regarding the practice environment and practice nurse characteristics (e.g. age, gender, education and experience); billing of Medicare service item number 10997, which covers 'provision of monitoring and support for a person with a chronic disease by a practice nurse or Aboriginal and Torres Strait Islander health practitioner' [25]; and the billing of Medicare mental health service item numbers (2702, 2710 and 2712), which covered preparation and review of mental health care plans by GPs.

Patient recruitment

Within participating practices, eligible patients were identified using the Pen Computer Systems Clinical Audit Tool (CAT). The CAT tool identified patients who had a diagnosis of depression listed in their medical history summary. This meant we were more likely to select patients who had experienced depression severe enough to warrant a diagnosis and ongoing monitoring or intervention, rather than patients with a milder, transient experience of 'feeling depressed' (which would be recorded in the general consultation notes). Eligible patients were aged between 18 and 75 years, regularly visited the practice (i.e. at least 3 times in the last 2 years), were not under regular psychiatric care, not pregnant, not living in a managed care facility and did not have a severe mental disorder or mental impairment (e.g. schizophrenia, bipolar disorder, or dementia). After recruitment, but prior to data analysis, eligibility criteria were further refined to exclude patients for whom less than 50% of their GP visits during the study period were to the participating practice (as indicated by Medicare billing of GP visit item numbers). Patients were asked for consent to access their medical records held by the participating general practice, Medicare Australia (the federal government department which organises and distributes payment for Australia's publically funded, universal health care system) and SA Health. There was no intervention within the study design. Sample size calculations estimated that 100 patients per model of care were required, details of calculations have been provided elsewhere [24].

Ethics approval was granted by the Human Research Ethics Committees of the University of Adelaide and SA Health (the South Australian Department of Health).

Data sources and data collection

Data were collected for the period between October 2007 and October 2010 from three sources: patient medical records held at general practices, Medicare Australia, and SA Health.

Patient medical records provided information on patient characteristics (e.g. age, gender, comorbidities), referrals to specialists and allied health professionals, prescriptions written, GP management plans prepared or reviewed, scores on any standardised assessment tools for depression and general medical notes. Record information was extracted from the practice and entered directly into a purpose built Access 2007 database (Microsoft Office 2007, Microsoft Corporation), with identifying information removed.

Medicare Australia provided data on out-of-hospital health service usage and costs, including GP visits, management plan preparation or review, psychological services provided under the Better Access Initiative, specialist visits, and prescriptions provided under the government subsidised Pharmaceutical Benefits Scheme (PBS). Unit costs were allocated as per the year incurred. SA Health provided information on public and private inpatient hospital services, to which 2008–09 average diagnosis related group (DRG) costs were applied. The evaluation took the perspective of the health-care system, thus only direct health-care costs were included.

Data from each source were cleaned, formatted and linked to create comprehensive individual patient records.

Classification of depression state

To track the progression of depression, the depression state of each patient needed to be categorised throughout the study period. Standardised assessment tools for depression, such as the DASS-21 or the Hamilton Rating Scale for Depression, were not routinely used or recorded within the obtained data, therefore proxy measures had to be developed.

A proposed model structure (Figure 1) for cost-effectiveness analyses of depression management includes six clinically and economically relevant depression-related states, based on the natural history of depression [23].

Howell [26] published a 'Case note audit form', which was used to identify relapse in depression patients from general practice medical records. The audit form contained detailed lists of depression symptoms, treatment options, depression-related medications and mental health services to which a patient could be referred. In a prior publication [23], we suggested a method of incorporating changes to treatment and GP notes as proxy

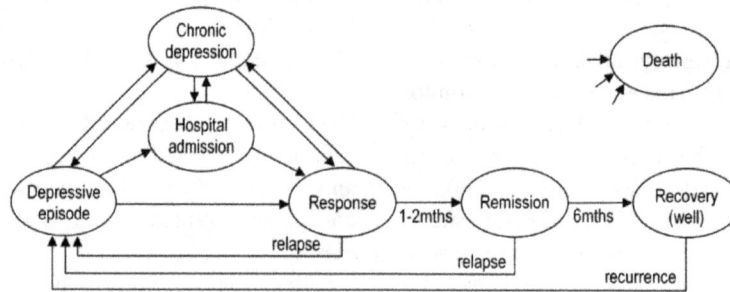

Figure 1 Depression model showing depressive states and transitions. Ovals indicate states, arrows indicate transitions between states. Patients may transition into the death state from any other state (i.e. all cause mortality). Adapted from [23].

measures from which to determine a range of depressive states beyond relapse. In practice the proposed method required simplification in order to apply, resulting in the following conceptualisation of the symptoms and timing of depressive states:

- Depressive episode – significant symptom intensity described, with impact on daily living.
- Chronic depression – low or moderate symptoms of depression are recorded and appear to have been present for two or more years.
- Hospital admission – where the reason for admission is depression-related. Reason for admission may be determined via general notes in the GP records, discharge summaries provided to the GP, or diagnosis related data provided by SA Health.
- Response – patient experiences a substantial reduction in depressive symptoms (e.g. symptoms appear to 'halve'). Response period is considered to last a minimum of eight weeks, but may last longer if symptoms remain reduced but do not fully abate.
- Remission – patient is symptom free or experiences very minimal symptoms. Remission is considered to last for six months following response.
- Recovery – a patient who remains asymptomatic and has spent six months in the remission state is considered to transition into the recovery state.

In addition to the symptom intensity and timing described above, antidepressant medications, psychology and psychiatry referrals, emergency department referrals or suicide attempts were also incorporated. Further details on the classification process are provided in the appendix (see Additional file 1).

While the analyses described in this paper ultimately required the classification of only two states – depression or depression-free – it was intended that the dataset would also be used to populate a decision analytic model based on the proposed model structure. Hence, it was important that the classification system be able to identify all six depressive states shown in Figure 1, and

that the proposed model structure was congruent with the observed data.

Analysis

All analyses were undertaken using STATA, Release 12 (StataCorp). The duration of a patient's participation in the study was calculated as the number of days between the first and last visits at which the patient's depressive state could be determined.

The number of depression-free days were calculated as the total number of days spent in either the remission or recovery states. In all other states, including response, the patient experienced some degree of depression. For each patient, the proportion of depression-free days (pDFDs) were calculated as the total number of depression-free days, divided by the number of days the patient participated in the study. Health service costs were calculated per patient for the participation period.

Both unadjusted and adjusted multiple regression analyses were undertaken to determine differences between models of care in the pDFDs experienced and health service costs. To adjust for potential confounders, propensity score weighted analyses were used [27]. Variables considered as potential covariates in the logistic regression model included: patient age, gender, marital status, socioeconomic status (based on postcode level census data (SEIFA score)), concessional status, relevant physical comorbidites (myocardial infarction, ischemic heart disease, congestive heart failure, stroke, cancer, diabetes, respiratory disease, musculoskeletal conditions and chronic pain), relevant psychological comorbidities (alcohol or drug abuse, gambling addiction, postnatal depression, anxiety disorder, post traumatic stress disorder, obsessive compulsive disorder, eating disorders, and social or other phobia), measures of practice loyalty (the length of time since the patient first attended the practice, the proportion of visits to a GP during the study that were at the participating practice, and the number of practices attended during the study), depression history (the length of time since the first recorded depressive episode (which may or may not have been prior to the study period), and the depressive state at the start of the study period) and the number of days the patient participated in the study.

The distribution of pDFD contained distinct peaks at both 0 and 1, and so a propensity weighted zero one inflated beta (ZOIB) model, with clustering of patients by practice, was used for the adjusted analysis [28,29]. This model contains three components: two separate logistic regression models to predict whether the proportion is equal to 0 or 1, and a beta model to predict proportions between 0 and 1. Variables considered as potential covariates included those listed above, as well as GP characteristics (age, gender, experience, and the number of training sessions in depression undertaken in the previous two years), practice characteristics (bulk billing behaviour, practice size as measured by the number of GPs, and the number of depression patients attending the practice (defined as the number of eligible depression patients identified during the patient recruitment CAT search)) and the model of care. Model fit was determined using the Ramsey RESET test.

Adjusted analyses of health service costs were undertaken, by fitting generalised linear models (GLMs), which allowed for weighting using average treatment effect (ATE) weights [27] and clustering by general practice. The same variables, as listed for the ZOIB model, were considered as potential covariates. Goodness of fit was determined using the modified Park test (for the GLM family) and the Pearson correlation test, the Pregibon link test, and the modified Hosmer and Lemeshow test (for the GLM link) [30]. Total costs were analysed including and excluding hospital costs, to determine whether hospital costs were an important driver of expenditure. A bootstrapping approach (one thousand bootstrap samples) was applied to represent the uncertainty around the mean outcome and cost estimates.

Results

Ten general practices with practice nurses were recruited to the PCSIP. One practice was later excluded as only one patient with depression could be recruited from this practice. On the basis of the practice nurse survey, six practices were allocated to the low level model of care and three to the high level model. Across the nine practices, 208 depression patients were initially recruited. The response rates were 33% (124 patients) and 30% (84 patients) for the low and high level models of care, respectively.

Depression state classification

During data extraction and the subsequent classification process, 54 of the 208 recruited patients (25 from the high level model, 29 from the low level model) were excluded from the study. Exclusions occurred as it became apparent from the extracted data that these patients did not meet the defined inclusion criteria (e.g. they were not depression patients but instead had a primary diagnosis of anxiety or had experienced symptoms indicative of psychosis, received regular psychiatric care, were living in managed accommodation, the participating practice was not the patients' main practice, or the first categorised visit was beyond the study period).

The level of detail provided in medical notes regarding the patients' experience of depression symptoms and their severity varied between practices and GPs. Chronic depression was particularly difficult to identify, while depressive episodes, having higher symptom intensity and greater functional impairment, appeared to be better documented. In instances where medical notes were less detailed, some states had to be inferred. An assumption was made that symptoms were not present if not recorded, however the reality may be that symptoms remained at lower levels. Where patients stated they had experienced 'long standing depression', details of the depression history were generally not provided, and we were unable to determine if the patient experienced episodes of depression interspersed with periods of wellness, or prolonged periods of depression with unremitting symptoms (i.e. chronic depression).

Where present, distressing life events (both current and historical) and comorbid conditions (such as anxiety, alcoholism, chronic pain or musculoskeletal injury) often appeared to interact with, exacerbate or share symptoms with depression. Thus it was challenging to differentiate the course of a comorbidity from the course of a depressive episode, particularly if, after initially noting concurrent depression, the medical notes focussed predominantly on the comorbidity.

While changes to antidepressant prescriptions provided a strong indicator of the course of a depressive episode, limitations applied. Despite being offered, some patients experiencing a depressive episode were unwilling to take antidepressant medications. Some antidepressants and mood stabilising medications were prescribed for non-depression-related reasons, for example amitriptyline for management of neuropathic pain or sodium valproate for epilepsy. Patient compliance varied, with some patients ceasing, decreasing or increasing dosages independent of medical advice. Medications could be ceased or dosages reduced due to side-effects or affordability, rather than symptom abatement, and reasons for changes were not always provided. These findings suggest that antidepressant prescriptions have limited use as a sole indicator of depressive state.

While most patients followed pathways congruent with the proposed depression model structure (Figure 1), three did not. One patient experienced a rapid onset of depression and anxiety symptoms due to life events, resulting in a transition directly from the recovery (well) state to a hospital admission. Two patients transitioned from a hospital admission to a depressive episode, rather than the response state as proposed. No patients died during the study period.

Practice, GP and practice nurse characteristics

Characteristics of practices and practice nurses are shown in Table 1. While no practice nurses reported specific qualifications in the field of mental health care, practice nurses in high level model practices attended significantly more training sessions for depression in the previous two years (1.33 sessions), compared with practice nurses in low level model practices (0.38 sessions, p = 0.04). No other significant differences in practice or practice nurse characteristics were found.

Patient characteristics

Patient characteristics for the 99 patients from low level model practices and 55 patients from high level model practices participating in the PCSIP are shown in Table 2. In the unweighted (before adjustment) analysis, significant differences (p < 0.05) existed between the models in

terms of the socioeconomic status of the patient, the duration of attendance at the participating practice, and duration of study follow-up.

The application of propensity weights reduced differences between the two models for all but two patient characteristics (gender, and whether the patient was in a depressive state at the start of the study) and attained standardised differences of less than 0.1, indicating negligible differences [31], for five of the twelve characteristics. The subsequent use of propensity weighted regression further controls for those variables with standardised differences greater than 0.1.

Outcomes and costs

Unadjusted analyses found no significant differences in the pDFDs between the high and low level models of care (Table 3). Medicare out-of-hospital costs were significantly higher for the high level model compared to the low level model (high level = $2039, low level = $1502, p = 0.005), as were total depression-related costs (high level = $2374, low level = $1750, p = 0.01).

Adjusted analyses found no significant difference in pDFDs or costs between the models of care (Table 3).

Table 1 Practice, GP and practice nurse characteristics by model of care

	Low level model	High level model	p value
Practice characteristics (mean)			
Number of practices in model	6	3	
Number of GPs	6.00	2.67	0.11
Total number of patients with depression	398.83	235.00	0.47
GP age (years)	45.70	46.11	0.94
GP experience (years)	19.04	20.89	0.77
GP gender (proportion male)	0.70	0.72	0.93
Number of depression-related training sessions attended by GPs in last 2 years	1.69	2.11	0.42
Practices bulk bill[1] (proportion):			
all patients	0.50	1.00	
concession/pension card patients only	0.50	0.00	0.13
Billing of Medicare mental health item numbers (items per patient year)[2]	0.37	0.34	0.78
Practice nurse (PN) characteristics (mean per practice)			
Number of PNs in model	13	3	
Number FTE[3] PNs per GP	0.24	0.27	0.70
PN age (years)	49.92	46.33	0.40
Experience working as a PN (years)	6.20	9.17	0.55
Experience working as a PN in the participating practice (years)	5.13	3.50	0.68
Number of depression-related training sessions attended by PNs in last 2 years	0.38	1.33	0.04
Billing of Medicare item number 10997 (items per patient year)[4]	0.08	0.06	0.64

[1]The Medicare benefit paid for the visit is accepted as the full fee, therefore there is no out of pocket expense for the patient. [2]Included mental health item numbers cover preparation of a GP mental health care plan by a medical practitioner (2702, 2710), and review of a GP Mental Health Treatment plan (2712). [3]FTE: full time equivalent. [4]Item number 10997 covers 'provision of monitoring and support to people with a chronic disease by a practice nurse or registered Aboriginal Health Worker on behalf of a GP'.

Table 2 Patient characteristics, before and after propensity score weighting

	Before adjustment			After adjustment[1]		
	Low level model[2]	High level model[2]	St. difference (p value)[3]	Low level model	High level model	St. difference (p value)
Age (years)	52.56	51.14	0.12 (0.49)	50.13	51.00	−0.07 (0.70)
Gender (male)	0.24	0.28	−0.11 (0.53)	0.19	0.25	−0.14 (0.37)
Married or defacto relationship	0.49	0.38	0.22 (0.20)	0.40	0.40	−0.001 (0.996)
Concessional patient	0.80	0.68	0.28 (0.10)	0.66	0.70	−0.10 (0.68)
SEIFA score[4]	854.24	905.08	−0.70 (0.00)	877.86	887.05	−0.13 (0.60)
Time since first recorded depressive episode (days)	824.91	1226.00	−0.32 (0.06)	1068.46	1135.63	−0.05 (0.78)
In a depressive state at start of study[5]	0.60	0.52	0.17 (0.31)	0.66	0.56	0.20 (0.26)
Pre-study chronic condition[6]	0.58	0.52	0.13 (0.43)	0.51	0.51	−0.01 (0.96)
Pre-study psychological condtion[7]	0.15	0.18	−0.10 (0.57)	0.16	0.17	−0.03 (0.89)
Time attending the practice (days)	816.58	1564.69	−0.65 (0.00)	1118.51	1280.96	−0.14 (0.52)
Percentage of GP visits in the study period to the participating practice	0.94	0.93	0.15 (0.39)	0.94	0.93	0.11 (0.50)
Time in study (days)	799.02	882.05	−0.38 (0.02)	812.96	843.78	−0.14 (0.54)

[1]Adjustment is based on propensity score weighted analysis. [2]Low level model includes 99 patients, high level model includes 55 patients. [3]Standardised difference is the difference between the means for the low and high level practices divided by the standard deviation (p value is for differences). [4]SEIFA is the Socio-Economic Index for Areas (lower scores indicate more disadvantage, Australia wide scores are standardised to a mean of 1000). [5]Depressive states include depressive episode, chronic depression, hospital admission for depression, or response. [6]Pre-study chronic conditions include myocardial infarction, ischemic heart disease, congestive heart failure, stroke, cancer (excluding skin cancer), diabetes, respiratory disease (e.g. asthma, COPD), musculoskeletal conditions (e.g. arthritis) and chronic pain. [7]Pre-study psychological conditions include alcohol or drug abuse, gambling addiction, postnatal depression, anxiety disorder, post traumatic stress disorder, obsessive compulsive disorder, eating disorders, and social or other phobia.

Based on the mean adjusted estimates of the primary cost measure (total depression-related costs) and outcome variable (proportion of depression-free days), the high-level practice nurse model of care was shown to cost more and resulted in 5% less depression-free days than the low level model. However, this result is highly uncertain. A bootstrapped sensitivity analysis generated a 95% confidence interval that ranged from 15% less to 5% more depression-free days for the high level model of care, with a cost difference ranging from minus $314.76 to $584.00 more.

A cost-effectiveness plane, showing five thousand bootstrapped samples, was generated to demonstrate the uncertainty (Figure 2). While the sampled values spread across all four segments of the plane, 62% are positioned in the north west quadrant, in which the high level model is more costly and less effective than the low level model.

Discussion

This study has reported on the application of a framework to classify depression-related states of health using

Table 3 Unadjusted and adjusted costs and outcomes per alternative models of care

Variables	Before adjustment				After adjustment[1]	
	Low level model	High level model	High level minus low level model mean difference (95% CI)	p value	High level minus low level model mean difference (95% CI)	p value
Proportion of depression-free days (mean)	0.55	0.51	−0.04 (−0.17 to 0.09)	0.54	−0.05 (−0.15 to 0.05)	0.31
Medicare out-of-hospital costs	$1502	$2039	$537 (165 to 909)	0.005	$33 (−270 to 337)	0.83
Total pharmaceutical[2] costs	$1185	$1389	$204 (−340 to 749)	0.46	$147 (−161 to 456)	0.35
Total depression-related pharmaceutical costs[3]	$156	$171	$14 (−50 to 79)	0.65	$41 (−7 to 89)	0.09
Total hospital costs	$1964	$1525	-$439 (−1513 to 636)	0.42	$181 (−742 to 1103)	0.70
Total depression-related hospital costs	$92	$164	$72 (−206 to 351)	0.61	—	—
Total costs	$4652	$4954	$302 (−1155 to 1760)	0.68	$574 (−487 to 1635)	0.29
Total depression-related costs[4]	$1750	$2374	$624 (150 to 1098)	0.01	$135 (−315 to 584)	0.56

[1]Adjustment is based on propensity score weighted analysis. [2]For all pharmaceuticals supplied under the Pharmaceutical Benefits Scheme (PBS). [3]Antidepressant medications supplied under the PBS. [4]Total depression-related costs = Medicare out-of-hospital costs + total depression-related pharmaceutical costs + total depression-related hospital costs.

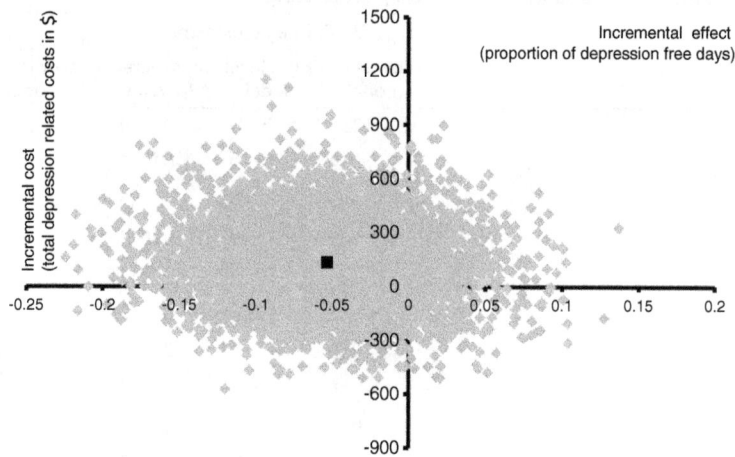

Figure 2 Cost-effectiveness plane. Incremental (high level minus low level model) costs and effects after adjustment. Black square shows mean values.

routinely collected clinical data from a range of sources. The resulting classifications informed a cost-effectiveness analysis of alternative levels of involvement of practice nurses in the care of patients with depression in an Australian primary health care setting.

The process of manually categorising depressive state was time consuming, but feasible using the protocol described. Almost all observed transitions between states followed pathways consistent with the proposed depression model, suggesting strong congruence between the proposed model structure and the observed data.

Variation in the level of detail provided in general practice medical notes may have been a source of potential bias, especially as it was necessary to assume that the absence of notes regarding depressive symptoms indicated the absence of symptoms. This is of particular concern for chronic depression, where persistent low to moderate level symptoms may be less likely to be recorded, especially by GPs who are providing a lower intensity of depression care.

In future applications, the inclusion of a measure of uncertainty for each classified state may be one way of quantifying bias in the classification process. For example, adding a notation on whether a state was allocated based on multiple indicators, a single indicator or via time-based assumptions only.

The classification framework expands on methods used in previous studies, which have classified depressive state based solely on the antidepressant prescription information available in routinely collected medical records [21,22]. For example, Sicras-Mainer et al. [22] defined patients as entering remission after completing six months of antidepressant therapy. Discontinuation of the antidepressant was not considered evidence of remission as patients may discontinue for other reasons, or continue treatment for prolonged periods despite

being asymptomatic. Comparing remission identified via antidepressant use and remission identified through a review of a random sample of patient medical records, Sicras-Mainer et al. found high concordance between the two measures. Details of how remission was determined in the medical record review were not supplied. Nordstrom et al. [21] determined depressive relapse on the basis of an antidepressant prescription received within one to six months of ceasing an antidepressant.

The PCSIP found that, while changes to antidepressant prescriptions provided an indication of depressive state, there were limitations to using them as a sole means of classification. For example, cross-referencing Medicare and general practice data found that not all prescriptions written were supplied under the PBS. Patient medical notes also indicated that not all antidepressant prescriptions were written to treat depressive symptoms. This is consistent with the findings of the Bettering the Evaluation and Care of Health (BEACH) programme [32], which continually surveys general practice activity across Australia. The BEACH programme found only 70% of antidepressant prescriptions were for depression. The remaining 30% were prescribed for other psychological issues, such as anxiety, phobias, or eating disorders, or for non-psychological issues, such as musculoskeletal and neurological problems.

Further work is required to validate the developed classification framework. This will require a comparison of classifications based on routinely collected data sources with classifications based on either diagnostic interview of patients or responses to standardised depression assessment tools taken independently of routine practice at regular time intervals. Threshold values on these tools are commonly used to define depression states (such as response, remission, recurrence) in RCT based modelling studies [33,34].

Strengths of the PCSIP include: the assessment of the level of practice nurse involvement, rather than assessing only the presence or absence of a practice nurse; the allocation of general practices to models of care based on existing differences, rather than through the imposition of an intervention, allowing the study to examine the real world impact; and the classification of depression state using the framework derived, rather than relying on medication changes alone.

The study was subject to some limitations, including: the relatively small sample size, particularly given the high level model did not reach the numbers indicated by the sample size calculation; the allocation of practices to models of care based on the subjective responses of practice nurses; and the observational study design which, despite the rigorous methods used to minimise bias due to observed confounders (i.e. combined use of propensity score weighting and regression analyses), still had an associated likelihood of unobserved confounding between the two models of care (for example, unknown differences in the number of previous depressive episodes, or occurrence of stressful life events). Unobserved differences in the characteristics of patients consenting and not consenting to participate in the study may have resulted in a selection bias, which would reduce the representativeness of the sample population to the general depression population. Cost values were not discounted over the three year time horizon and Medicare costs remained in the unit cost of the year incurred, rather than being re-estimated for a single base year. Given the relatively short time horizon of the study, the consistency in cost allocation methods across the models of care and the small difference in costs found, this is unlikely to have had a significant effect on the findings of the study.

In interpreting the finding of no significant difference in costs and outcomes between the models of care it is pertinent to consider that, although practice nurses in the high level model attended more depression related training sessions, none of the practice nurses in the study had formal qualifications in mental health care or experience working in a mental health nurse role. Information was not collected on the duration of training sessions attended, however, at the time of the study, the majority of training sessions for practice nurses were provided by the ANDGP. These consisted of evening education sessions lasting approximately two and a half hours (ANDGP, personal communication, 17 May 2011). Therefore, the actual difference in the number of hours of training may equate to as little as two and a half hours over the two years. Thus, the result may reflect similar, low levels of mental health training across both models of care. Although the study did not include a 'no practice nurse' model of care, the findings imply that

practice nurses with low levels of training in mental health have a limited effect on the outcomes of patients with depression.

Existing evidence indicates that the inclusion of case managers, who are often nurses, in collaborative care for depression is effective [5-7] and cost-effective [8]. However, it is vitally important that nurses engaged in this role receive adequate training and ongoing support [5,7]. Effectiveness is further improved if the nurse is able to provide psychological therapies as a part of enhanced care [6]. For example, the IMPACT method includes 4 days of training, 30 sessions with 'training patients' and 15 supervised sessions with videotape review. The nurse is then able to provide patient education, discuss treatment options, conduct follow-up and deliver a 6 to 8 session psychotherapy based intervention [35]. The TrueBlue study, which translates the IMPACT methodology to the Australian setting, provides 2 days of training, though this covers chronic disease management for diabetes and heart disease, as well as depression care (screening and counselling). Practice nurses were also given case management templates that provided written protocols for "gold-standard" depression management, as well as ongoing expert and peer support [14-16]. Since 2007, the Mental Health Nurse Incentive Program (MHNIP) has provided incentives for Australian general practices, private psychiatry practices and Indigenous health services to employ a credentialed mental health nurse [36]. In 2012, there were 1,153 credentialed mental health nurses in Australia and the MHNIP had been taken up by 470 organisations [37]. Unfortunately, none were employed in the ANDGP area at the time of the PCSIP to enable comparison with generalist practice nurses.

Despite the limitations, and in line with previous studies, the PCSIP findings suggest that practice nurses involved in the management of patients with depression require specific training in mental health. They suggest that without focused training and support, it is not an efficient use of scarce nursing time to promote greater involvement of generalist nurses in the care of depressed patients. Training may range from two days (the TrueBlue study) to a university awarded postgraduate qualification with additional work experience (mental health nurse credential required to receive the MHNIP). Other RAC-E studies have shown that greater practice nurse involvement in the care of patients with diabetes and obesity is cost-effective [19,20]. Thus, in primary care settings where no specific framework for mental health training and support has been provided, practice nurse time might be better targeted towards diabetic or obese patient groups.

The general methods used in the PCSIP, including the application of the RAC-E methodology and the depression state classification framework, demonstrate the feasibility of evaluating real world interventions in the primary care setting. The non-significant differences found in outcomes and costs illustrate the value of such evaluations, particularly for those involved in policy and planning decisions, such as expansion or redirection of financial incentives.

Conclusions

This study has shown that it is feasible to classify depression status based on routinely collected clinical data collated from multiple sources. Further research is required to validate the described classification process, and findings should be interpreted with some caution until this has been done.

This paper used data from a retrospective observational study based on routinely collected data. It has reported small and non-significant differences in health service costs and proportions of depression-free days between patients attending general practices in which practice nurses were defined as having a high level of involvement in the clinical care of depression patients, and practices with a low level of practice nurse involvement. Further research might focus on the costs and effects of different levels of training and support for practice nurses in a mental health role and the use of specialist mental health nurses in routine general practice.

Abbreviations

AD: Antidepressant; ANDGP: Adelaide Northern Division of General Practice; ATE weights: Average treatment effect; DRG: Diagnosis related group; ED: Emergency department; FTE: Full time equivalent; GLM: Generalised linear model; GP: General practitioner; MHNIP: Mental Health Nurse Incentive Program; PBS: Pharmaceutical Benefits Scheme; PCSIP: Primary Care Services Improvement Project; pDFDs: Proportion of depression-free days; PN: Practice nurse; RAC-E: Risk adjusted cost-effectiveness; RCT: Randomised controlled trial; SA Health: The South Australian Department of Health; SEIFA: Socio-Economic Index for Areas; St. difference: Standardised difference; ZOIB: Zero one inflated beta.

Competing interests

There are no known competing interests for any of the authors in relation to the work presented in this paper.

Authors' contributions

All authors contributed to study design, interpretation of results and drafting of manuscript. In addition: JK was responsible for study conception and organisation; JG performed data extraction; HH conducted the classification of model of care; HH and JG designed the classification framework and performed depression state classification; JG performed the statistical analysis, advised by JK and HH; JG completed the first draft of the manuscript. All authors read and approved the final manuscript.

Acknowledgements

This research was funded by grants from the Australian Research Council (ARC) and our research partners, SA Health and the Central Northern Adelaide Health Service. We received strong support from the ANDGP, in particular CEOs Barbara Magin and Deb Lee and the eHealth Data Support Officer, Jodie Pycroft. Statistical advice was provided by Professor Phil Ryan and Thomas Sullivan, and general advice was provided by Wendy Sutton, manager of the GP Plus Health Care Centre in Elizabeth. We would like to thank the general practices and patients who participated, and acknowledge the support of Woolworths in supplying discounted gift cards which were offered to patients during recruitment.

Author details

[1]Discipline of Public Health, The University of Adelaide, Adelaide, South Australia. [2]Faculty of Health Sciences, The University of Adelaide, Adelaide, South Australia. [3]Discipline of General Practice, The University of Adelaide, Adelaide, South Australia. [4]Office for Research Development, Health System Performance Division, SA Health, Adelaide, South Australia.

References

1. Paykal ES, Brugha T, Fryers T: Size and burden of depressive disorders in Europe. Eur Neuropsychopharmacol 2005, 15:411–423.
2. Australian Bureau of Statistics (ABS): National Survey of Mental Health and Wellbeing: Summary of results, Australia 2007. Canberra; 2008.
3. Department of Health and Ageing (DoHA): Programs - beyondblue - the National Depression Initiative. http://www.health.gov.au/internet/main/publishing.nsf/content/mental-beyond.
4. Britt H, Miller GC, Charles J, Henderson J, Bayram C, Pan Y, Valenti L, Harrison C, O'Halloran J, Zhang C, et al: General practice activity in Australia 2010–11. Sydney: Sydney University Press; 2011.
5. Bower P, Gilbody S, Richards D, Fletcher J, Sutton A: Collaborative care for depression in primary care. Making sense of a complex intervention: systematic review and meta-regression. Br J Psychiatry 2006, 189:484–493.
6. Christensen H, Griffiths KM, Gulliver A, Clack D, Kljakovic M, Wells L: Models in the delivery of depression care: a systematic review of randomised and controlled intervention trials. BMC Fam Pract 2008, 9:25.
7. Thota AB, Sipe TA, Byard GJ, Zometa CS, Hahn RA, McKnight-Eily LR, Chapman DP, Abraido-Lanza AF, Pearson JL, Anderson CW, et al: Collaborative care to improve the management of depressive disorders: a community guide systematic review and meta-analysis. Am J Prev Med 2012, 42(5):525–538.
8. Gilbody S, Bower P, Whitty P: Costs and consequences of enhanced primary care for depression: systematic review of randomised economic evaluations. Br J Psychiatry 2006, 189:297–308.
9. Jacob V, Chattopadhyay SK, Sipe TA, Thota AB, Byard GJ, Chapman DP: Economics of collaborative care for management of depressive disorders: a community guide systematic review. Am J Prev Med 2012, 42(5):539–549.
10. Medicare Australia: Practice Nurse Incentive Program (PNIP). http://www.medicareaustralia.gov.au/provider/incentives/pnip.jsp.
11. Carne A, Moretti C, Smith B, Bywood P: Summary Data Report of the 2009–10 Annual Survey of Divisions of General Practice. Adelaide: Primary Health Care Research & Information Service, Discipline of General Practice, Flinders University, and Australian Government Department of Health and Ageing; 2011.
12. Commonwealth of Australia: Parlimentary Debates: House of Representatives, Questions in Writing, Practice Incentives Program: Practice Nurse Incentive, Question 118, p526-7 (Ms Nicola Roxon, Minister for Health and Ageing); 2011 http://www.aph.gov.au/binaries/hansard/reps/dailys/dr100211.pdf.
13. Keleher H, Joyce CM, Parker R, Piterman L: Practice nurses in Australia: current issues and future directions. Med J Aust 2007, 187(2):108–110.
14. Morgan M, Dunbar J, Reddy P, Coates M, Leahy R: The TrueBlue study: is practice nurse-led collaborative care effective in the management of depression for patients with heart disease or diabetes? BMC Fam Pract 2009, 10:46.
15. Morgan MA, Coates MJ, Dunbar JA, Reddy P, Schlicht K, Fuller J: The TrueBlue model of collaborative care using practice nurses as case managers for depression alongside diabetes or heart disease: a randomised trial. BMJ Open 2013, 3(1):1–11.

16. Schlicht K, Morgan MA, Fuller J, Coates MJ, Dunbar JA: Safety and acceptability of practice-nurse-managed care of depression in patients with diabetes or heart disease in the Australian TrueBlue study. *BMJ Open* 2013, **3**(4):1–6.

17. Stables RH: Observational research in the evidence based environment: eclipsed by the randomised controlled trial? *Heart* 2002, **87**:101–102.

18. Karnon J, Caffrey O, Pham C, Grieve R, Ben-Tovim D, Hakendorf P, Crotty M: Applying risk adjusted cost-effectiveness (RAC-E) analysis to hospitals: estimating the costs and consequences of variation in clinical practice. *Health Econ* 2013, **22**(6):631–42.

19. Haji Ali Afzali H, Gray J, Beilby J, Holton C, Banham D, Karnon J: A risk adjusted economic evaluation of alternative models of involvement of practice nurses in management of type 2 diabetes. *Diabet Med* 2013, **30**(7):855–63.

20. Karnon J, Haji Ali Afzali H, Gray J: A risk adjusted cost-effectiveness analysis of alternative models of nurse involvement in obesity management in primary care. *Obesity* 2013, **21**(3):472–9.

21. Nordstrom G, Despiegel N, Marteau F, Danchenko N, Maman K: Cost effectiveness of escitalopram versus SNRIs in second-step treatment of major depressive disorder in Sweden. *J Med Econ* 2010, **13**(3):516–526.

22. Sicras-Mainar A, Navarro-Artieda R, Blanca-Tamayo M, Gimeno-de la Fuente V, Salvatella-Pasant J: Comparison of escitalopram vs. citalopram and venlafaxine in the treatment of major depression in Spain: clinical and economic consequences. *Curr Med Res Opin* 2010, **26**(12):2757–2764.

23. Haji Ali Afzali H, Karnon J, Gray J: A proposed model for economic evaluations of major depressive disorder. *Eur J Health Econ* 2012, **13**(4):501–510.

24. Haji Ali Afzali H, Karnon J, Gray J, Beilby J: Evaluation of collaborative models of care in management of patients with depression - protocol and progress. *Ment Health Fam Med* 2012, **9**(2):91–97.

25. Department of Health and Ageing (DoHA): *Medicare Benefits Schedule - Item 10997.* http://www9.health.gov.au/mbs/fullDisplay.cfm?type=item&q=10997.

26. Howell CA: *Study of a primary care depression relapse prevention program: "Keeping the blues away",* PhD thesis. Adelaide: University of Adelaide, Discipline of General Practice; 2009.

27. Guo S, Fraser MW: *Propensity score analysis: Statistical methods and application.* California: Sage Publications; 2010.

28. Buis ML: Analyzing Proportions. In *Eighth German Stata Users Group Meeting.* Berlin; 2010. http://www.stata.com/meeting/germany10/germany10_buis.pdf.

29. Buis ML: *ZOIB.* http://maartenbuis.nl/software/zoib.html.

30. Glick HA, Doshi JA, Sonnad SS, Polsky D: *Economic Evaluation in Clinical Trials.* Oxford: Oxford University Press; 2007.

31. Austin P: An introduction to propensity score methods for reducing the effects of confounding in observational studies. *Multivariate Behav Res* 2011, **46**(3):399–424.

32. Henderson J, Harrison C, Britt H: Indications for antidepressant medication use in Australian general practice patients [letter]. *Aust N Z J Psychiatry* 2010, **44**(9):865.

33. Sobocki P, Ekman M, Ovanfors A, Khandker R, Jonsson B: The cost-utility of maintenance treatment with venlafaxine in patients with recurrent major depressive disorder. *Int J Clin Pract* 2008, **62**(4):623–632.

34. Sullivan P: A comparison of the direct costs and cost effectiveness of serotonin reuptake inhibitors and associated adverse drug reactions. *CNS Drugs* 2004, **18**(13):911–932.

35. Unützer J, Katon W, Williams JW Jr, Callahan CM, Harpole L, Hunkeler EM, Hoffing M, Arean P, Hegel MT, Schoenbaum M, *et al*: Improving primary care for depression in late life: the design of a multicenter randomized trial. *Med Care* 2001, **39**(8):785–799.

36. The Australian College of Mental Health Nurses Inc (ACMHN): *Mental Health Nurse Incentive Program: achieving through collaboration, creativity and compromise.* Deakin West, ACT: ACMHN; 2011 http://www.acmhn.org/career-resources/mhnip/mhnip-review.

37. Healthcare Management Advisors Pty Ltd (HMA), Department of Health and Ageing (DoHA): *Evaluation of the mental health nurse incentive program, final report.* Adelaide: HMA; 2012.

2

To what extent do primary care practice nurses act as case managers lifestyle counselling regarding weight management?

Sonja ME van Dillen* and Gerrit J Hiddink

Abstract

Background: In this review study, we are the first to explore whether the practice nurse (PN) can act as case manager lifestyle counselling regarding weight management in primary care.

Methods: Multiple electronic databases (MEDLINE, PsycINFO) were searched to identify relevant literature after 1995. Forty-five studies fulfilled the inclusion criteria. In addition, all studies were judged on ten quality criteria by two independent reviewers.

Results: Especially in the last three years, many studies have been published. The majority of the studies were positive about PNs' actual role in primary care. However, several studies dealt with competency issues, including disagreement on respective roles. Thirteen studies were perceived as high quality. Only few studies had a representative sample. PNs' role in chronic disease management is spreading increasingly into lifestyle counselling. Although PNs have more time to provide lifestyle counselling than general practitioners (GPs), lack of time still remains a barrier. In some countries, PNs were rather ambiguous about their role, and they did not agree with GPs on this.

Conclusion: The PN can play the role of case manager lifestyle counselling regarding weight management in primary care in the UK, and wherever PNs are working under supervision of a GP and a primary health care team is already developed with agreement on roles. In countries in which a primary health care team is still in development and there is no agreement on respective roles, such as the USA, it is still the question whether the PN can play the case manager role.

Keywords: Primary care, Systematic review, Obesity, Nutrition education, Communication

Background

In recent years, general practitioners (GPs) have faced a heavy workload. This led to a call for more practical support. The emergence of primary care practice nurses (PNs) came in a period of increasing awareness of chronic disease management [1]. In the UK, chronic disease services have shifted from secondary care to general practice and from GPs to practice nurses (PNs). A new UK GP contract requires adherence to chronic disease

management tools, and facilitating self-management is recognized as an important component [2]. In the Netherlands, PNs are specially trained to be employed in GP practices: currently three quarters of all practices have a PN at their disposal [1]. Besides chronic disease management PNs provide an increasing proportion of preventive lifestyle advice. PNs work under supervision of GPs, which means that PNs cannot refer patients or prescribe medicines without permission of a GP. In the UK, the Netherlands, Sweden, Finland, Australia and New Zealand, such a collaborative system has been implemented [3]. A review revealed that lifestyle advice provided by GPs was rather general [4]. Moreover,

* Correspondence: sonja.vandillen@wur.nl
Strategic Communication, Section Communication, Philosophy and Technology, Centre for Integrative Development (CPT-CID), Wageningen University, P.O. Box 8130, 6700 EW Wageningen, the Netherlands

research showed that GPs perceive barriers in lifestyle counselling [5]. To overcome these barriers, PNs can partially take over lifestyle counselling [6]. There is evidence that supports effectiveness of lifestyle interventions delivered by PNs to affect positive changes on outcomes associated with prevention of chronic disease, including weight and dietary and physical activity behaviors [7]. Moreover, a Cochrane review suggests that appropriately trained PNs can produce as high quality care as GPs and achieve as good health outcomes for patients [8].

The obesity epidemic is escalating and creating enormous disease burdens. Nearly 1.5 billion adults were overweight in 2008, and of these half a billion were clinically obese – almost double the rates of 1980 [9]. A large proportion will need help with weight management: the primary health care team (such as GPs and PNs) have an important role in the identification, assessment and management of overweight and obese adults and children [10]. GPs and PNs should advise patients on weight, diet, and physical activity to motivate patients to change. However, it is not known what is PNs' actual role in lifestyle counselling in primary care at present. A clear overview of studies performed in the field is missing. A solid description of the current situation in terms of PNs' attitudes and their perceived barriers, as well as their lifestyle counselling practices is needed.

Furthermore, PNs have to work together with other health professionals in primary care and public health, such as GPs, practice assistants, and dieticians. In an interdisciplinary model, different members of a primary health care team take appropriate and complementary roles to increase treatment effectiveness and health care system efficiency, as well as coordination with resources outside primary care setting [11]. In the Netherlands, the core primary health care team consists of a GP, PN and practice assistant. The practice assistant is responsible for administrative duties, while the PN supports the GP in the care for chronically ill people [1]. PNs are actually generalists, while competent in several different fields, but in integrated care they might cooperate with other professionals, such as dieticians who are specialized in the area of nutrition. Assessment of the contribution that various health professionals in primary care can make is relevant to explicating role responsibilities. Understanding of collaborative practice is needed, as well as comparison of the outcomes of their individual lifestyle counseling practices in terms of patients' satisfaction, lifestyle behavior and health. In some countries, shift in extended care of PNs might cause tension. For example, GPs and PNs in the USA do not agree about their respective roles in delivery of primary care [12]. In other countries, such as the Netherlands, it runs relatively smoothly.

It is important that one professional has the lead and overview; this is indicated as case management. Case managers manage collaborative process of assessment, planning, facilitation and advocacy for options and services to meet individual's health needs through communication and available resources to promote quality cost-effective outcomes [13]. Coordination of care, patient education and counselling, and monitoring of health outcomes, are all integral part of nurse case management. For example, Dutch lifestyle interventions in primary care were primarily undertaken by case managers like lifestyle advisors or PNs under supervision of GPs [14,15]. Other potential case managers are GPs themselves, dieticians, diabetes educators, exercise specialists, and psychologists. We wonder whether the PN can play the role of case manager lifestyle counselling regarding weight management in primary care. To our knowledge, no systematic review has been performed in this field before. Since we are specifically interested in the case manager role, we will not take into account any regulatory issues as well as patients' perceptions. However in case of intervention studies, we are interested in the lifestyle behavior and health outcomes for patients.

Therefore, the aim of this review is to describe PNs' actual role in lifestyle counselling in primary care and their cooperation with other health professionals.

The underlying research questions are:

- What is known about the main outcomes of studies conducted regarding PNs' actual role in lifestyle counselling in primary care?
- What is known about how PNs' role in lifestyle counselling relates to the role of other health professionals in primary care and public health?

This review will provide an overview of the state of the art with respect to PNs' involvement in lifestyle counseling in primary care, and we will use this as a first approach to discuss for the near future whether the PN can act as case manager lifestyle counselling regarding weight management in primary care.

Methods
Search strategy

A computerized literature search of multiple electronic databases was performed (MEDLINE, PsycINFO) with EBSCO-host as resource for relevant papers published between 1 January 1995 and 1 July 2013, using the following keywords as search strategy in the title or abstract (Table 1). The year 1995 was chosen, because PNs were introduced into primary health care in the nineties. This review is a first approach for carefully examining the role of PN as case manager lifestyle counselling regarding weight management, based on an overview about the description of the actual role of PNs in lifestyle counselling and its cooperation with other health

Table 1 Search strategy of electronic databases MEDLINE and PsycINFO with EBSCO-host

Search strategy	
Step 1	Practice nurse OR nurse practitioner OR primary nursing care OR primary care nurse OR primary health care nurse OR PHC nurses
Step 2	Guidance OR counselling OR communication OR advice OR health education OR health promotion OR prevention OR lifestyle behaviour OR chronic disease OR chronic illness
Step 3	Nutrition OR diet OR food OR physical activity OR exercise OR physical fitness OR weight OR overweight OR obesity OR adiposity OR corpulence
Step 4	Role OR position OR task OR duty OR responsibility OR competency OR skill OR expertise OR mission OR profession OR contribution OR lifestyle advisor OR case manager OR case management
Step 5	Cooperation OR collaboration OR teamwork OR alliance OR referral OR interdisciplinary OR multidisciplinary OR network OR delegation
Combine search 1, 2 and 3	
Combine search 1, 2 and 4	
Combine search 1, 2 and 5	

professionals. We also checked Cochrane library for relevant reviews.

Inclusion criteria

Studies had to be peer-reviewed journal articles, which addressed PNs' involvement in lifestyle counselling in primary care. Only studies published in English language and original papers were included, of which full text was available. The review excluded studies that were based in hospitals, studies among children, and studies about patients' perceptions.

Study selection

After the electronic database search by one reviewer (SvD), reference lists of articles and reviews were screened for other potentially relevant papers. Figure 1 shows the flow chart for study selection.

Data extraction

Data extraction of main characteristics was performed, namely:

- Author, year of publication, country;
- Study design: cross-sectional/longitudinal; randomized controlled trial (RCT)/interview/ questionnaire;
- Sample: random sampling, number of PNs or GPs;

- Main outcomes for studies about PNs' actual role in lifestyle counselling in primary care;
- Main outcomes for studies about PNs' cooperation in the field of lifestyle counselling with other health professionals in primary care and public health.

Assessment of study quality

Two reviewers (SvD and GH) independently assessed study quality of selected studies. The studies were judged on the following quality criteria, which were applied before in a review study among GPs [4]:

- Clear description of study aim (e.g. consistency in research questions, measurement instrument, results and conclusions);
- Appropriate size of study population (e.g. report of rationale for sample size);
- Sound selection of study population (e.g. random, stratified);
- Representative sample (e.g. no over-representation of female PNs, no over-representation of older PNs);
- Good response rate (e.g. > = 80% for phone or face-to-face interviews, > = 50% for mail questionnaires or classroom papers, > = 30% for Internet questionnaires) or low refusal rate/drop-out;
- Efforts were undertaken to optimize response rate (e.g. personalized letters, postage paid return envelope, reminders, incentive/gifts, simple and short measurement instrument, inclusion of group new respondents);
- Measurement instrument was well-developed (e.g. based on validated measures, prior research or reviewed literature);
- Measurement instrument was tested before use (e.g. pilot-test, pre-test for clarity, test-retest);
- Appropriate measurement instrument (e.g. distinguishable answer categories, Likert scales);
- Suitable report of study limitations and shortcomings (e.g. to overcome bias).

A maximum score of ten plusses could be achieved. Studies with eight plusses or more were seen as high quality. Studies with five, six or seven plusses were considered as medium quality studies, and studies with four or less plusses were considered as low quality studies. Although arbitrary, this quality assessment was done by two independent researchers, who compared results and reached consensus.

Conditions for acting as case manager in primary care

The results were viewed against conditions for acting as case manager lifestyle counselling regarding weight management in primary care [15]:

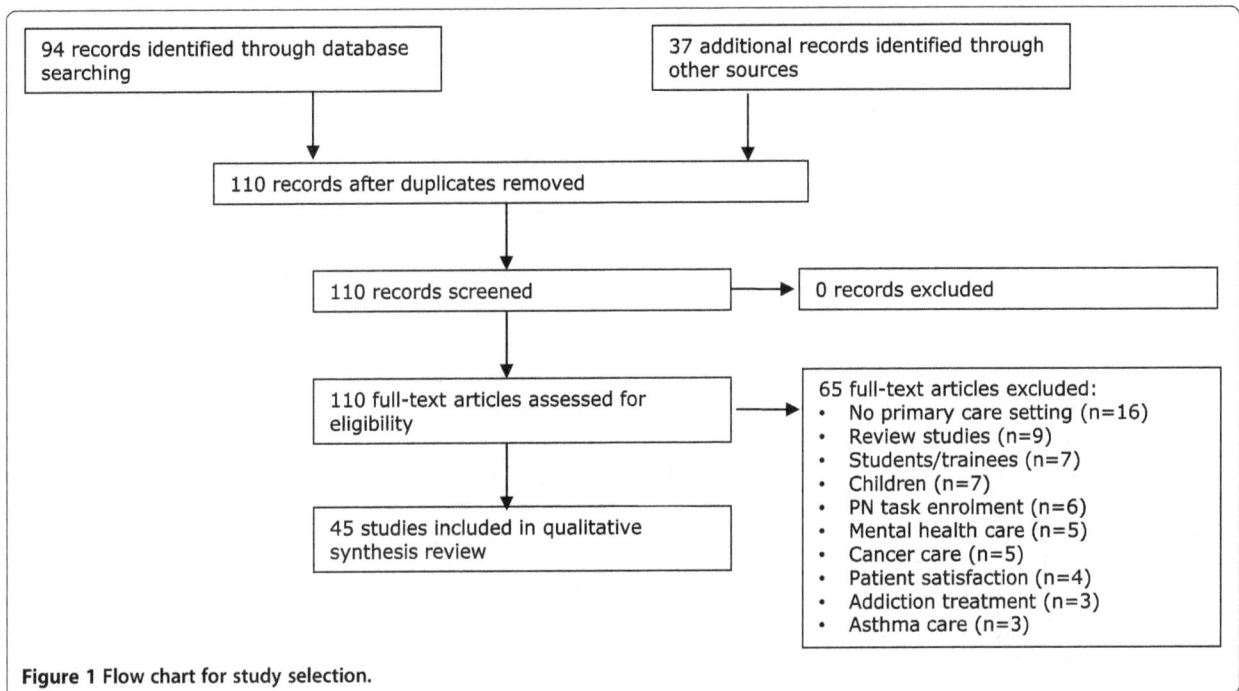

Figure 1 Flow chart for study selection.

- Time;
- Money;
- Interest;
- Perceived expertise;
- Competences;
- Type of intervention activity

Results and discussion
Main characteristics of studies
An additional file shows the main characteristics in more detail [see Additional file 1]. Thirty-three studies were performed in Europe, specifically in the UK (18 studies) and the Netherlands (10 studies). Six studies were done in Australia and five studies in the USA.

Our review delivered a wealth of studies (45 in total), which all concerned cross-sectional studies. The cross-sectional study of Philips et al. (2009) [16] was also accompanied by a longitudinal study. Both qualitative and quantitative studies were found, with slightly more quantitative studies. Twelve RCTs were found and four national surveys. Next to mail questionnaires, we also found observations, focus groups, and interviews. This order of scientific rigidity will be followed in the evaluation and discussion of the results.

Samples ranged between 1 [17] and 606 PNs [18]. Most studies were published after 2000, especially in the last three years.

Main outcomes for studies about PNs' actual role in lifestyle counselling in primary care
All 45 studies found were indeed discussing PNs' actual role in lifestyle counselling in primary care. Outcomes of these studies were classified into three categories: positive, neutral, and negative. In order to be evaluated as "positive", the study should show that PNs' role in lifestyle counselling is warranted. An additional file shows in more detail that the majority of studies were positive about PN's actual role in lifestyle counselling in primary care [see Additional file 1]. Twenty-six studies demonstrated that PNs' role in lifestyle counselling is warranted. Furthermore, 10 out of 12 RCTs with an intervention by PNs resulted in positive outcomes. Six intervention studies in the UK and the Netherlands showed that PNs can achieve equally good health outcomes as GPs for different kinds of diseases [19-24]. More intensive interventions initiated the most changes [25]. Three other intervention studies revealed that consultations with PNs were significantly longer than those of GPs, and patients were significantly more satisfied with PNs' care [26-28]. Two surveys showed that British PNs reported high levels of physical activity counselling [29,30] and three other surveys revealed that physical activity counselling increased in recent years in the USA [18,31,32]. Two observational studies comparing PNs' and GPs' counselling practices showed that Finnish and Dutch PNs more often discussed diet and physical activity than GPs [33,34]. In the UK, PNs and GPs agreed

that PNs have main responsibility to cardiovascular health promotion [35], and weight management was considered as just one aspect of the busy and diverse role of the PN [36]. Australian PNs performed at least six roles, often alternating rapidly between them [16].

However, eight studies were neutral about PNs' actual role in lifestyle counseling in primary care. According to these studies, parts of the role of PNs in lifestyle counselling in primary care are debatable. A survey among PNs and GPs in Ireland showed that there is some congruence in opinion regarding current role of the PN [37]. Although British PNs were more likely to raise weight issues than GPs, only 9% self-reported to present solutions or discuss health promotion [38], and weight management seems to be based on brief opportunistic intervention undertaken mainly by PNs [39]. Interviews with American PNs identified that realities of PN practice were often different from idealized practice, role identity was considered as ambiguous, and a need to blend medical and nursing models [40].

Moreover, eleven studies were negative about PNs' actual role in lifestyle counseling in primary care. These studies showed that PNs' role in lifestyle counselling in primary care seems to be limited. Two RCTs found no outcomes of a intervention by PNs. A RCT showed that adding nurse practitioners (NPs) to Dutch general practice teams did not reduce GPs' workload, implying that NPs are used as supplements, rather than substitutes [41]. Another RCT showed that follow-up by PNs in the UK does not necessarily translate into better care or clinical outcomes [42]. Results from a national survey in Australia showed that PNs are a clinically experienced workforce whose skills are not optimally harnessed to improve care of growing number of people with chronic conditions [43]. Another national survey among American GPs and PNs indicated that they do not agree about their respective roles in delivery of primary care for complex chronic conditions [12]. The majority of Australian PNs agreed in a survey that PNs' role could be expanded to include autonomous functioning, while most GPs were amenable to some extension of nursing practice [44]. Regarding weight management, PNs in the UK self-reported that they mainly offer general nutrition and exercise advice [45], and GPs and PNs in another British survey showed diversity with respect to their own relative importance in weight management [46].

Main outcomes for studies about PNs' cooperation in the field of lifestyle counselling with other health professionals in primary care and public health

Fourteen studies were found to answer the second research question. In all these studies, the relationship with GPs was described. In six studies, it was explicitly mentioned that PNs worked under supervision of a GP

[16,22,23,34,44,47]. In a Dutch intervention study for example, NPs intensively guided behavioral change process, while GPs oversaw patients' progress [22]. A national survey showed that for all referrals made to medical specialists, a GP was involved in the nurse-patient encounter [47]. They concluded that greater flexibility in PNs' role will maximize efficient use of nurses' skills in primary health care context in Australia. In Ireland, over 85% of PNs and GPs surveyed appear to have an agenda in chronic disease management, and strong primary care teams are under development [37]. Most GPs in the UK seem to refer obese patients to their PN instead of using external sources of support [39]. NPs interviewed in Canada described their expectation in collegial partnerships with GPs, but in reality they work in more traditional hierarchical relationships [48]. Besides GPs, cooperation with dieticians was discovered in eight studies [22,23,34,36,39,46,49,50]. Collaboration with several disciplines in general practice, like dietician, was perceived as an important facilitator in interviews with Dutch PNs and GPs [49]. Australian PNs were reluctant to cross professional boundaries: they often refer to "not being a dietician", when explaining the scope of their own practice [50]. Another collaboration partner appeared to be the practice assistant (two studies). An observational study in Australia showed that PNs spent 45% of their time in contact with patients and 16% in contact with other general practice staff, including bridging the gap between clinical and administrative staff [16]. Interviewed PNs in the UK felt that health care assistants encroached their territory [51].

Study quality

Studies in this review were assigned six plusses on average. Thirteen studies were perceived as high quality, 20 studies were considered as medium quality studies, and 12 studies were judged as low quality.

All studies had a clear description of study aim, and the majority had a well-developed or appropriate measurement instrument, suitable report of limitations, and an appropriate size of study population. Less than half of the studies had a good response rate, took efforts to optimize response rate, tested the measurement instrument before use, or had a sound selection of study population. Only few studies were representative.

All 45 papers discussed PNs' actual role in lifestyle counselling in primary care, and addressed the first research question. Of these, 26 were positive, 8 were neutral, and 11 were negative. The 26 studies considered as positive, were of high or medium quality. Not all papers addressed PNs' cooperation with other health professionals. Fourteen studies were found for answering the second research question. The studies found were of medium quality.

Analysis on the basis of conditions for acting as case manager in primary care

No study explicitly discussed PNs' role as case manager in primary care. Conditions for acting as case manager in primary care were found in 27 studies.

With respect to the condition time (in relation to task), four studies showed that PNs have more time to provide lifestyle counselling than GPs [23,33,34,39] and that frequency of PNs' lifestyle counselling has increased in recent years [32]. However, six studies discussed time as a barrier for providing lifestyle counselling, of which five lack of time [40,50,52-54], but the majority of PNs in the study of Steptoe et al. (1999) [35] disagreed with the statement that they had no time for health promotion.

Regarding money, six studies identified funding as barrier for lifestyle counselling [18,31,32,40,43,52]. According to PNs in the study of Donelan et al. (2013) [12], they should be paid equally for the same clinical service. However, PNs did not rank adequate reimbursement as being as important as GPs in influencing their decision to counsel [54].

According to the factor interest, PNs were generally positive towards lifestyle counselling. However, motivation of PNs to continue implementation of a Dutch lifestyle intervention was lower compared with GPs or physiotherapists [55].

Regarding expertise, six studies were found. Grimstvedt et al. (2012) [32] concluded that PNs were knowledgeable. An Australian national survey confirmed the generalist role with PNs seeing patients who have a wide range of chronic conditions [47]. However, there is clearly a tension among PNs and GPs to remain generalists and pressure to become primary care specialists in care of people with diabetes or coronary heart disease (CHD) [56]. Provision of simple lifestyle information and advice was predominant strategy used by PNs [53]. PNs self-reported they would benefit from further training about nutrition knowledge and obesity [36]. In the survey of Hankey et al. (2003) [46] both PNs and GPs felt that dieticians should hold specialist posts in weight management.

Moreover, nine studies dealt with competency issues. PNs were rather ambiguous about their role [43,51]. Furthermore, both PNs and GPs did not agree on the PNs' role [12,16,44,46,49] or showed only some congruence in opinion [37]. Australian PNs felt competent at providing basic nutrition care [50]. However, PNs had better interpersonal skills than GPs [16]. The review of Horrocks et al. (2002) [57] showed that NPs may have superior interpersonal skills than doctors.

With respect to type of intervention activity, the majority of studies reported on lifestyle counselling, while only eight included weight management [20,22,23,36,38,39,45,46].

Conclusion

Our review about PNs' actual role in lifestyle counselling in primary care reveals that we might be just at the beginning of understanding how PNs can contribute to lifestyle counselling or how PNs best fit into the primary health care team. A variety of studies have been found, ranging from differences in self-reported roles between PNs and GPs to intervention studies and observations of real-life counselling. We will elaborate on four main outcomes.

First, in some countries, such as the UK, the Netherlands, and Scandinavian countries, PNs can play the role of case manager lifestyle counselling regarding weight management in primary care. They are supervised by GPs, within primary health care team different roles are considered as clear, and cooperation is going well. Lifestyle counselling regarding weight management can be seen as the first step in the right direction in order to manage even more cases. In countries in which a primary health care team is still in development and there is no agreement on respective roles, such as the USA, it is still the question whether the PN can play the case manager role, because they need to agree on their roles in primary health care team and feel this teamwork is feasible, attractive and satisfactory.

Moreover, PNs' role in chronic disease management is spreading increasingly into lifestyle counselling. Already in 2001, Katon et al. [58] suggested that GPs diagnose and initiate treatment and lifestyle counselling, whereas PNs monitor treatment outcome, provide counselling and support for behavior change, and offer follow-contacts. Patients themselves were generally satisfied with PNs' lifestyle counselling [59,60], and perceived that PN have more available time [61,62].

Furthermore, we found that PNs experience the same barriers for lifestyle counselling as GPs. PNs have more time than GPs to provide lifestyle counselling, and frequency increased in recent years. Nevertheless, lack of time was still an important barrier. The review of Tulloch et al. (2006) [63] including 19 studies suggested that non-physician providers may be better suited for providing physical activity counselling due to an ability to provide a more intensive intervention. Moreover, the review of Fokkens et al. (2011) [64] including 10 studies indicated that interventions in which the nurse fulfils the role of the primary care provider result in larger effects on clinical outcomes.

Finally, a variety of PNs' competences are required for effective lifestyle counselling. The review of Smith (2011) [65] including 11 studies found that nurses can expect to experience substantial role ambiguity and role conflict. In the Counterweight Project Team (2004) [39] for example, PNs were trained dieticians, who received competence training with respect to communication skills and behavioral change.

A strength of this study is the systematic way in which an electronic literature search was performed in order to provide state of the art on main outcomes of studies about PNs' actual role in lifestyle counselling in primary care and cooperation with other health professionals.

A possible limitation is the grey area with (yet?) unpublished literature. Moreover, we found a lot of studies published after 2010, so some studies might still be in the pipeline. Unfortunately, we did not have access to the CINAHL database, so we might miss some specific nursing papers. Definition and education level of PNs differed between countries, as well as the primary health care systems and variety of variables, resulting in a heterogeneous mix of studies. Furthermore, the quality of studies was not very high. Due to the low number of (national) representative studies, caution is warranted for making comparisons.

Practice implications

Further training is required before case management of chronic diseases in primary care becomes an integral part of the role of PNs in Ireland [37]. The majority of American NPs are interested in receiving additional training to aid in providing physical activity counselling [32]. Competency training in both general communication skills and motivational interviewing skills are recommended.

According to Frank (1998) [66], shifting the major responsibility to non-physician professionals may offer the most promising therapeutic opportunities for obesity management. A review including 11 studies showed that there is potential in primary care nursing to help patients manage obesity [67]. Recently, a study suggested that PNs are well placed to perform two key roles in obesity management, namely counselling patients who have obesity-related co-morbidities and identification of patients who are overweight and healthy [68]. Recently, an observational study identified that PNs' goal setting could be improved [69]. The quality of PNs' weight loss counselling might be increased by routinely providing assistance in addressing barriers and securing support, and routinely reaching agreement with collaboratively set goals [70]. A multidisciplinary team approach to weight management is preferable, with training of PNs and specialized dieticians to address this issue [46]. Closer liaison with dietetic services could allow dietician expertise regarding weight management to be utilized more fully [36].

It seems to be crucial that members of the primary health care team agree on their respective roles, and feel this teamwork is feasible, attractive, and satisfactory. Monitoring these roles with quantitative studies is recommended.

In conclusion, because of the heterogeneity of the studies, the lack of (national) representative studies and the differences between countries (among other factors), there is no definite answer to the question whether or not the PN can act as case manager lifestyle counselling regarding weight management in primary care. It depends on the context of the situation and the country.

Abbreviations
PN: Practice nurse; GP: General practitioner; RCT: Randomized controlled trial; NP: Nurse practitioner; CHD: Coronary heart disease.

Competing interests
The authors declare that they have no competing interests.

Authors' contributions
SvD and GH contributed to study design. SvD conducted the computerized literature search. SvD and GH read the selected studies and independently assessed study quality of selected studies. They compared results and reached consensus. SvD wrote the first draft. Both authors reviewed and contributed to the final manuscript. Both authors read and approved the final manuscript.

References
1. Heiligers PJM, Noordman J, Korevaar JC, Dorsman S, Hingstman L, Van Dulmen AM, De Bakker DH: *Praktijkondersteuners in de huisartspraktijk (POH's), klaar voor de toekomst? [Practice nurses in general practice, ready for the future?].* NIVEL: Utrecht; 2012.
2. Macdonald W, Rogers A, Blakeman T, Bower P: **Practice nurses and the facilitation of self-management in primary care.** *J Adv Nurs* 2008, **62:**191–199.
3. Bourgueil Y, Marek A, Mousquès J: *The participation of nurses in primary care in six European countries, Ontario and Quebec. Health Economics Letter, no. 95.* Paris: Institute for Research and Information in Health Economics (IRDES); 2005.
4. Van Dillen SME, Van Binsbergen JJ, Koelen MA, Hiddink GJ: **Nutrition and physical activity guidance practices in general practice: a critical review.** *Patient Educ Couns* 2013, **90:**155–169.
5. Hiddink GJ, Hautvast JGAJ, Van Woerkum CMJ, Fieren CJ, Van 't Hof MA: **Driving forces for and barriers to nutrition guidance practices of Dutch primary care physicians.** *J Nutr Educ* 1997, **29:**36–41.
6. Fransen GAJ, Hiddink GJ, Koelen MA, Van Dis SJ, Drenthen AJM, Van Binsbergen JJ, Van Woerkum CMJ: **The development of a minimal intervention strategy to address overweight and obesity in adult primary care patients in The Netherlands.** *Fam Pract* 2008, **25:**i112–i115.
7. Sargent GM, Forrest LE, Parker RM: **Nurse delivered lifestyle interventions in primary health care to treat chronic disease risk factors associated with obesity: a systematic review.** *Obes Rev* 2012, **13:**1148–1171.
8. Laurant M, Reeves D, Hermens R, Braspenning J, Grol R, Sibbald B: **Substitution of doctors by nurses in primary care.** *Cochrane Database Syst Rev* 2004, **2:**CD001271.
9. Swinburn BA, Sacks G, Hall KD, McPherson K, Finegood DT, Moodie ML, Gortmaker SL: **The global obesity pandemic: shaped by global drivers and local environments.** *Lancet* 2011, **378:**804–814.
10. National Institute on Health and Clinical Excellence (NICE): *Obesity: the prevention, identification, assessment and management of overweight and obesity in adults and children.* London: NICE; 2006.
11. Whitlock EP, Orleans T, Pender N, Allan J: **Evaluating primary care behavioural counselling interventions: an evidence-based approach.** *Am J Prev Med* 2002, **22:**267–284.

12. Donelan K, DesRoches CM, Dittus RS, Buerhaus P: Perspectives of physicians and nurse practitioners on primary care practice. *New Engl J Med* 2013, 368:1898–1906.

13. Case Management Society of America (CMSA): What is a case manager? [http://www.cmsa.org/Consumer/FindaCaseManager/WhatisaCaseManager/tabid/276/Default.aspx]

14. Helmink JH, Meis JJ, De Weerdt I, Visser FN, De Vries NK, Kremers SPJ: Development and implementation of a lifestyle intervention to promote physical activity and healthy diet in the Dutch general practice setting: the BeweegKuur programme. *Int J Behav Nutr Phys Act* 2010, 7:49.

15. Duijzer G, Jansen SC, Haveman-Nies A, Van Bruggen R, Ter Beek J, Hiddink GJ, Feskens EJM: Translating the SLIM diabetes prevention intervention into SLIMMER: implications for the Dutch primary health care. *Fam Pract* 2012, 29:i145–i152.

16. Philips CB, Pearce C, Hall S, Kljakovic M, Sibbald B, Dwan F, Porritt J, Yates R: Enhancing care, improving quality: the six roles of the general practice nurse. *Med J Aus* 2009, 191:92–97.

17. Marsh GN, Dawes ML: Establishing a minor illness nurse in a busy general practice. *BMJ* 2000, 30:778–780.

18. Burns KJ, Camaione DN, Chatterton CT: Prescription of physical activity by adult nurse practitioners: a national survey. *Nurs Outlook* 2000, 48:28–33.

19. Campbell NC, Thain J, Deans HG, Ritchie LD, Rawles JM, Squair JL: Secondary prevention clinics for coronary heart disease: randomized trial of effect on health. *BMJ* 1998, 316:1434–1437.

20. Ter Bogt NCW, Bemelmans WJE, Beltman FW, Broer J, Smit AJ, Van der Meer K: Preventing weight gain: one-year results of a randomized lifestyle intervention. *Am J Prev Med* 2009, 37:270–277.

21. Koelewijn-Van Loon MS, Van der Weijden T, Ronda G, Van Steenkiste B, Winkens B, Elwyn G, Grol R: Improving lifestyle and risk perception through patient involvement in nurse-led risk management: a cluster-randomized controlled trial in primary care. *Prev Med* 2010, 50:35–44.

22. Vermunt PWA, Milder IEJ, Wielaard F, De Vries JHM, Van Oers HAM, Westert GP: Lifestyle counselling for type 2 diabetes risk reduction in Dutch primary care: results of the APHRODITE study after 0.5 and 1.5 years. *Diab Care* 2011, 34:1919–1925.

23. Voogdt-Pruis HR, Van Ree JW, Gorgels APM, Beusmans GHMI: Adherence to a guideline on cardiovascular prevention: A comparison between general practitioners and practice nurses. *Int J Nurs Stud* 2011, 48:798–807.

24. Driehuis F, Barte JCM, Ter Bogt N, Smit AJ, Van der Meer K, Bemelmans WJE: Maintenance of lifestyle changes: 3-year results of the Groningen Overweight and Lifestyle study. *Patient Educ Couns* 2012, 88:249–255.

25. Little P, Dorward M, Gralton S, Hammerton L, Pillinger J, White P, Moore M, McKenna J, Payne S: A randomized controlled trial of three pragmatic approaches to initiate increased physical activity in sedentary patients with risk factors for cardiovascular disease. *Br J Gen Pract* 2004, 54:189–195.

26. Kinnersley P, Anderson E, Parry K, Clement J, Archard L, Turton P, Stainthorpe A, Fraser A, Butler CC, Rogers C: Randomised controlled trial of nurse practitioner versus general practitioner care for patients requesting "same day" consultations in primary care. *BMJ* 2000, 320:1043–1048.

27. Shum C, Humphreys A, Wheeler D, Cochrane MA, Skoda S, Clement S: Nurse management of patient with minor illnesses in general practice: multicentre, randomised controlled trial. *BMJ* 2000, 320:1038–1043.

28. Venning P, Durie A, Roland M: Randomised controlled trial comparing cost effectiveness of general practitioners and nurse practitioners in primary care. *BMJ* 2000, 320:1048–1053.

29. McDowell N, McKenna J, Naylor PJ: Factors that influence practice nurses to promote physical activity. *Br J Sports Med* 1997, 31:308–313.

30. Douglas F, Torrance N, Van T, Meloni S, Kerr A: Primary care staff's views and experiences related to routinely advising patients about physical activity. A questionnaire survey. *BMC Pub Health* 2006, 6:138.

31. Buchholz SW, Purath J: Physical activity and physical fitness counselling patterns of adult nurse practitioners. *J Am Acad Nurs Pract* 2007, 19:86–92.

32. Grimstvedt ME, Der Ananian C, Keller J, Woolf K, Sebren A, Ainsworth B: Nurse practitioner and physician assistant physical counseling knowledge, confidence and practices. *Prev Med* 2012, 54:306–318.

33. Poskiparta M, Kasila K, Kiuru P: Dietary and physical activity counselling on Type 2 diabetes and impaired glucose tolerance by physicians and nurses in primary healthcare in Finland. *Scand J Prim Health Care* 2006, 24:206–210.

34. Noordman J, Koopmans B, Korevaar JC, Van der Weijden T, Van Dulmen S: Exploring lifestyle counselling in routine primary care consultations: the professionals' role. *Fam Pract* 2013, 30:332–340.

35. Steptoe A, Doherty S, Kendrick T, Rink E, Hilton S: Attitudes to cardiovascular health promotion among GPs and practice nurses. *Fam Pract* 1999, 16:158–163.

36. Green SM, McCoubrie M, Cullingham C: Practice nurses' and health visitors' knowledge of obesity assessment and management. *J Hum Nutr Diet* 2000, 13:413–423.

37. McCarthy G, Cornally N, Moran J, Courtney M: Practice nurses and general practitioners: perspectives on the role and future development of practice nursing in Ireland. *J Clin Nurs* 2012, 21:2286–2295.

38. Michie S: Talking to primary care patients about weight: A study of GPs and practice nurses in the UK. *Psych Health Med* 2007, 12:521–525.

39. The Counterweight Project Team: Current approaches to obesity management in UK Primary Care: the Counterweight Programme. *J Hum Nutr Diet* 2004, 17:183–190.

40. Hernandez J, Anderson S: Storied experiences of nurse practitioners managing prehypertension in primary care. *J Am Acad Nurs Pract* 2012, 24:89–96.

41. Laurant MGH, Hermens RPMG, Braspenning JCC, Sibbald B, Grol RPTM: Impact of nurse practitioners on workload of general practitioners: randomised controlled trial. *BMJ* 2004, 328:927.

42. Moher M, Yudkin P, Wright L, Turner R, Fuller A, Schofield T, Mant D: Cluster randomized controlled trial to compare three methods of promoting secondary prevention of coronary heart disease in primary care. *BMJ* 2001, 322:1338–1342.

43. Halcomb EJ, Davidson PM, Salamonson Y, Ollerton R, Griffiths R: Nurses in Australian general practice: implications for chronic disease management. *J Clin Nurs* 2008, 17:6–15.

44. Patterson E, Del Mar C, Najman C: Nursing's contribution to general practice: general practitioners' and practice nurses' views. *Collegian* 1999, 6:33–39.

45. Hoppé R, Ogden J: Practice nurses' beliefs about obesity and weight related interventions in primary care. *Int J Obes* 1997, 21:141–146.

46. Hankey CR, Eley S, Leslie WS, Hunter CM, Lean MEJ: Eating habits, beliefs, attitudes and knowledge among health professionals regarding the links between obesity, nutrition, and health. *Pub Health Nutr* 2003, 7:337–343.

47. Joyce CM, Piterman L: The work of nurses in Australian general practice: A national survey. *Int J Nurs Stud* 2011, 48:70–80.

48. Bailey P, Jones L, Way D: Family practitioner/nurse practitioner: stories of collaboration. *J Adv Nurs* 2006, 53:381–391.

49. Geense WW, Van de Glind IM, Visscher TLS, Van Achterberg T: Barriers, facilitators and attitudes influencing health promotion activities in general practice: an explorative pilot study. *BMC Fam Pract* 2013, 14:20.

50. Cass S, Ball L, Leveritt M: Australian practice nurses' perceptions of their role and competency to provide nutrition care to patients living with chronic disease. *Aus J Prim Health* 2013, 20:203–208.

51. McDonald R, Campbell S, Lester H: Practice nurses and the effects of the new general practitioners contract in the English National Health Service: The extension of a professional project? *Soc Sci Med* 2009, 68:1206–1212.

52. Lambe B, Collins C: A qualitative study of lifestyle counselling in general practice in Ireland. *Fam Pract* 2010, 27:219–223.

53. Jansink R, Braspenning J, Van der Weijden T, Elwyn G, Grol R: Primary care nurses struggle with lifestyle counseling in diabetes care: a qualitative analysis. *BMC Fam Pract* 2010, 11:41.

54. Mitchell LJ, MacDonald-Wicks L, Capra S: Nutrition advice in general practice: the role of general practitioners and practice nurses. *Aus J Prim Health* 2011, 17:202–208.

55. Helmink JHM, Kremers SPJ, Van Boekel LC, Van Brussel-Visser FN, De Vries NK: Factors determining the motivation of primary health care professionals to implement and continue the 'Beweegkuur' lifestyle intervention programme. *J Eval Clin Pract* 2012, 18:682–688.

56. Williams R, Rapport F, Elwyn G, Lloyd B, Rance J, Belcher S: The prevention of type 2 diabetes: general practitioner and practice nurse opinions. *Br J Gen Pract* 2004, 54:531–535.

57. Horrocks S, Anderson E, Salisbury C: **Systematic review of whether nurse practitioners working in primary care can provide equivalent care to doctors.** *BMJ* 2002, **324**:819–823.

58. Katon W, Von Korff M, Lin E, Simon G: **Rethinking practitioner roles in chronic illness: the specialist, primary care physician, and the practice nurse.** *Gen Hosp Psych* 2001, **23**:138–144.

59. Duaso MJ, Cheung P: **Health promotion and lifestyle advice in a general practice: what do patients think?** *J Adv Nurs* 2002, **39**:473–479.

60. Wilson PM, Brooks F, Procter S, Kendall S: **The nursing contribution to chronic disease management: A case of public expectation? Qualitative findings from a multiple case study design in England and Wales.** *Int J Nurs Stud* 2012, **49**:2–14.

61. Hayes E: **Nurse practitioners and managed care: Patient satisfaction and intention to adhere to nurse practitioner plan of care.** *J Am Acad Nurs Pract* 2007, **19**:418–426.

62. Mahomed R, St John W, Patterson E: **Understanding the process of patient satisfaction with nurse-led chronic disease management in general practice.** *J Adv Nurs* 2012, **68**:2538–2549.

63. Tulloch H, Fortier M, Hogg W: **Physical activity counselling in primary care: Who has and who should be counselling?** *Patient Educ Couns* 2006, **64**:6–20.

64. Fokkens AS, Wiegersma PA, Reijneveld SA: **Organization of diabetes primary care: a review of interventions that delegate general practitioner tasks to a nurse.** *J Eval Clin Pract* 2011, **17**:199–203.

65. Smith AC: **Role ambiguity and role conflict in nurse case managers: an integrative review.** *Prof Case Man* 2011, **16**:182–197.

66. Frank A: **A multidisciplinary approach to obesity management: the physician's role and team care alternatives.** *J Am Diet Ass* 1998, **10**:S44–S48.

67. Brown I, Psarou A: **Literature review of nursing practice in managing obesity in primary care: developments in the UK.** *J Clin Nurs* 2007, **17**:17–28.

68. Philips K, Wood F, Kinnersley P: **Tackling obesity: the challenge of obesity management for practice nurses in primary care.** *Fam Pract* 2014, **31**:51–59.

69. Van Dillen SME, Noordman J, Van Dulmen S, Hiddink GJ: **Examining the content of weight, nutrition and physical activity advices by Dutch practice nurses in primary care: analysis of video-taped consultations.** *Eur J Clin Nutr* 2014, **68**:50–56.

70. Van Dillen SME, Noordman J, Van Dulmen S, Hiddink GJ: **Quality of weight-loss counseling by Dutch practice nurses in primary care: an observational study.** *Eur J Clin Nutr* 2014, doi:10.1038/ejcn.2014.129.

71. Kiuru P, Poskiparta M, Kettunen T, Saltevo J, Liimatainen L: **Advice-giving styles by Finnish nurses in dietary counselling concerning type 2 diabetes care.** *J Health Com* 2004, **9**:337–354.

72. Goetz K, Szecsenyi J, Campbell S, Rosemann T, Rueter G, Raum E, Brenner H, Miksch A: **The importance of social support for people with type 2 diabetes – a qualitative study with general practitioners, practice nurses and patients.** *GMS Psychosoc Med* 2012, **9**:1–9.

3

Practice nurse chlamydia testing in Australian general practice: a qualitative study of benefits, barriers and facilitators

Rebecca Lorch[1*], Jane Hocking[2], Rebecca Guy[1], Alaina Vaisey[2], Anna Wood[2], Dyani Lewis[2], Meredith Temple-Smith[3] and on behalf of the ACCEPt consortium

Abstract

Background: Chlamydia infection is a significant public health issue for young people; however, testing rates in Australian general practice are low. Practice nurses (PNs) could have an important role in contributing to increasing chlamydia testing rates. The Australian Chlamydia Control Effectiveness Pilot (ACCEPt), a large cluster randomised control trial of annual testing for 16 to 29 year olds in general practice, is the first to investigate the role of PNs in maximising testing rates. In order to assess the scope for PN involvement, we aimed to explore PN's views in relation to involvement in chlamydia testing in general practice.

Methods: Semi structured interviews were conducted between June 2011 and April 2012 with a purposive sample of 23 PNs participating in ACCEPt. Interview data was thematically analysed using a conventional content analysis approach.

Results: The participants in our study supported an increased role for PNs in chlamydia testing and identified a number of patient benefits from this involvement, such as an improved service with greater access to testing and patients feeling more comfortable engaging with a nurse rather than a doctor. An alleviation of doctors' workloads and expansion of the nurse's role were also identified as benefits at a clinic level. Time and workload constraints were commonly considered barriers to chlamydia testing, along with concerns around privacy in the "small town" rural settings of the general practices. Some felt negative GP attitudes as well as issues with funding for PNs' work could also be barriers. The provision of training and education, streamlining chlamydia testing pathways in clinics and changes to pathology ordering processes would facilitate nurse involvement in chlamydia testing.

Conclusion: This study suggests that PNs could take a role in increasing chlamydia testing in general practice and that their involvement may result in possible benefits for patients, doctors, PNs and the community. Strategies to overcome identified barriers and facilitate their involvement must be further explored.

Keywords: Australia, Chlamydia, Clinical nursing research, General practice, Primary health care, Qualitative research

Background

Chlamydia trachomatis (hereafter referred to as chlamydia) is a significant public health concern for young people. Chlamydia continues to be the most frequently reported notifiable condition in the United States (US), Europe and Australia. In 2012, around 1.4 million new chlamydia diagnoses were reported in the US, over 350,000 in 25 European Union member states and over 82 000 in Australia. The greatest burden of infection is in young people aged 15–29 years [1-3]. In young women, about 10% with untreated chlamydia will develop pelvic inflammatory disease [4], placing them at increased risk of serious reproductive morbidity including infertility and ectopic pregnancy [5,6]. Since most cases of chlamydia are asymptomatic [6], many infections go undetected.

A number of countries including the USA, Sweden, Denmark and New Zealand recommend yearly chlamydia screening in young adults; however, only England

* Correspondence: rlorch@kirby.unsw.edu.au
[1]The Kirby Institute, University of New South Wales, Sydney, NSW, Australia
Full list of author information is available at the end of the article

currently implements an organized chlamydia screening program [7,8], with screening programs planned for some European countries in the future [9]. An opportunistic program of chlamydia testing in general practice is currently being piloted – the Australian Chlamydia Control Effectiveness Pilot (ACCEPt) [10]. Over 85% of women and nearly two thirds of young men aged 16–29 years attend a general practice each year, making it an ideal setting for increased testing. Current Australian guidelines for general practitioners (GPs) recommend annual testing of this age group [11], but testing rates are low - 12.1% in women and 4.8% in men [12].

Practice nurses (PNs) are an integral part of general practice in Australia, the UK and other countries. With increasing pressures being placed on GPs' time and workload, PNs could play an important role in contributing to increasing chlamydia testing rates. PNs have a well-established role in sexual health in countries such as the UK [13], but studies specifically examining PN involvement in chlamydia testing and management are scarce. A pilot study of chlamydia testing in general practice in New Zealand reported an increase in chlamydia testing when led by PNs [8,14] and a PN-led partner notification strategy in the UK was found to have similar effectiveness and costs to referral to a specialist health adviser [15]. To our knowledge, this is the first qualitative study exploring chlamydia testing and the role of PNs specifically in general practice. We aimed to explore PN's views and opinions in relation to involvement in chlamydia testing in general practice.

Methods
Setting
This study was undertaken as part of ACCEPt. ACCEPt is the world's first cluster randomised controlled trial (RCT) of an organised programme of yearly chlamydia testing in general practice and aims to determine whether annual chlamydia testing of 16–29 year old men and women can reduce the prevalence of chlamydia. ACCEPt is being conducted in 54 rural areas of four Australian states (Victoria, New South Wales, Queensland and South Australia). The risk of contamination between control and intervention sites was minimised by conducting ACCEPt in rural and regional areas and making the unit of randomisation the town, or postcode. By recruiting every clinic within a rural area, the possibility of patients attending non-participating in clinics was reduced. Towns were eligible to participate if they had a minimum population of 500 16–29 year olds, were at least 150 kilometers away from a capital city and had up to seven general practice clinics. Clinics varied considerably in size, with some solo GP-based clinics through to large clinics with over 20 GPs on staff.

A total of 143 general practice clinics have been enrolled and randomised to either receive a multifaceted intervention designed to facilitate increased testing or to continue with usual care. ACCEPt practices in towns randomised to the intervention arm could choose for PNs to become more involved in testing and management and receive PN specific education and training, plus financial incentives payable to the clinic. ACCEPt is the first large-scale chlamydia testing RCT to investigate the potential role of the PN in chlamydia testing.

Sexual and reproductive health in rural areas of Australia is largely provided by general practice as there are few specialist sexual health or family planning clinics available. General practice clinics (hereafter referred to as practices) in Australia are small businesses that receive most of their income via "fee per service", with ~85% directly billed to the Australian government through the Medicare rebate system [16]. Until recently practices were also able to receive rebates for PN involvement in a narrow range of specific duties including immunisations, Pap smears and wound dressings. PNs' work was thus often focused on and influenced by these income generating areas [17]. However, recent restructuring of PN funding under the Practice Nurse Incentive Program (PNIP), sees most task specific funding now replaced with a single funding stream. This change aims to support an enhanced role for PNs, allowing them more flexibility to undertake a broader range of activities in areas including preventative health [18] and aligning their role more closely to PNs in the UK [17].

Sample
In-depth telephone interviews were conducted at the beginning of the trial and prior to randomisation with PNs employed in 23 different rural practices participating in ACCEPt. Purposive sampling [19] was used to maximize diversity and to provide the broadest representation of PNs. Selection was based on a number of characteristics that may influence chlamydia testing rates - size of clinic from data collected during clinic recruitment into ACCEPt; remoteness of area based on Australian Bureau of Statistics remoteness classification [20] and the PNs' prior experience in chlamydia testing, as reported in cross sectional surveys completed by the PNs during ACCEPt recruitment. PNs were contacted by telephone by one of the authors (RL), and oral consent obtained for a telephone interview to be conducted at a later date.

Interview schedule
A semi structured interview guide was drafted, reviewed by ACCEPt study staff and further refined. After the initial interviews ACCEPt study staff (RL, MTS) reviewed the

transcripts to ensure comprehension of the questions, and quality of responses. Some minor changes were made to the interview guide following these initial interviews. The semi structured interviews covered the following domains: PNs' current role in chlamydia testing and management, opinions on a PN role in chlamydia testing and management and perceived barriers and facilitators to this role. Participants also completed 12 structured questions capturing demographic, educational and employment history data (See Table 1).

Interview procedure
The interviews were undertaken by one of the authors (RL), an ACCEPt research officer with a background in nursing and midwifery practice both in Australia and the UK. Close supervision and support was provided by MTS, a qualitative researcher with extensive experience in the area of sexual health and general practice. Interviews were conducted via telephone, recorded and transcribed verbatim. Interviews were undertaken until no new themes or insights were observed to be emerging i.e. data saturation was achieved [19].

Analysis
NVivo qualitative data analysis software (QSR International Pty Ltd. Version 10, 2012) was used to organize and code the interview data. To ensure confidentiality during analysis, interview participants were assigned and identified by numbers prior to interview data being transferred into the data analysis software. Conventional content [21] and thematic analysis was undertaken, with interim analysis of early interviews occurring whilst the others were ongoing, to allow

inclusion of unanticipated themes as prompts in subsequent interviews. After multiple readings, the transcripts were initially coded using a list of broad themes derived from the main categories of the interview schedule. Blocking, grouping and labelling of data was followed by secondary analysis to identify emerging themes. Analyst triangulation was utilised; all interviews were coded by one author (RL) and a sub-set of 12 interviews was coded separately by MTS. Consensus on both codes and themes was reached following comparison of analysis.

Ethical approval
ACCEPt received ethical approval from the Royal Australian College of General Practitioners National Research and Evaluation Ethics Committee, the Aboriginal Health and Medical Research Council Ethics Committee and the University of Melbourne Human Research Ethics Committee.

Results
A total of 23 interviews with PNs were completed between June 2011 and April 2012. The majority of the participants were female, aged 30–59 years and had been working in general practice for less than 10 years (See Table 2 for participant characteristics).

The themes and sub-themes that arose from the interviews can be viewed in Table 3.

Current role – chlamydia testing and management
Most of the PNs were involved at some level with chlamydia testing and management at their practices. Many

Table 1 Interview guide for ACCEPt baseline practice nurse interviews

Domain	Questions
Participant characteristics	• Age and sex
	• Duration of nursing practice
	• Duration of employment in general practice
	• Employment status (Full/part time or casual)
	• Postgraduate qualifications
	• Education/training in sexual health
Current involvement in sexual health/chlamydia testing	• What is your role in relation to preventive health care with young men and women aged less than 30 years?
	• What is your involvement in the area of sexual health within the practice?
Opinions on PN involvement in chlamydia testing	• Can you tell me what you think about practice nurses taking an increased role in chlamydia testing in general practice?
	• What might be some of the benefits of practice nurses taking an increased role in chlamydia testing?
Barriers and facilitators to PN involvement in testing	• What could make it difficult for practice nurses to take an increased role in chlamydia testing?
	• What would make it easier for practice nurses to take an increased role in chlamydia testing?

Table 2 Participant characteristics (n = 23)

Characteristic	n (%)
Sex	
Female	22 (96)
Male	1 (4)
Age group (years)	
30–44	10 (43)
45+	12 (53)
>60	1 (4)
Location of general practice	
New South Wales	10 (44)
Victoria	7 (30)
Queensland	4 (17)
South Australia	2 (9)
Size of practice	
Small (<3 GPs)	6 (26)
Medium (3–5 GPs)	9 (39)
Large (>5 GPs)	8 (35)
Years since qualification	
<15	6 (26)
15–29	13 (57)
30 -45	4 (17)
Years working in any general practice	
<5	13 (56)
5–10	8 (35)
11-20	2 (9)
Past women's health training	
Yes	14 (61)
Past sexual health training	
Yes	6 (26)
Chlamydia testing experience	
Yes	12 (51)

provided safe sex advice and discussed sexual health issues with patients whilst collecting specimens for GPs or prior to referring to doctors for chlamydia testing.

"The doctor might have ordered a series of tests for chlamydia and HIV and all those sorts of things. So obviously there has been an issue...I ask them do they practice safe sex. I will often have discussions with young people about making sure that they are trying to do the right thing." PN22

"Basically it is an advisory role as much as anything. I don't have obviously any prescribing role or anything like that or I can't order pathology and stuff, so if they had unprotected then I suggest that they consider seeing the doctor." PN16

Of the PNs who initiated *and* carried out testing, most were doing so during Pap smear consultations and thus testing mostly women and very small numbers of young men. However, one of these PNs described how she sometimes saw both sexes:

"Within the realms of just offering Pap smears and breast checks here I have also been able to address sexual health and offer chlamydia testing as well. Often I am the first port of call and for the females sometimes they say, "Can I bring my partner in as well?" So therefore I have had the chance to talk to both." PN12

Very few nurses reported the widespread routine testing of young people, which was described by one nurse:

"Anyone that is sexually active that comes into our clinic we recommend a chlamydia screen, an STI overall screen. And we just get them to do a urine sample and nearly everyone is willing to do it. We have a pretty good success rate in doing the screening." PN6

A number of PNs also reported some involvement in partner notification, although this was seen as a role of the GP by some.

"I like the idea of the doctor actually speaking to someone and saying, "Right you need to think about your partners in this one as well." So we leave it to the doctors." PN9

Increased PN role in chlamydia testing and management
The majority of participants were supportive of having increased involvement in chlamydia testing and management, feeling PNs were suited to the role.

"I am all for it. I think that we are often the first person the patient sees especially in that age group and we have an ideal opportunity to offer that." PN18

"Yeah I think it is a great idea...Well I think in general nurses are a little bit more in tune with primary health care and preventative health" PN25

Benefits of PN involvement
Patient benefits
The PNs felt that their involvement in testing could lead to increased access to testing, diagnosis and treatment for young people, thus benefitting the community.

Table 3 Themes/sub-themes arising from ACCEPt baseline practice nurse interviews

Domain	Themes
PNs current role in sexual health/chlamydia testing	Advice and discussion
	Referral to/specimen collection for GP
	Complete consultation – women's health
	Testing all young people as normal practice
Opinion around PN involvement in chlamydia testing	Support
	PNs suitability for role
Benefits of PN involvement in chlamydia testing	Patient benefits:
	• Increased access to testing
	• Patients prefer PNs
	• Patient empowerment
	GP benefits:
	• Ease workload
	PN benefits:
	• Role expansion – job satisfaction
Barriers to PN involvement in chlamydia testing	Time and workload
	Small town concerns:
	• Privacy and confidentiality
	GP attitudes:
	• Role conflict and handing over power
	Pathology ordering:
	• GP involvement and nurse autonomy
	Remuneration:
	• General practice as a business
	• Revenue attracting work
Facilitators to PN involvement in chlamydia testing	Education and training:
	• Knowledge and skills acquisition
	• Confidence and empowerment
	Change to pathology ordering
	Organisation of chlamydia testing:
	• Testing pathways
	Funding for PN chlamydia testing:
	• Item numbers for PN testing and PNIP

"Hopefully more (tests) actually being done for young people ...patients can access practice nurses more easily and freely." PN1

"We are not even touching on it here; it is generally not bought up in a conversation with a doctor in a consultation... so I think if it we could make it more available then there would be a lot more testing." PN12

"Well definitely it would benefit the community, (we) would be able to pick up chlamydia earlier, inform people earlier about it and information like that would be of obvious benefit." PN20

A number of PNs felt that patients preferred a consultation with the PN as they were more approachable and easier to talk to than the GP, especially for females.

"Look I think young people feel a lot more comfortable speaking to a nurse...I think they feel a lot more at ease." PN6

"I think it is better for practice nurses to be doing that, the one-on-one situation, the confidentiality is there and with the women I think they feel more comfortable speaking to another woman rather than to males." PN19

One nurse felt her interactions with the patients empowered them to feel more confident to discuss sexual health matters with the GP.

> "...sometimes if they go to see a doctor without seeing me, the doctor will just discuss with them the doctor's preference not the patient's preference...So by seeing me, having the information, they can ask questions and then this encourages the doctors to be more open." PN12

GP benefits

The majority of PNs thought that their involvement could benefit GPs by easing their workload and that chlamydia testing was an easy role to hand over to PNs, who may have more time to provide patient education.

> "It certainly takes the emphasis off the doctors having to do things like that. It is not a difficult test so if somebody else can do it for them I think that would be beneficial." PN19

> "Well I think a practice nurse can have a little bit more time (than doctors) therefore a bit more time with the education and answering questions if required." PN4

PN benefits

Finally, some felt that PNs themselves could benefit, with job satisfaction resulting from role expansion into chlamydia testing

> "And I guess I love doing anything new so anything that adds interest to your job too is good and keeps you a bit on your toes and keeps you a bit more current." PN21

Barriers to an increased PN role in chlamydia testing
Time and workload

Time and workload constraints were commonly raised as an important barrier by many in our sample. At busy times chlamydia testing would take a lower priority than acute cases.

> "...time constraints for practice nurses. Their workload is pretty heavy and pretty varied too...And certainly you have to prioritise what you can do. If you have got chest pain it is a priority over asking someone about chlamydia." PN9

However, the barrier was not insurmountable for some.

> "There is really no barrier other than a time barrier... Our own time constraints are fairly big...we never have time to scratch ourselves so from that point of view that is a definite constraint. As far as it is us fitting it into our days which could be a problem, there would be a way around it." PN16

"Small town" concerns

Many nurses spoke about the experience of living in a "small town", linking this to patients' and their own concerns about confidentiality and testing.

> "...it is a small town and you sort of know everybody but you try and explain to patients about confidentiality but I suppose it is still in the back of their mind." PN14

> "One of the biggest barriers I guess for this town is that is a really small tight knit community. I have children the same age; my kids went to the school here so they are the same age as the guys that are young coming in here all the time...So as far as I am concerned I guess they might feel a bit uncomfortable I guess." PN8

GP attitudes

A number of PNs felt that GP attitudes towards PN involvement in testing could act as a barrier, with issues such as role conflict and GP concerns about handing over "power" to PNs identified.

> "When I worked in other clinics there were a lot of issues with me having that knowledge and me being able to do that. It is a case of 'that is our role', but then (the doctors) didn't want to do it either. The doctors are just threatened I think, threatened that you will take over a role that they can do. If you are working with doctors who treat you as a hand maiden it is very difficult then to come forward and say, 'Well actually I think (PNs) can do this or this'." PN8

> "I actually think there is a role for practice nurses in that and I suppose the one difficulty might be how doctors feel about it...Oh you know sometimes depending who you work for some of them like to be the ones to instigate things. ... GP Management Plans, 'well just don't do it, let me see them first and if I decide their GP Management Plan then I will let you know to do it'. Do you know what I mean?" PN22

> "We are realising that we can do more and more and offer more that complements the doctors but (we need to) bridge that understanding that we are not in competition with them" PN12

Pathology ordering

The ordering of pathology for chlamydia testing was identified as a barrier by a number of PNs. In Australia federal legislation requires that when diagnostic pathology investigations attract a charge against Medicare (as is the case in general practice) the request form must be signed by a medical practitioner *before* the service is provided [22], requiring direct input from a GP who is often too busy to do this or uncomfortable with the nurse managing the process independently.

"I think one of the things is addressing the pathology side of things. Like at this stage most doctors would want to be involved if there is any discussion on chlamydia. They wouldn't feel comfortable just handing that straight over to the nurses. At this stage I think the doctors would be, from what I have seen, reluctant to let us have that sort of freedom." PN12

"They have to be seen by a doctor to order the pathology and generally our doctors are sort of they are reasonably booked up on a day to day basis." PN18

Remuneration for PN testing

The issue of funding for PN activities was raised by some as an important barrier. These PNs felt that GPs run businesses and so it was desirable for PNs to be undertaking activities that attract revenue. Prior to the introduction of the PNIP (when some of these interviews took place), some nurse activities such as Pap smears were funded specifically, whereas chlamydia testing was not.

"The principal, he is paying us good wages, well my boss does. He pays us good wages so if we are going to do more and more testing, this is my management hat coming back on now, if I am doing more and more testing for chlamydia he doesn't get a cent to pay my wages." PN2

Facilitators to an increased PN role in chlamydia testing
Education and training

By far, the most significant facilitator for the PNs was the provision of education and training, which would not only provide knowledge and skills, but empower the nurses in their role as chlamydia testers.

"That would come, I think, with the education. And the knowledge and awareness to have the confidence to approach and talk to people about it." PN9

"There is nothing more embarrassing than someone asks you a question and you can't answer it. So it is important we are trained." PN13

"I think nurses need to be educated and part of that is about increasing their self-esteem and their recognition that they have the power to make a difference with these things." PN3

Changes to pathology processes

Some PNs suggested changes to systems of pathology ordering as facilitators to increase PN involvement in testing.

"Basically what we need is pre-signed forms from the doctor... if someone came and the moment arose then you could say, "Well look here is the form just slip it back to the pathology with the specimen of urine." It just makes it very simple rather than having to involve a doctor to get that testing done" PN12

Organisation of chlamydia testing

Changes to the organisation of chlamydia testing within practices could facilitate increased PN chlamydia testing, with strategies to streamline the process, set up "testing pathways" and include other staff suggested by some.

"Doing chlamydia screens certainly isn't a huge time spender so if we could find a way of trying to identify the young people that are coming into the clinic and try to capture them and give them a cup and a path form. It is fairly straight forward after that isn't it?" PN6

"I have spoken to the doctors and they are happy ... when those patients come through the girls at the front desk, we have to give them the responsibility of looking at their ages and they will then redirect them through to the nurses." PN13

Funding for PN testing

A system for reimbursing the cost of PN involvement in chlamydia testing, such as a Medicare nurse item number, was identified as a facilitator by some nurses.

"...so I don't know is there anything that can be done like your Pap smear incentive number...because then that would then pay for some of the ongoing costs" PN2

"...it possibly helps us to be a little bit more pro-active some sort of incentive number payment I think...if you are busy you think, "Oh well I won't do the chlamydia, I haven't go time to talk about the chlamydia today."" PN4

In later interviews, the change in PN funding with the introduction of the PNIP was seen a facilitator.

"Because the whole funding for practice nurses has changed that is probably a benefit if you were looking at introducing chlamydia testing because... the practice gets compensated from the government for the hours the nurse works not for who they see in that time frame, so that could actually work to the benefit of nurses doing chlamydia testing." PN12

Discussion

This first qualitative study specifically exploring PNs and chlamydia testing and management in general practice suggests that PNs could take a role in chlamydia testing. The PNs in our study demonstrated support for an increased role in testing and identified important benefits of increased involvement for patients, PNs, GPs, and the community. The PNs raised a number of barriers to PN involvement in testing, but also some practical ways to overcome them.

Issues concerning living in a "small town" were commonly raised by our PNs. It has been suggested that young people accessing local services for sexual health care have fears around confidentiality and anonymity and in small rural towns these problems may be even more acute due to their high visibility and the "interconnectedness" of the community [23,24]. Possible personal links with health professionals, as highlighted by some of our PNs, may act as a further barrier [23]. However, during a cross-sectional chlamydia prevalence survey carried out as part of ACCEPt, 70% of young people approached agreed to chlamydia testing, with 86% reporting that they were attending their local practice [25]. This suggests that whilst young people in rural towns may not commonly ask for chlamydia testing, they are happy to accept it, if offered. Although PN themselves did not suggest ways to overcome "small town" concerns, the issues could be minimized by PNs reinforcing their duty of confidentiality to young patients, along with normalization of chlamydia testing into routine primary healthcare for this population to reduce stigma [23,26].

GP attitudes towards a PN role in testing were seen as a key barrier by some PNs. Other studies have suggested reluctance among some GPs in Australia in handing over responsibility for aspects of care to PNs, whilst the hierarchical structure and medical dominance that exists in some practices may prevent collaboration between health professionals and limit PNs' scope of practice [27,28]. However, as has occurred in the UK, the extension of PN roles into areas such as preventative health and screening may alleviate some of the increasing pressures on GPs driven by shortages in workforce and an increase in the burden of disease attributable to chronic conditions [29,30]. In light of this, GPs may therefore find it acceptable for PNs to increase their involvement in chlamydia testing and management. Validation and promotion of the role of the PN in sexual health may also have an effect on the attitudes of GPs and positive work in this area is already being done by state based organisations in Australia [31]. It is also interesting to note there may be some disparity between PNs' perception of GP attitudes and the actual attitudes of GPs. In a series of qualitative interviews with 44 GPs undertaken as part of ACCEPt, the vast majority supported the concept of PN chlamydia testing, identifying similar benefits to their involvement as were raised by the PNs in this study [32].

PNs raised barriers to their involvement relating to the logistics of testing, such as being unable to order chlamydia investigations for patients without consultation with a GP. As mentioned earlier, most diagnostic pathology investigations undertaken in Australian general practice are claimed through Medicare. Currently, nurse initiated pathology which attracts a Medicare charge is only possible for eligible nurse practitioners and "appropriately qualified and experienced midwives" [33]. Furthermore, the signing of "blank" request forms by GPs, a facilitator suggested by the PNs, or signing *after* a service has taken place is a breach of federal legislation [22], although there is anecdotal evidence that this has happened [34]. It can be argued that in cases where chlamydia testing is clinically indicated, such as for sexually active patients aged 16–29 years, ordering a chlamydia test, independent of immediate GP involvement, is well within the scope of practice of an appropriately trained PN. Systems that permit PNs to initiate chlamydia testing, along with modifications to clinic testing pathways so young people were seen by the PN first, without direct input from a GP, could also address the barrier of time and workload pressures, which was commonly raised and consistent with earlier GP studies on chlamydia testing in the United Kingdom [35,36] and Australia [37,38]. The provision of education and training was a major facilitator for our PNs and the in-depth interviews not only confirmed the importance of the ACCEPt PN training session and education pack as a central component of the ACCEPt PN intervention but also informed its content. The ACCEPt PN education package includes discussion around and suggestions for chlamydia testing pathways that could be used in clinics, along with strategies to employ to minimize time spent and simplify testing consultations. Such strategies include providing "scripts" for PNs to use when offering tests with examples demonstrated for the PNs via DVD [39], checklists to ensure essential elements of the consultation are covered and educational resources for patients to take away.

Funding to cover PN involvement in testing was another identified barrier/facilitator, with a number of PNs suggesting a rebate similar to those previously provided for specific PN tasks such as immunisations. However, as mentioned previously, a number of the interviews took place before the introduction of the new PN funding mechanism, the PNIP. This new arrangement may allow PNs to expand their roles beyond those determined by specific MBS item numbers and include sexual health and chlamydia testing, whilst also addressing the funding for these activities. Resources are available to inform Australian GPs of the rationale and practicalities of PN involvement in sexual health care under the PNIP, and to assist PNs to "make their case" for an expanded role in this area [40]. Formal evaluation of the PNIP is currently being undertaken and aims to identify if the changed funding mechanism has had any impact on the role and function of PNs [41].

The strengths of this study include the recruitment of participants from a diverse range of clinics and from a range of locations across Australia. There are also some limitations. The PNs interviewed reflect those who were selected by their clinics to possibly be involved in chlamydia testing if randomised to the intervention arm of ACCEPt. Thus these PNs may represent a biased sample of PNs who are more "interested" in sexual health. Also, the sample was drawn from clinics in rural and regional areas and some findings such as the issue of 'small town concerns' may therefore be context specific.

Conclusion

Chlamydia infection is an important public health issue for young people and general practice is ideally placed to implement widespread chlamydia testing. However, testing rates must increase to sufficient levels to impact on the burden of chlamydia in this population. As Australia investigates the feasibility, acceptability, efficacy and cost-effectiveness of an organised programme of annual chlamydia testing in general practice and as other countries plan the implementation of screening programmes, our study suggests that PNs could emerge as a potentially valuable resource in contributing to increasing chlamydia testing rates. However, barriers exist that may impede the development of the PN role into this area. Strategies to overcome these barriers and facilitate PN involvement, along with further research into the effectiveness and acceptability of PN chlamydia testing are warranted and should be explored.

Abbreviations
ACCEPt: Australian control effectiveness pilot; GP: General practitioner; PN: Practice nurse; PNIP: Practice nurse incentive program; RCT: Randomised controlled trial; UK: United Kingdom; US: United States.

Competing interests
The authors declare that they have no competing interests.

Authors' contributions
RL devised the research question, analysed the data and drafted the manuscript. JH, RG, MTS contributed to the study design, supervised data analysis and writing of the manuscript. AV, AW, DL contributed to development of study instruments, administered study instruments and contributed to writing of the manuscript. All authors read and approved the final manuscript.

Acknowledgements
This survey was conducted as part of the Australian Chlamydia Control Effectiveness Pilot (ACCEPt). We would like to thank the ACCEPt research staff for their hard work in recruiting the PNs, and the PNs who kindly donated their time in participating in these interviews.

Author details
[1]The Kirby Institute, University of New South Wales, Sydney, NSW, Australia. [2]Melbourne School of Population and Global Health, University of Melbourne, Melbourne, VIC, Australia. [3]Department of General Practice, University of Melbourne, Melbourne, VIC, Australia.

References
1. European Centre for Disease Prevention and Control. Annual epidemiological report 2013. Reporting on 2011 surveillance data and 2012 epidemic intelligence data. Stockholm; 2013.
2. The Kirby Institute. HIV, Viral Hepatitis and Sexually Transmissible Infections in Australia Annual Surveillance. Report 2014. Sydney: The University of New South Wales; 2014.
3. Centres for Disease Control and Prevention. Reported STDs in the United State 2012. [http://www.cdc.gov/nchhstp/newsroom/docs/STD-Trends-508.pdf]
4. Oakeshott P, Kerry S, Aghaizu A, Atherton HHS, Taylor-Robinson D, Simms I, et al. Randomised controlled trial of screening for Chlamydia trachomatis to prevent pelvic inflammatory disease: the POPI (prevention of pelvic infection) trial. BMJ (Clinical research ed). 2010;340:c1642.
5. Haggerty CL, Gottlieb SL, Taylor BD, Low N, Xu F, Ness RB. Risk of sequelae after Chlamydia trachomatis genital infection in women. J Infect Dis. 2010;201 Suppl 2:S134–55.
6. Peipert JF. Genital Chlamydial infections. N Engl J Med. 2003;349(25):2424–30.
7. Hocking JS, Guy R, Walker J, Tabrizi SN. Advances in sampling and screening for chlamydia. Future Microbiol. 2013;8(3):367–86.
8. Azariah S, McKernon S, Werder S. Large increase in opportunistic testing for chlamydia during a pilot project in a primary health organisation. J Prim Health Care. 2013;5(2):141–5.
9. Low N, Cassell JA, Spencer B, Bender N, Martin Hilber A, van Bergen J, et al. Chlamydia control activities in Europe: cross-sectional survey. Eur J Public Health. 2012;22(4):556–61.
10. Hocking JS, Low N, Guy R, Matthew Law, Basil Donovan, John Kaldor, et al. 12 PRT 09010: Australian Chlamydia Control Effectiveness Pilot (ACCEPt): a cluster randomised controlled trial of chlamydia testing in general practice (ACTRN1260000297022). [http://www.thelancet.com/protocol-reviews/12PRT-9010]
11. Royal Australian College of General Practitioners. Guidelines for preventive activities in general practice, 8th edn. East Melbourne; 2012.
12. Kong FGR, Hocking J, Merritt T, Pirotta M, Heal C, Bergeri I, et al. Australian general practitioner chlamydia testing rates among young people. Med J Aust. 2011;194(5):249.
13. Stokes T, Mears J. Sexual health and the practice nurse: a survey of reported practice and attitudes. Br J Fam Plann. 2000;26(2):89–92.
14. Lawton BA, Rose SB, Elley CR, Bromhead C, MacDonald EJ, Baker MG. Increasing the uptake of opportunistic chlamydia screening: a pilot study in general practice. J Prim Health Care. 2010;2(3):199–207.
15. Low N, McCarthy A, Roberts TE, Huengsberg M, Sanford E, Sterne JA, et al. Partner notification of chlamydia infection in primary care: randomised controlled trial and analysis of resource use. BMJ (Clinical research ed). 2006;332(7532):14–9.
16. Saunders C, Tierney L. A Guide to Understanding and Working with General Practice in NSW. Sydney: General Practice NSW; 2011.
17. Joyce CM, Piterman L. The work of nurses in Australian general practice: a national survey. Int J Nurs Stud. 2011;48(1):70–80.

18. King JWI, Brewerton R. Developing a Business Case for An Enhanced Practice Nurse Role under the Practice Nurse Incentive Program (PNIP). Auckland: Australian Practice Nurse Association (APNA); 2011.

19. Richards L, JM M. Read Me First For a Users Guide To Qualitative Research Methods. 3rd ed. Los Angeles, USA: Sage; 2013.

20. Australian Bureau of Statistics. Remoteness Structure. [http://www.abs.gov.au/websitedbs/D3310114.nsf/home/remoteness+structure#Anchor2c]

21. Hsieh HF, Shannon SE. Three approaches to qualitative content analysis. Qual Health Res. 2005;15(9):1277–88.

22. Guidelines on Nurse and Midwife Initiated Diagnostic Investigations. NSW Nurses and Midwives Association. [http://www.nswnma.asn.au/wp-content/uploads/2013/07/Guidelines-on-Nurse-and-Midwife-Initiated-Diagnostic-Investigations.pdf]

23. Garside R, Ayres R, Owen M, Pearson VA, Roizen J. Anonymity and confidentiality: rural teenagers' concerns when accessing sexual health services. J Fam Plann Reprod Health Care. 2002;28(1):23–6.

24. Quine S, Bernard D, Booth M, Kang M, Usherwood T, Alperstein G, et al. Health and access issues among Australian adolescents: a rural–urban comparison. Rural Remote Health. 2003;3(3):245.

25. Yeung AH, Temple-Smith M, Fairley CK, Vaisey AM, Guy R, Law MG, et al. Chlamydia prevalence in young attenders of rural and regional primary care services in Australia: a cross-sectional survey. Med J Aust. 2014;200(3):170–5.

26. Rose SB, Smith MC, Lawton BA. "If everyone does it, it's not a big deal." Young people talk about chlamydia testing. N Z Med J. 2008;121(1271):33–42.

27. Pearce C, Phillips C, Hall S, Sibbald B, Porritt J, Yates R, et al. Following the funding trail: financing, nurses and teamwork in Australian general practice. BMC Health Serv Res. 2011;11:38.

28. Phillips CB, Pearce C, Hall S, Kljakovic M, Sibbald B, Dwan K, et al. Enhancing care, improving quality: the six roles of the general practice nurse. Med J Aust. 2009;191(2):92–7.

29. Parker R, Keleher H, Forrest L. The work, education and career pathways of nurses in Australian general practice. Aust J Prim Health. 2011;17(3):227–32.

30. Parker R, Walker L, Hegarty K. Primary care nursing workforce in Australia: a vision for the future. Aust Fam Physician. 2010;39(3):159–60.

31. Abbott P, Dadich A, Hosseinzadeh H, Kang M, Hu W, Bourne C, et al. Practice nurses and sexual health care: enhancing team care within general practice. Aust Fam Physician. 2013;42:729–33.

32. Lorch R, Hocking J, Guy R, Vaisey A, Wood A, Donovan B, et al. Do Australian general practitioners believe practice nurses can take a role in chlamydia testing? A qualitative study of attitudes and opinions. BMC Infect Dis. 2015;15:31.

33. Health Legislation Amendment (Midwives and Nurse Practitioners) Bill. 2010. [http://www.aph.gov.au/Parliamentary_Business/Bills_Legislation/Bills_Search_Results/Result?bld=r4151]

34. Submission from the Australian Nurse Practitioner Association to the National Health and Hospitals Reform Commission. 2009. [https://acnp.org.au/sites/default/files/docs/014_australian_nurse_practitioners_association_submission.pdf]

35. McNulty CA, Freeman E, Howell-Jones R, Hogan A, Randall S, Ford-Young W, et al. Overcoming the barriers to chlamydia screening in general practice–a qualitative study. Fam Pract. 2010;27(3):291–302.

36. Perkins E, Carlisle C, Jackson N. Opportunistic screening for Chlamydia in general practice: the experience of health professionals. Health Soc Care Community. 2003;11(4):314–20.

37. Hocking JS, Parker RM, Pavlin N, Fairley CK, Gunn JM. What needs to change to increase chlamydia screening in general practice in Australia? The views of general practitioners. BMC Public Health. 2008;8:425.

38. Merritt TD, Durrheim DN, Hope K, Byron P. General practice intervention to increase opportunistic screening for chlamydia. Sex Health. 2007;4(4):249–51.

39. McNulty CA, Hogan AH, Ricketts EJ, Wallace L, Oliver I, Campbell R, et al. Increasing Chlamydia Screening Tests in General Practice: A Modified Zelen Prospective Cluster Randomised Controlled Trial Evaluating A Complex Intervention Based On The Theory Of Planned Behaviour, Sexually transmitted infections. 2013.

40. Australian Medicare Local Alliance. PNIP and Sexual Health. [http://www.iwsml.org.au/images/allied_health_services_directory/Sexual_Health_2014013_1info_FINAL.pdf]

41. Australian Medical Association. Evaluation of the Practice Nurse Incentive Program. [https://ama.com.au/ausmed/evaluation-practice-nurse-incentive-program]

4

Measuring empathic, person-centred communication in primary care nurses: validity and reliability of the Consultation and Relational Empathy (CARE) Measure

Annemieke P. Bikker[1*], Bridie Fitzpatrick[1], Douglas Murphy[2] and Stewart W. Mercer[1]

Abstract

Background: Empathic patient-centred care is central to high quality health encounters. The Consultation and Relational Empathy (CARE) Measure is a patient-rated experience measure of the interpersonal quality of healthcare encounters. The measure has been extensively validated and is widely used by doctors in primary care but has not been validated in nursing. This study assessed the validity and reliability of the CARE Measure in routine nurse consultations in primary care.

Methods: Seventeen nurses from nine general medical practices located in three Scottish Health Boards participated in the study. Consecutive patients (aged 16 years or older) were asked to self-complete a questionnaire containing the CARE Measure immediately after their clinical encounter with the nurse. Statistical analysis included Spearman's correlation and principal component analysis (construct validity), Cronbach's alpha (internal consistency), and Generalisability theory (inter-rater reliability).

Results: A total of 774 patients (327 male and 447 female) completed the questionnaire. Almost three out of four patients (73 %) felt that the CARE Measure items were very important to their current consultation. The number of 'not applicable' responses and missing values were low overall (5.7 and 1.6 % respectively). The mean CARE Measure score in the consultations was 45.9 and 48 % achieved the maximum possible score of 50. CARE Measure scores correlated in predicted ways with overall satisfaction and patient enablement in support of convergent and divergent validity. Factor analysis found that the CARE Measure items loaded highly onto a single factor. The measure showed high internal consistency (Cronbach's alpha coefficient = 0.97) and acceptable inter-rater reliability ($G = 0.6$ with 60 patients ratings per nurse). The scores were not affected by patients' age, gender, self-perceived overall health, living arrangements, employment status or language spoken at home.

Conclusions: The CARE Measure has high face and construct validity, and internal reliability in nurse consultations in primary care. Its ability to discriminate between nurses is sufficient for educational and quality improvement purposes.

Keywords: Empathy, CARE Measure, Practice nurses, Validation, Reliability, Primary care

* Correspondence: Annemieke.Bikker@glasgow.ac.uk
[1]General Practice and Primary Care, Institute of Health and Wellbeing, University of Glasgow, 1 Horselethill Road, Glasgow G12 9LX, UK
Full list of author information is available at the end of the article

Background

Patients consistently score empathy and the human aspects of care as top priorities in their health care [1–4]. Research has linked empathic care to higher levels of patient satisfaction [5–7], enablement [8–10] and improved health outcomes [8, 10–14]. Its importance is emphasised in healthcare policies [15–17] and professional codes of conduct [18, 19]. Healthcare practitioners are increasingly expected to demonstrate their interpersonal skills in terms of empathic, patient-centred care in practice and training [20, 21]. Measurement is crucial to evaluate this aspect of quality of care and to obtain feedback on individual practitioners.

The Consultation and Relational Empathy (CARE) Measure is a patient-assessed measure of the quality of the encounter with healthcare professionals [3, 21]. Ten items ask patients' perception of the practitioner's 'relational empathy', defined as the healthcare practitioner's ability to:

a) understand the patient's situation, perspective and feelings (and their attached meanings);
b) communicate that understanding and check its accuracy, and
c) act on that understanding with the patient in a helpful (therapeutic) way [3, 21].

The development of the measure was based on a review of existing measures and qualitative interviews with patients, and their feedback on the individual items in order to create a measure that was meaningful regardless of the patients' socioeconomic status [21]. We did this by assessing the views of patients living in areas of high or low socioeconomic deprivation and, in an iterative process, developed, validated and tested the CARE Measure in primary care consultations with general practitioners (GPs) [21, 22].

Since its development and validation with general practitioners (GPs) in the UK [21], the measure has been extensively validated with a range of physician groups in primary and secondary care [22–26]. It has been widely used nationally (including in GP appraisal and revalidation) and internationally, and has been translated and validated in various languages [23, 24, 27]. However, to date nurses have not been included in this expanding body of work on the CARE Measure. Given the increasing role of nurses in primary care in many countries, it would seem timely to asses whether the CARE Measure is valid and reliable in this professional group. It would be scientifically wrong to assume that a measure developed primarily for use with GPs will also be valid and reliable with nurses. The role of nurses in primary care is distinct from that of GPs; in the United Kingdom (UK), practice nurses are employed by GPs to carry out routine annual reviews of a limited number of single chronic disease, and some also do minor illness clinics. GPs, on the other hand, deal with a wide range of clinical issues, including the management of most mental health problems and patients with complex multimorbidity of chronic diseases.

In carrying out the current study we have a number of hypotheses to be tested based on our previous work on empathy and the CARE Measure:

1. We would expect the CARE measure to be relevant to most consultations with practice nurses, as we have found for primary care and secondary care doctors [22, 25, 26].
2. Since the CARE measure reflects patients' views on generic interpersonal skills, we would expect it to be valid and reliable in primary care nurses, similar to what we have found for GPs and other doctor groups [22, 25, 26].
3. We would expect the CARE measure to load onto a single factor in factor analysis as found in other studies [22, 24–26].
4. As in this previous work [22, 24–26], we would predict the CARE Measure would show convergent validity with patient satisfaction but divergent validity with patient enablement, since the latter is a construct quite distinct from satisfaction [28].
5. We would also predict that the CARE Measure would be related to factors such as consultation length and continuity, as shown in our previous work with doctors [22, 25, 26].

Methods

Sampling, data collection and ethics

Ten out of 55 randomly selected GP Practices within a 40 mile radius of the study office responded positively to an invitation to participate in the study. The Practices represented three Scottish Health Board areas and combined provided the opportunity to collect data on the consultations of 20 nurses (19 practice nurses and 1 nurse practitioner). The aim was to collect self-completed patient questionnaires for 50 consecutive consultations with each participating nurse. The sampling strategy ensured that patients from a range of socioeconomic levels would be included in the study, but we did not have sufficient funding to specifically sample from high and low deprivation areas as we did in our original validation work [21, 22]. The consultation number was based on previous work that demonstrated the required sample size to effectively discriminate between GPs [22].

Practice receptionists gave consecutive adult patients (16 years or older) a questionnaire when they checked in for their appointment with a participating nurse. This is the same approach that we have used in our previous validation studies with GPs [21, 22]. Patients completed the questionnaire immediately after the consultation and placed it in a sealed box in the waiting room. The questionnaire contained:

- The 10 item CARE Measure [21]
- A question on the importance of the CARE Measure items to their consultation (rated on a 4 point scale from 1 = not important to 4 = very important) which we have used previously [22].
- An overall satisfaction question (rated on a Likert scale from 1 = completely satisfied to 7 = completely dissatisfied). This was included because perceived empathy is known to be an important determinant of patient satisfaction and thus would be predicted to correlate positively with CARE measure scores, and thus provide evidence of convergent validity [5–7].
- The six items contained in the Patient Enablement Instrument (PEI) [28]. The PEI was included because although enablement is related to satisfaction and CARE measure scores, it is a different construct. It would be predicted to correlate less strongly with the CARE measure than patient satisfaction, and thus provide evidence of divergent validity.
- Questions we have used previously [12, 22, 28] on relational continuity (how well the patients knows the nurse, rated on a Likert scale from 1 = don't know at all to 5 = know very well), whether or not previously seen by nurse, consultation length, satisfaction with consultation length (from 1 = very poor to 6 = excellent)
- Socio-demographic details (self-perceived overall health, age, gender, living arrangements, employment status and language spoken at home).

Data were collected between September 2012 and October 2013.

Scoring of the CARE Measure
The 10 CARE Measure items are rated on a 5-item response scale from 1 = poor to 5 = excellent. The overall score is the sum of the ten items with 10 being the lowest possible score and 50 the highest. Up to two not applicable (N/A) responses or missing values are allowed and these are replaced by the average item score.

As we wanted to directly compare the findings of the current study with our previous work with GPs [21, 22] we did not attempt to 'weight' the scores.

Ethics
Ethical approval was obtained from the National Research Ethics Service (NRES) Committee North West,

Preston (Reference 12/NW0607, on 2/8/2012). All nurses who participated in the study provided written informed consent. Informed consent was not required from the patients who decided to complete the questionnaire, because the questionnaire was anonymous and did not ask for identifiable information. Completion of the questionnaire was voluntary and the optional nature of the study was explained in the information on the front of the questionnaire.

Analysis
The data were analysed using SPSS (version 21) and urGENOVA software via its associated wrapper program GS4 for the reliability analyses [29, 30] as was done in our previous studies [25, 26]. Descriptive methods were used to describe the sample, calculate the CARE Measure and PEI scores, and check the variability in the data. As data distributions were skewed, differences between groups were assessed through non-parametric tests. The perceived relevance and face validity of the CARE Measure was assessed by analysing the number of not applicable and missing values for each of its 10 items as well as the patients' rating of the importance of the 10 items, as in previous studies [22–27]. Construct validity was examined through factor analysis (principal component analysis with varimax rotation and Kaiser normalisation) and correlations (Spearman' rho) between the CARE Measure items, and PEI and the overall satisfaction measure. The internal reliability of the CARE Measure was assessed through Cronbach's alpa. The ability of the measure to discriminate between nurses was assessed using Generalisability-theory (G-Theory) and associated Decision D studies [22, 25, 26].

Results
One practice with three nurses withdrew from the study, thus 17 nurses took part. Completed questionnaires were obtained for 774 practice nurse consultations (37–55 per nurse). Consultations included appointments for clinics for chronic disease management such as diabetes, coronary heart disease and chronic obstructive pulmonary disease. One nurse provided acute care only. The age of patients attending these consultations ranged from 16 to 93 years (mean age = 54.9 years, SD = 18.2), 447 patients (57.8 %) were female, and 391 patients (51 %) rated their overall health as good or very good (Table 1).

In terms of consultation characteristics, the length of consultations ranged from 1 to 50 min (mean consultation length = 13 min, SD = 7.6 min). Around three-quarter of patients (76 %) reported a previous consultation with the nurse and half the patients (50 %) reported that they knew the practice nurse quite well or very well. CARE Measure scores were weakly correlated with how well patients knew the nurse (Spearman's rho

Table 1 Demographic data of participating patients

	Sample size (n)	% of total sample
Gender		
Male	290	37.5
Female	447	57.8
Missing values	37	4.8
Age group		
16–29 years	87	11.2
30–44 years	105	13.6
45–65 years	298	38.5
>65 years	234	30.2
Missing values	50	6.5
Overall Health Status		
Very good/ good	394	50.9
Fair	239	30.9
Bad/ very bad	103	13.4
Missing values	38	4.9
Living arrangements		
With Partner/Spouse	453	58.5
Not with Partner/Spouse	281	36.3
Missing Values	40	5.2
Language Spoken at Home		
English	729	94.2
Other	6	0.8
Missing Values	39	5.0
Employment status		
Employed (full- or part-time, including self-employed)	279	36.0
Unemployed (looking for work)	41	5.3
Unfit to work	92	11.9
Retired	265	34.2
Looking after home/family	19	2.4
In education	19	2.5
Other	18	2.1
Missing	41	5.3
Help with Questionnaire		
Yes	64	8.3
No	681	88.0
Missing Values	29	3.7

218, $p = 0.000$) and with consultation length (rho 0.123, $p = 0.001$).

Relevance to current consultation

Overall, almost three-quarters of patients (73 %) perceived the CARE Measure items as very important to their current consultation. Older patients and patients

with worse self-reported overall health tended to score the importance of the items higher than younger patients ($p = 0.000$) and patients with better health status ($p = 0.033$) (Table 2). No statistical differences were found for the other patient characteristics.

'Not applicable' responses in the CARE Measure amounted to only 6 % of the total possible 'not applicable' responses (444/7740 items; see Table 3). For CARE Measure items 1 to 8, the average number of not applicable responses was 3 % ($n = 181$), ranging from 0.6 % for item 1 to 5 % for item 2. The highest number of "not applicable" responses were recorded for items 9 ($n = 112$, 15 %) and 10 ($n = 151$, 20 %), which relate to 'taking control' and 'making a plan of action' respectively. The total number of responses for which there was missing data was 124, representing less than 2 % of the total possible number of missing responses (i.e. 124/7740). The missing responses were evenly distributed across the CARE Measure items.

Three or more 'not applicable' or missing responses were given by 76 (9.8 %) patients. Patients with worse self-reported health had less occurrences of three or more 'not applicable' or missing responses than patients with better self-reported health status ($\chi^2 = 5.860$, $p = 0.53$). No statistical associations were found for the other patient characteristics (results not shown).

Performance of the CARE Measure

The overall mean CARE Measure score for all practice nurses was 45.9 (SD 5.9) and the mean CARE Measure scores per practice nurse ranged from 42.6 to 47.9 ($p = 0.005$). Individual patient scores ranged from 20 (minimum possible score being 10) to the maximum score of 50. Nearly half of practice nurse consultations (48 %) received the maximum possible score. The distribution of the scores showed a skew of −1.5 and a kurtosis of 1.8.

Explanatory factor analysis on the CARE Measure items, PEI and satisfaction questions showed three factors with the CARE Measure items on one factor with high loadings (0.883-0.967), indicating a robust internal structure of the CARE Measure (Table 4). The PEI items loaded on the second factor, and the satisfaction measures on the third factor. The three factors explained 83 % of the variance.

Correlations between the CARE Measure scores and patient enablement and overall satisfaction supported construct (convergent) validity in relation to overall satisfaction (Spearman's rho 0.54, $p = 0.000$), and as expected less (divergent) with patient enablement (Spearman's rho 0.19, $p = 0.000$).

The CARE Measure showed weak but significant positive relationships with consultation length (Spearman's rho 0.12, $p = 0.002$) and how well patients knew the nurse (Spearman's rho 0.22, $p = 0.000$). The patient

Table 2 Patients' perceived importance of the CARE Measure items to their consultation

	Little or No Importance (%)	Moderate Importance (%)	Very Important (%)	p- value
All Consultations	39 (5.1)	137 (17.7)	562 (72.6)	
Age group				0.000
29	12 (14.1)	26 (30.6)	47 (56.3)	
30–44	7 (6.8)	28 (27.2)	68 (66.0)	
45–65	12 (4.1)	43 (14.7)	237 (81.2)	
> 65	5 (2.2)	33 (14.8)	185 (83.05)	
Gender				ns
Male	20 (7.1)	40 (14.3)	220 (78.6)	
Female	17 (3.9)	93 (21.4)	325 (74.7)	
Overall Health Status				0.033
Very good/good	22 (5.7)	86 (22.5)	275 (71.8)	
Fair	10 (4.3)	38 (16.5)	182 (79.1)	
Bad/very bad	5 (5.0)	10 (9.9)	86 (85.1)	
Living arrangements				ns
With Partner/Spouse	23 (5.3)	76 (17.4)	338 (77.3)	
Not with Partner/Spouse	12 (4.5)	52 (19.4)	204 (76.1	
Language Spoken at Home				ns
English	37 (5.2)	132 (18.6)	539 (76.1)	
Other	0 (0)	1 (16.7)	6 (83.3)	
Employment Status				0.081
Employed (full- or part-time, including self-employed)	18 (6.8)	56 (21.1)	192 (72.2)	
Unemployed (looking for work)	5 (12.5)	8 (20.0)	27 (67.5)	
Unfit to work	5 (5.7)	12 (13.8)	70 (80.5)	
Retired	5 (2.0)	41 (16.1)	208 (81.9)	
Looking after home/family	1 (5.9)	3 (17.6)	13 (76.5)	
In education	1 (5.0)	6 (30.0)	13 (65.0)	
Other	1 (6.3)	1 (6.3)	14 (87.5)	
Help with Questionnaire				ns
Yes	2 (3.2)	6 (9.5)	55 (87.3)	
No	35 (5.4)	125 (19.2)	492 (75.5)	

Table 3 Applicability and missing values by CARE Measure items

CARE Measure item	Not Applicable responses (%)	Missing values (%)
item 1 Making you feel at ease	5 (0.6)	11 (1.4)
item 2 Letting you tell your story	42 (5.4)	11 (1.4)
item 3 Really listening	16 (2.1)	12 (1.6)
item 4 Being interested in you as a whole person	14 (1.8)	13 (1.7)
item 5 Fully understand your concerns	41 (5.3)	13 (1.7)
item 6 Showing care and compassion	15 (1.9)	12 (1.6)
item 7 Being positive	22 (2.8)	15 (1.9)
item 8 Explain things clearly	26 (3.4)	11 (1.4)
item 9 Helping you to take control	112 (14.5)	12 (1.6)
item 10 Making a plan of action with you	151 (19.5)	14 (1.8)
Total	444 (5.7)	124 (1.6)

characteristics of age, gender, self-perceived overall health, living arrangements, employment status and language spoken at home were unrelated to the CARE Measure score.

In terms of the CARE Measures ability to discriminate between nurses a moderate level of agreement (inter-rater reliability) between patients was found with 50–60 patient ratings per nurse (Table 5). As expected, the reliability of the measure increased with the number of completed questionnaires per practice nurse.

The measure showed high internal reliability (Cronbach's alpha coefficient 0.97). Removal of any item weakened this internal reliability (results not shown).

Discussion

This study aimed to determine the reliability (internal and inter-rater) and validity (face and construct) of the CARE Measure as an outcome measure of routine primary care nursing consultations. The results suggested that overall the patients viewed the CARE Measure items as highly relevant to their consultations with nearly three quarters rating the items as 'very important' to their consultation. The low number of 'not applicable' responses and missing values in the CARE Measure items further suggests that the CARE Measure is relevant to primary care nursing consultations and supports the face validity of the measure.

Construct validity of the CARE Measure was demonstrated by a moderate/strong correlation with overall satisfaction (convergent validity) and a weaker correlation with patient enablement (divergent validity). The factor analysis further supported the construct validity as the CARE Measure items loaded highly on one factor showing that they capture the same concept, which was different from overall satisfaction and patient enablement.

In the present study mean CARE Measure scores per nurse were generally high and this restriction in range, caused by the ceiling effect of high scores within the studied cohort of nurses, limited variation between nurses. Despite this phenomenon, the measure could still effectively discriminate between the nurses with 60 questionnaires per nurse with an acceptably high level of stability ($G = 0.6$). While this inter-patient reliability is short of the commonly accepted level of 0.8 for a stand-alone 'high stakes' assessment [31], the results are consistent with other tools, such as Objective Structured Clinical Examinations (OSCE), commonly used to inform summative decisions in other contexts [32]. For 'low stakes' assessments, the CARE Measure is likely to be useful even at much lower numbers of patients per nurse. Furthermore, a larger number of nurses in a more diverse range of practices may have yielded more variation between nurses and thus higher G scores, and further research on a larger and more diverse sample may be useful to determine this. The Cronbachs alpha coefficient of 0.97 indicated high internal reliability. Moreover, the mean CARE Measure scores were not

Table 4 Factor analysis of the CARE Measure, PEI, and satisfaction items

	Factor 1	Factor 2	Factor 3
1. Making you feel at ease	.889	.185	.028
2. Letting you tell your story	.954	.127	.019
3. Really listening	.968	.145	.006
4. Being interested in you as a whole person	.966	.148	.007
5. Fully understand your concerns	.967	.118	.014
6. Showing care and compassion	.967	.144	.008
7. Being positive	.883	.102	.008
8. Explain things clearly	.912	.134	−.009
9. Helping you to take control	.937	.036	−.006
10. Making a plan of action with you	.890	.007	.001
PEI 1 Ability to cope with life	−.182	.794	−.065
PEI 2 Ability to understand illness	−.234	.844	−.029
PEI 3 Ability to cope with illness	−.214	.885	−.001
PEI 4 Ability to keep self health	−.217	.890	.051
PEI 5 Confidence about health	−.196	.869	.052
PEI 6 Ability to help self	−.208	.887	.038
Overall satisfaction	−.039	−.015	.786
Rating consultation time	.039	.061	−.781

Table 5 Reliability of the CARE Measure in differentiating between nurses in relation to number of questionnaires

Number of Completed per Practice Nurse	Reliability(G-Theory Analysis)
37	0.479
50	0.554
60	0.598
100	0.713

affected by any of the measured patients' characteristics and this gives some confidence that the measure can be used in different primary care nursing settings.

Relationship to literature

Overall, the mean CARE Measure score for all practice nurses (45.9) was somewhat higher than in the primary care setting with GPs (40.9) [22]. Additionally, the primary care nurses required a slightly higher number (60) of completed CARE Measures than the GPs for whom 50 CARE Measure scores were sufficient to estimate reliably the mean CARE Measure score for an individual GP [22]. The reason for the higher number of required patient questionnaires for practice nurses is that the practice nurses had less variability in the data. The high level of perceived importance of the CARE Measure items to everyday practice nurse consultations in this study (73 %) was similar to those with general practitioners (76 %) [22]. In the latter, it was also found that older patients and patient with worse health status (in terms of long-standing illness, psycho-social or emotional problems) tended to rate the items as more relevant. The high perceived relevance of the measure to clinical encounters has also been found in similar studies outside primary care [25, 26] and in international settings [24, 27]. The finding that most "not applicable" responses were given to item 9 (helping you to take control) and item 10 (making a plan of action with you) was also in agreement with previous studies [22–26]. As the majority of consultations were routine nursing appointments it could be the case that within that context empowerment and shared-decision making were perceived as less relevant by some patients. Finally, the significant but weak positive associations between estimated consultation length, how well patients know the nurse and CARE Measure scores were similar to those shown in previous studies [22, 25]

Strengths and weaknesses

A strength of the study was that it builds on earlier work on the CARE Measure and adds to the body of knowledge on its reliability and validity across healthcare disciplines. It was also a reasonably large number of patients, though the number of nurses was lower than we had hoped for. The study had some limitations.

First, the participating nurses were volunteers and the study may have been open to sampling bias. This could have led to the high consultation scores and limited the range in performance and the resulting reliability of the inventory. Secondly, one practice withdrew from the study (due to circumstances unrelated to the study) and this reduced the number of participating nurses from 20 to 17. A larger sample size, as employed in previous studies [22, 25, 26], may have captured a wider potential spectrum of possible population performance among nurses and may have found it easier to discriminate between different nurses and demonstrate higher levels of reliability. Another limitation was that it was underestimated how many patients would not return the questionnaires. This resulted in some nurses having collected less than 50 questionnaires even though more than 50 questionnaires had been handed out to patients.

Implications for practice and future studies

As the CARE Measure was originally developed and validated in primary care with GPs, the findings of this study suggest that the CARE Measure can be used reliably with primary care practice nurses as well. Practice nurses working in general practice tend to have serial consultations with patients allowing them to establish ongoing relationships with them. In this study, most patients felt that they knew the nurse quite well or very well. Further work is required across nursing to establish if the CARE Measure is also reliable, valid, acceptable and feasible in other nursing settings, such as secondary care or acute care community clinics such as sexual health, and also in allied healthcare professionals such as physiotherapists, occupational therapists, podiatrists, and so on.

Although capturing patients' views on health professionals' interpersonal skills is now widely regarded as an important feature of high quality health care systems, the evidence that such feedback in itself leads to change in professionals consulting behaviour (and thus improves scores) is equivocal [33]. In order to support healthcare practitioners to improve or maintain their CARE Measure scores and/or the ability to provide an empathic service, earlier work developed [34, 35] and piloted [36] the CARE Approach framework. This interdisciplinary resource is derived from the CARE Measure and wider literature and covers the four interactive components of Connecting, Assessing, Responding and Empowering with the aim of fostering empathy and patient-centredness in clinical encounters [34, 35]. The use of the CARE Measure as well as the CARE Approach feeds into current healthcare policies and professional codes of conduct on maintaining, enhancing and monitoring empathic, person-centred care [15–19].

Conclusion

Research shows that an emphatic, person-centred approach to care is linked with improved experiences of care, higher patient enablement and better health outcomes. The CARE Measure appears relevant to, valid and reliable in routine practice nurse consultations. Completed CARE Measures from 60 patient consultations are required to provide a stable enough view on which to base feedback for educational and quality improvement purposes in relation to relational empathy. As patients' demographics did not affect the CARE Measure scores, it can be used in different primary care settings. In conclusion, the results underpin the CARE Measure as a useful tool to facilitate the patients' voice in providing feedback to practice nurses on their relational empathy.

Competing interests
Stewart Mercer and Annemieke Bikker co-authored the book 'Embracing Empathy in the Health care Encounter [34] and both receive royalties from the sale of the book.

Authors' contributions
AB contributed to the data collection, analysis and interpretation, and the drafting of the article. BF contributed to the conception and design of the study, data collection and the interpretation of the data. DM contributed to the analysis and interpretation of the data. SM contributed to the conception and design of the study, and the interpretation of data. All authors contributed to the revision of the article, and read and approved the final manuscript.

Acknowledgements
Thanks to the nurses who participated in this study and the patients who completed the questionnaires. The study was funded by the Scottish Government.

Author details
[1]General Practice and Primary Care, Institute of Health and Wellbeing, University of Glasgow, 1 Horselethill Road, Glasgow G12 9LX, UK. [2]School of Medicine, University of Dundee, Mackenzie Building, Kirsty Semple Way, Dundee DD2 4BF, UK.

References
1. Stewart M, Brown JB, Weston WW, McWhinney I, McWilliam C, Freeman T. Patient-centered medicine: transforming the clinical method. 3rd ed. Abingdon: Radcliffe Medical Press; 2013.
2. Wensing M, Jung HP, Mainz J, Olesen F, Grol R. A systematic review of the literature on patient priorities for general practice care. Part 1: description of the research domain. Soc Sci Med. 1998;47:1573–88.
3. Mercer SW, Reynolds WJ. Empathy and quality of care. Br J Gen Pract. 2002;52(Suppl):S9–S12.
4. Mercer SW, Cawston PG, Bikker AP. Quality in general practice consultations: a qualitative study of the views of patients living in an area of high socio-economic deprivation in Scotland. BMC Fam Pract. 2007;8:22.
5. Neumann M, Bensing J, Mercer S, Ernstmann N, Ommen O, Pfaff H. Analyzing the "nature" and "specific" effectivesness of clinical empathy: a theoretical overview and contribution towards a theory-based research agenda. Pat Educ Couns. 2009;74:339–46.
6. Griffin SJ, Kinmonth AL, Veltman MW, Gillaard S, Grant J, Stewart M. Effect on health-related outcomes of interventions to alter the interaction between patients and practitioners: a systematic review of trials. Ann Fam Med. 2004;2:595–608.
7. Lelorain S, Brédart A, Dolbeault S, Sultan S. A systematic review of the associations between empathy measures and patient outcomes in cancer care. Psychooncology. 2012;21(12):1255–64.
8. Bikker AP, Mercer SW, Reilly D. A pilot prospective study on consultation and relational empathy, patient enablement, and health changes over 12 months in patients going to the Glasgow Homoeopathic hospital. J Alt Comp Med. 2005;11(4):591–600.
9. Mercer SW, Jani B, Wong SY, Watt GCM. Patient enablement requires physician empathy: a cross-sectional study of general practice consultations in areas of high and low socioeconomic deprivation in Scotland. BMC Fam Pract. 2012;13:6.
10. Price S, Mercer SW, MacPherson H. Practitioner empathy, patient enablement and health outcomes: a prospective study of acupuncture patients. Patient Educ and Couns. 2006;63(1–2):239–45.
11. Rakel DP, Hoeft TJ, Barrett BP, Chewning BA, Craig BM, Min Niu MS. Practitioner empathy and the duration of the common cold. Fam Med. 2009;41(7):494–501.
12. Mercer SW, Howie JGR. CQI-2: a new measure of holistic, interpersonal care in primary care consultations. BJGP. 2006;56(525):262–8.
13. Mercer SW, Neumann M, Wirtz W, Fitzpatrick B, Vojt G. General practitioner empathy, patient enablement, and patient-reported outcomes in primary care in an area of high socio-economic deprivation in Scotland: a pilot prospective study using structural equation modelling. Patient Educ Couns. 2008;73(2):40–245.
14. Yu J, Kirk M. Measurement of empathy in nursing research: systematic review. J Adv Nurs. 2008;64(5):440–54.
15. World Health Organisation. Primary care: putting people first in the world health report 2008: primary health care, now more than ever. Geneva: WHO; 2008.
16. The Scottish Governmen. The healthcare quality strategy for NHS Scotland. Edinburgh: The Scottish Government; 2010.
17. Department of health [England]. Equity and excellence: liberating the NHS. London: Department of Health; 2010.
18. Nursing & Midwifery Council. The Code. 2008. http://www.nmc-uk.org/Documents/Standards/The-code-A4-20100406.pdf Accessed 19 Jan 2015.
19. British Medical Council. Good Medical Practice. 2013. http://www.gmc-uk.org/guidance/good_medical_practice.asp Accessed 19 Jan 2015.
20. Campbell SM, Roland MO, Buetow S. Defining quality of care. Soc Sci Med. 2000;51:1611–25.
21. Mercer SW, Watt GCM, Maxwell M, Heaney DH. The development and preliminary validation of the Consultation and Relational Empathy (CARE) Measure: an empathy-based consultation process measure. Fam Pract. 2004;21(6):699–705.
22. Mercer SW, McConnachie A, Maxwell M, Heaney DH, Watt GCM. Relevance and performance of the Consultation and Relational Empathy (CARE) Measure in general practice. Fam Pract. 2005;22(3):328–34. F.
23. Neumann M, Wirtz M, Bollschweiler E, Mercer SW, Warm M, Wolf J, et al. Determinants and patient-reported long-term outcomes of physician empathy in oncology: a structural equation modelling approach. Patient Educ Couns. 2007;69(1–3):63–75.
24. Fung C, Hua A, Tam L, Mercer SW. Reliability and validity of the Chinese version of the CARE Measure in a primary care setting in Hong Kong. Fam Pract. 2009;26(5):398–406.
25. Mercer SW, Murphy DJ. Validity and reliability of the CARE Measure in secondary care. Clin Gov. 2008;13:261–83.
26. Mercer SW, Hatch DJ, Murray A, Murphy DJ, Eva HW. Capturing patients' views on communication with anaesthetists: the CARE Measure. Clin Gov. 2008;13(2):128–37.
27. Aomatsu M, Abe H, Yasui H, Suzuki T, Sato J, Ban N, et al. Validity and reliability of the Japanese version of the CARE Measure in a general medicine outpatient setting. Fam Pract. 2014;31(1):118–26l.
28. Howie JGR, Heaney DJ, Maxwell M, Walker JJ. A comparison of a Patient Enablement Instrument (PEI) against two established satisfaction scales as outcome measure of primary care consultations. Fam Pract. 1998;15(2):165–71.
29. Brennan R. urGENOVA http://www.education.uiowa.edu/centers/casma/computer-programs. Accessed 11 March 2015.
30. Bloch R, Norman N. 2011. G String IV http://fhsperd.mcmaster.ca/g_string/download/g_string_4_manual_611.pdf Accessed 11 March 2015.
31. Streiner DL, Norman GR. Health measurement scales (3rd ed.). Oxford: Medical Publications; 2003.

Measuring empathic, person-centred communication in primary care nurses: validity and reliability...

39

32. Brannick MT, Erol-Korkmaz HT, Prewett M. A systematic review of the reliability of objective structured clinical examination scores. Med Educ. 2005;45:1181–9.

33. Reinders ME, Ryan BL, Blankenstein AH, van der Horst HE, Stewart MA, van Marwijk HW. The effect of patient feedback on physicians' consultation skills: a systematic review. AcadMed. 2011;86:1426–36.

34. Bikker AP, Cotton P, Mercer SW, Embracing Empathy in Healthcare. A universal approach to person-centred, empathic healthcare encounters. London: Radcliffe; 2014. ISBN-13: 978 190936 8187.

35. Bikker AP, Mercer SW, Cotton P. Connecting, assessing, responding and empowering (CARE): a universal approach to person-centred, empathic healthcare encounters. Educ Primary Care. 2012;23(6):454–7.

36. Fitzgerald NM, Heywood S, Bikker AP, Mercer SW. Enhancing empathy in healthcare: mixed-method evaluation of a pilot project implementing the CARE Approach in primary and community care settings in Scotland. J Compassionate Health Care. 2014;1:6. doi:10.1186/s40639-014-0006-8.

Experiences of nurse practitioners and medical practitioners working in collaborative practice models in primary healthcare in Australia

Verena Schadewaldt[1][*] ⓘ, Elizabeth McInnes[2], Janet E. Hiller[3,4] and Anne Gardner[5,6]

Abstract

Background: In 2010 policy changes were introduced to the Australian healthcare system that granted nurse practitioners access to the public health insurance scheme (Medicare) subject to a collaborative arrangement with a medical practitioner. These changes facilitated nurse practitioner practice in primary healthcare settings. This study investigated the experiences and perceptions of nurse practitioners and medical practitioners who worked together under the new policies and aimed to identify enablers of collaborative practice models.

Methods: A multiple case study of five primary healthcare sites was undertaken, applying mixed methods research. Six nurse practitioners, 13 medical practitioners and three practice managers participated in the study. Data were collected through direct observations, documents and semi-structured interviews as well as questionnaires including validated scales to measure the level of collaboration, satisfaction with collaboration and beliefs in the benefits of collaboration. Thematic analysis was undertaken for qualitative data from interviews, observations and documents, followed by deductive analysis whereby thematic categories were compared to two theoretical models of collaboration. Questionnaire responses were summarised using descriptive statistics.

Results: Using the scale measurements, nurse practitioners and medical practitioners reported high levels of collaboration, were highly satisfied with their collaborative relationship and strongly believed that collaboration benefited the patient. The three themes developed from qualitative data showed a more complex and nuanced picture: 1) Structures such as government policy requirements and local infrastructure disadvantaged nurse practitioners financially and professionally in collaborative practice models; 2) Participants experienced the influence and consequences of individual role enactment through the co-existence of overlapping, complementary, traditional and emerging roles, which blurred perceptions of legal liability and reimbursement for shared patient care; 3) Nurse practitioners' and medical practitioners' adjustment to new routines and facilitating the collaborative work relied on the willingness and personal commitment of individuals.

Conclusions: Findings of this study suggest that the willingness of practitioners and their individual relationships partially overcame the effect of system restrictions. However, strategic support from healthcare reform decision-makers is needed to strengthen nurse practitioner positions and ensure the sustainability of collaborative practice models in primary healthcare.

Keywords: Nurse practitioners, Primary health care, Physician-nurse-relation, Health policy, Collaboration

* Correspondence: verena.schadewaldt@myacu.edu.au
[1]Faculty of Health Sciences, School of Nursing Midwifery and Paramedicine, Australian Catholic University, Melbourne, Australia
Full list of author information is available at the end of the article

Background

Over the last 15 years, nurse practitioners (NPs) have become part of the Australian primary health care (PHC) sector. While the USA and Canada have utilised NPs in the healthcare system since 1965 the first NPs in Australia were formally authorised to practice in 2000 [1]. By March 2015 there were 1214 endorsed NPs, reflecting modest diffusion through the health care system [2]. Australian NPs are registered nurses with a minimum educational level of a Master's degree [3] and endorsement is regulated through the Australian Health Professional Regulation Agency (AHPRA). This endorsement includes the ability to prescribe. While endorsement is regulated through a national body, state-level legislation *regulates* prescribing rights [4].

A systematic review of US-based studies identified that NPs in PHC settings achieve excellent outcomes for their patients in regard to risk factor management, patient satisfaction, functional health status and hospitalisation rates [5]. A broader literature review including Australian and international literature confirmed that nurses and NPs in PHC can effectively and safely provide healthcare to patients [6]. Consequently they can contribute to solutions for current healthcare service delivery issues, which have occurred from escalating demands with an ageing population, an overall population growth, a rise in chronic diseases, an increase of healthcare service costs and workforce shortages [7]. However, a recent World Health Organisation (WHO) report on the healthcare workforce highlighted the underutilisation of advanced health practitioners, such as NPs, in addressing current healthcare issues world wide [8]. A review of NP implementation processes internationally highlighted a number of reasons for the underutilisation of NPs, such as a lack of knowledge of the NPs' scope of practice, non-recognition of their skills and lack of financial and organisational support for their implementation [9].

Primary healthcare in Australia offers the first point of contact for patients in the community and is based on a mixed funding model that includes funding from government programmes, direct payments from patients and private health funds [10]. Medicare, the government-funded public health insurance scheme subsidises a wide range of health services listed on the Medicare Benefits Schedule (MBS) and prescription medicines listed on the Pharmaceutical Benefits Scheme (PBS) [11]. Designated healthcare providers such as MPs, NPs, radiologists and allied health professionals can choose to charge the government-subsidised fee or charge an additional fee that the patient has to pay privately. Healthcare costs for PHC services in Australia account for 36.1 % of the total healthcare expenditure [11].

Since 2010, policy amendments to the National Health Act 1953 authorised NPs in Australia to prescribe medication as listed in the PBS and access the MBS [12, 13], which facilitated their implementation as PHC providers. Similar to some states in the USA [14], it is a prerequisite by Australian law for NPs to enter a collaborative arrangement with a MP in order to access Medicare subsidy schemes [15]. Table 1 presents four options of determining a collaborative arrangement and the frequency of their occurrence in practice.

National and international empirical evidence from interviews and surveys of NPs indicate that NP positions evolve where they receive support from MPs [16–18]. Support from MPs for the implementation of NPs is crucial with the requirement of collaborative arrangements [17, 19]. However, multiple factors can hinder or enable the establishment of collaborative practice models. An integrative review of collaboration between NPs and MPs in PHC identified numerous barriers to successful and satisfying collaborative work arrangements globally [20]. These barriers included interpersonal differences, system structures such as legislation and organisational protocols, a lack of clarity as to professional roles and financial aspects of collaboration [20]. The review identified no published Australian studies.

Collaboration is influenced and shaped by system structures, organisational arrangements and interpersonal relationships [21]. At the level of system structures, American economists identified the introduction of NPs to healthcare systems as a "disruptive innovation" [22, 23]. Disruptive innovations offer "cheaper, simpler, more convenient [...] services" ([22], p. 2). Nurse practitioners fulfil these criteria because they are able to diagnose and treat patients and provide cheaper healthcare

Table 1 Collaborative Arrangements - forms and occurrence in practice

Forms of collaborative arrangements[a]	Percentage of collaborative arrangements (ACNP member survey) [93]
(1) a written agreement about collaborative practice between the NP and the MP exists, or	51.0 %
(2) the NP is employed or engaged by a MP or an institution that employs or engages MPs, or	37.8 %
(3) a patient is referred to the NP by a MP, or	8.1 %
(4) an agreement about collaborative care for an individual patient is stated in the patient's clinical notes by the NP.	2.7 %

[a]National Health (Collaborative Arrangements for Nurse Practitioners) Determination [15], enabled by the *Health Insurance Regulations 1975*, section 2 F

NP Nurse Practitioner, *MP* Medical Practitioner, *ACNP* Australian College of Nurse Practitioners

services without compromising on quality and thus appeal to customers with unmet healthcare needs [23]. As a consequence, NPs offer services that have traditionally been regarded as part of a medical practitioner's work spectrum and "disrupt" existing service structures [22].

The addition of NPs to PHC creates an overlap of the scope of practice with MPs requiring the renegotiation of professional boundaries and roles [24], which can affect interpersonal relationships. Historically the relationship between nurses and medical practitioners has been hierarchical [25, 26]. Conditions that foster power imbalances between nurses and MPs and a "structural embeddedness of medical dominance" ([27], p. 482) continue to exist in healthcare systems of North America and the UK [28]. In Australia, the slow implementation of NPs was in part ascribed to "behind-the-scenes influence" ([29], p. 428) of the medical profession.

The outcomes of international research confirm the complexity of collaboration and therefore the findings cannot be transferred from one setting to another without understanding these complexities. Anecdotally there is controversy around collaborative arrangements and NP access to funding schemes in Australia [30–32]. The consequences of policy amendments regarding collaborative arrangements between NPs and MPs as a prerequisite for NP access to Medicare subsidy schemes are under researched in Australia [33]. This study is the first to report on experiences of Australian NPs and MPs who work together in collaborative practice models.

The aim of this study was to identify the experiences and perceptions of NPs and MPs working collaboratively in PHC settings in Australia following amendments to existing policies. The specific research questions were: What are Australian NPs' and MPs' experiences and perceptions of collaborative practice in PHC under new legal policies? What factors enable collaborative practice models to function?

Methods

This research comprised multiple case studies employing mixed methods research. A case study design was chosen because it is highly suitable for identifying the particularities and complexities of a phenomenon in everyday contexts [34, 35]. For an investigation of collaboration between NPs and MPs the contextual conditions in which collaboration occurred were considered very important to capture, as they might influence how collaborative practice models were realised. The inclusion of multiple cases in this study served to generate a more comprehensive understanding of the issue under investigation and provide a more powerful and robust basis for conclusions than a single case study [36, 37].

Within the multiple case study design mixed methods research (MMR) was applied [38] to triangulate methods and data sources for data enrichment, corroboration or identification of contradictions [39, 40]. This study was based on a qualitative core component including interviews, non-participant observations and documentary data that was supported with a quantitative component comprising a questionnaire [41].

Considering the available evidence from international research two models of collaboration provided a theoretical framework to inform some questions of the interview schedule and parts of the data analysis. These models were selected on the basis that the *Conceptual Model of Collaborative Nurse-Physician Interaction* was the only model to specifically focus on collaboration between nurses and MPs [42]; and the *Structuration Model of Collaboration* was based on extensive research and applied in multidisciplinary PHC settings [43]. The models present influencing factors of collaboration between health professionals including interpersonal, organisational and systemic dimensions. Table 2 presents the 17 combined dimensions of both models and shows where dimensions overlap and complement each other.

Table 2 Dimensions of the Structuration Model of Collaboration and the Model of Nurse-Physician Interaction

	Dimension	Model
1	Mutual trust and respect	C, S
2	Formalisation tools (policies, protocols, agreements)	C, S
3	Communication/behaviour tendencies/Information exchange	C, S
4	Compatible role perceptions/mutual acquaintanceship	C, S
5	Joint goal setting and decision making	C, S
6	Complementary management of influencing variables/ Client-centred orientation vs other allegiances	C, S
7	Conditions of power symmetry	C
8	Traditions of professionalization	C
9	Traditional gender/role norms	C
10	Personal attitudes	C
11	Complexity of care environment (the higher, the more collaboration)	C
12	Prevalent social reality	C
13	Nursing/medical school curricula	C
14	Support for innovation	S
15	Connectivity (opportunities for discussion and adjustment of coordination problems, for example information and feedback systems, meetings, committees etc.	S
16	Centrality (authorities that provide clear directions that foster collaboration, inherits a strategic and political role)	S
17	Leadership (local person)	S

C Conceptual Model of Collaborative Nurse-Physician Interaction [42]
S Structuration Model of Collaboration [43]

Recruitment and selection of sites

Recruitment of sites occurred from August 2012 to May 2013 through emailing a research invitation to members of nursing and medical organisations, calling potential PHC sites where NPs worked with MPs, and through publicising the study at NP workshops. Throughout the recruitment phase a snowball sampling technique was applied to identify further potential study sites [44] by asking NPs and MPs to promote the study to interested nursing and medical colleagues.

Potential sites were screened against selection criteria (Table 3). Once eligibility was confirmed, a telephone conference was undertaken with potential site staff to identify site characteristics such as practice size, practice type (public or private) location (urban or remote), PHC specialty and type of collaborative arrangement. Sites were purposefully selected considering maximum variation of these site characteristics. Data saturation was ensured by successively recruiting cases to the study. Following data collection at each site, preliminary analysis was initiated before the next site was visited for data collection. Once information and preliminary themes became repetitive, no further sites were recruited to the study. Prior to data collection written informed consent was sought from all study participants.

Data collection and analysis

Data collection was undertaken in three phases involving four data sources. Details about data collection methods and analysis have been reported previously [45] and are summarised here.

1. Non-participant observations of NPs and MPs were undertaken to capture collaborative behaviour and

Table 3 Selection criteria

Inclusion criteria

- Primary healthcare setting
- NP and MP registered with AHPRA for at least 6 months
- NP endorsed as NP for at least 6 months
- NP and MP working together for at least 6 months for at least 1 day per week
- Both NP and MP needed to be willing to participate in the study

Exclusion criteria

- Secondary/tertiary healthcare setting
- Sites with practice nurses or NP candidates who were not endorsed as NPs yet
- Participants who have not worked together for a minimum of 6 months
- Sites with complicated travelling logistics that would have exceeded the study budget

NP Nurse Practitioner, *MP* Medical Practitioner, *AHPRA* Australian Health Practitioner Regulation Agency

interactions; communication patterns and organisational and clinical context.

2. Nurse practitioners and MPs were asked to complete a questionnaire to collect demographic information. The questionnaire included three validated scales. Two scales were based on a provider collaboration survey, developed for NP-MP collaboration in Canadian primary healthcare settings to measure the experience with collaboration (9 items, 6-point Likert scale) and satisfaction with the collaborative relationship (15 items, 6-point Likert scale) [46]. In this study we used the expanded and modified versions by Donald et al. [47]. Both scales were pilot-tested for content validity, relevance and understandability by the original authors [46] in Canadian PHC settings. The modified versions by Donald et al. F Donald [47] were also tested for construct validity by comparing each of the scales with a single general question. This resulted in Spearman's $r = 0.89$, $p < 0.001$ for the scale measuring experience with current collaboration and $r = 0.91$, $p < 0.001$ for the scale on satisfaction with collaboration [47], indicating very good construct validity.

The third scale measured beliefs in the benefits of collaboration (5 items, 5-point Likert scale) developed as part of a survey to identify interprofessional processes in teams [48]. The scale had high reliability (Cronbach's α coefficient of 0.91). Factor analysis showed sufficient loading of the items on a single factor confirming high construct validity [48].

Higher scores indicated stronger perceptions of collaboration on all three scales. Permission to use the scales was granted from the original authors. The questionnaire was pilot-tested by a group of health academics, NPs and MPs.

3. Individual face-to-face interviews were conducted with NPs and MPs using a semi-structured interview guide (see Additional files 1, 2 and 3) to identify personal experiences of barriers and facilitators to collaborative working, perceptions on shared decision-making, autonomy and supervision as well as views on the legal requirement of collaborative arrangements. Where these positions existed, practice managers (PMs) were asked to participate in an interview to capture their perspective on the collaboration between NP and MP.

4. Throughout the data collection period at each site, practice documents stating the collaborative arrangements, the scope of practice of the NP and flyers for patients explaining the NP role within the practice were collected to gain further insights in

work mechanisms and roles that were defined in writing in these documents.

Data analysis occurred in several stages. Index scores of scales and demographic data were analysed using descriptive statistics. After consultation with a statistician statistical analysis was limited to descriptive statistics, which is a minor revision to the protocol [45]. Analysis of qualitative data was informed by the thematic analysis approach suggested by Braun and Clarke [49]. QSR International NVivo 10 software was used to assist data management and analysis. Braun and Clarke distinguish 'data-driven' (inductive) or 'theory-driven' (deductive) coding, which was preferable for this study to generate codes based on participant meaning first and then allow for comparison with the current theoretical models [49].

The inductive approach of qualitative data analysis identified new codes inherent to the participants and sites of this study. To allow comparison of the participants' views (interviews), the researcher's observations and documents describing the collaborative practice (practice documents), the three data types were coded separately and collapsed into thematic categories. Thematic categories from interviews and observations were compared through triangulation and summarised in themes. Reasons for differences and commonalities of codes are reported in the narrative of the developed themes. We drew on codes from the document analysis when they were useful to clarify or support themes. In a second step of triangulation, questionnaire results were woven together with themes at the point of data interpretation and are highlighted where they supported or contradicted qualitative findings [50].

A theory-driven and deductive approach of data analysis then assisted with determining how close the data set of this study was to existing international models by comparing the 17 combined dimensions of influence of collaboration [42, 43] (Table 2) with the empirically derived codes and categories in NVivo.

Ethics approval for this study was granted by the Human Research Ethics Committee of the Australian Catholic University (No. 2012 207 V). Stringent quality measures were applied to establish credibility and trustworthiness of findings [51]. These included the adherence to a research protocol [45], the use of a research diary, data triangulation, and comparison with existing theoretical frameworks. Potential influences of researchers on the study process were discussed to minimise bias. All authors are health services researchers, three with a nursing background.

Results

Of 13 eligible sites, five were selected including 22 participants comprising six NPs, 13 MPs and three PMs

considering variation of site characteristics and availability within the study period (Table 4). Site locations included country towns with a population under 2000, larger towns with 200,000-300,000 residents and cities with populations ranging from 1 to 4 million. Four sites were privately owned practices while the community centre was publicly funded. In total, data collection included 143 h of non-participant observation (varying from 3 to 10 days per site), a return of 18 questionnaires (95 % return rate), compilation of 12 practice documents and 21 interviews ranging from 16 to 60 min in duration.

The organisational context and working structures differed at each site. Practice size ranged from large practices at several locations and more than 20 MPs to small practices with 2 MPs at one location. At some sites NPs worked most of the time in the community whereas other NPs worked in consulting rooms at the practice. Practice managers managed the four private practices. At the community centre the NP ran the centre in her position as nurse unit manager and MPs were not consistently present on site but visited on a daily basis. Not all MPs in larger practices worked with the NP and not all MPs were participants in this study.

In general, separate healthcare consultations of NPs and MPs prevailed at all sites with NPs and MPs operating as autonomous health professionals. The collaborative character of the practice models only emerged when mutual patients were discussed or referred to another health professional. Information exchange about patient care occurred through meetings, internal messaging systems, phone calls and referral letters. Face-to-face contact

Table 4 Study Sample Characteristics

Sites	
Practices	4 private practices, 1 community centre
Locations	New South Wales, South Australia, Tasmania, Victoria
NPs per practice	1–2
MPs per practice	2–20
Individual participants	
Nurse Practitioners	6, all female
NP specialties	PHC, cardiology, aged care, drug and alcohol withdrawal
Working as NP (median, range)	2.0 years (0.5–11.5)
Medical Practitioners	13, four female
MP specialties	General practice/PHC, cardiology, gerontopsychology
Experience in PHC (median, range)	NPs: 8.75 years (1.2–15)
	MPs: 13.0 years (2.3–34)
Practice Managers	3, all female

NP Nurse Practitioner, MP Medical Practitioner, PHC Primary Healthcare

between NPs and MPs at sites ranged from daily to weekly encounters.

Questionnaire results

High scores on all scales indicated positive perceptions in the descriptive analysis. Median index scores of the three scales showed 1) NP and MP groups strongly believed that collaboration was beneficial for patients; 2) they experienced high levels of collaboration and 3) were highly satisfied with their collaborative relationship (Table 5).

The data revealed a greater variation among MP responses reflected in a wider range for all three scales. Instead of interquartile ranges, the minimum and maximum are presented for all scales to reflect the full range of responses in this small sample.

Results from thematic analysis of interview and non-participant observation data are presented in three main themes.

Influence of system structures

This theme reports challenges of working in collaborative practice models due to healthcare system structures, policies and also infrastructure at practice level. One of the major constraints to establish and maintain collaborative practice models was the way Medicare reimbursed NPs. While NPs, MPs and PMs valued NPs' access to Medicare, they critiqued the current reimbursement rates and available MBS items for NPs as insufficient and unfair. Nurse practitioners in private practice can use four professional attendance MBS items for patient consultations and a limited number of diagnostic test items [13]. For example, electrocardiography is a common investigation for NPs caring for cardiac patients, but it would incur the patient a private fee if ordered by the NP rather than the MP. In these cases, care needed to be escalated to the MP for ordering the investigations once the NP completed the initial patient assessment. *"Why do I see it not as equal? Because... [...] they [MPs] have the capacity to request more investigations than we do. I think, our practice [services that are covered by MBS items] is somewhat restricted by what Medicare says" (NP)*. Another example refers to 'Chronic disease management plans' for a joint approach to patient care that required MPs to sign off on care plans,

resulting in reimbursement going to MPs. However, typically the NP spent most of the time with the patient for assessment and planning.

In general, NPs and MPs commented that the fee-for-service (FFS) structure of Medicare lacked adequate financial compensation for health professionals discussing mutual patients. These discussions were common occurrences and considered important for a complementary approach to a person's care. *"If there needs to be feedback to [NP name] or [NP name] needs to talk to me we have to do that in our own time. And that can be a significant amount of time during the day you don't get paid for" (MP)*.

In addition to Medicare policies, the legal determination of collaborative arrangements impacted on collaborative practice between NPs and MPs. In our study, four of five practice settings had a written agreement [52]. In the community centre, no written arrangement existed but the legal determination was fulfilled because the organisation for which the NP worked sub-contracted MPs.

Some NPs and MPs perceived collaborative arrangements as positive because they considered it a safety net, which supported NP practice when a patient scenario required a second opinion or transfer of care through the availability of a MP. *"I do find it helpful. I think it's safe. I think that's the biggest issue, the fact that you know you've always got that backup" (NP)*. On the other hand, NPs critiqued the legal formalisation of collaboration. They considered it common sense to consult with another health professional when they needed a second opinion. Collaborative arrangements are *"a sore point that nurse practitioners fought not to have formal [legally required], because we feel we would refer anyway if we find something outside our scope" (NP)*. One NP reported that she was unable to establish a NP-led clinic because MPs declined to engage in a collaborative arrangement.

These policies and regulations weakened the NPs' position as legitimate healthcare providers within the collaborative practice. Difficulties in generating income decreased their chances of finding a practice that was willing to employ them. *"In a private GP practice, at this stage, [we] couldn't make enough money to fund ourselves or make it worthwhile for them [MPs] to fund us" (NP)*. The NP's limited ability to contribute to practice income reinforced uncertainty about the financial sustainability of NPs, which may impede the establishment of collaborative practice models because potential loss of income prompted MPs' concerns. Nurse practitioners reported that they were not entitled to demand their own office because they could not contribute sufficient income to the practice. Consequently, existing healthcare system regulations created a hierarchical, as opposed to balanced, professional

Table 5 Index Scores of three Scales (Median and Range)

Index scores	Median[a] [Range]	
	NPs	MPs
Beliefs in the benefits of collaboration	5.0 [4.2–5.0]	4.7 [3.3–5.0]
Experience with current collaboration	4.9 [4.7–5.3]	5.4 [2.7–6.0]
Satisfaction with current collaboration	5.1 [4.2–5.5]	5.4 [2.6–6.0]

[a]Median of means of individual responses, *NP* Nurse Practitioner, *MP* Medical Practitioner

relationship and contradicted the definition of ideal collaboration that emphasises equality, shared power and interdependency [53, 54].

At a practice level, a major challenge mentioned by NPs and MPs was a lack of dedicated time to actually collaborate, that is, discuss shared patient cases, which was also identified in the questionnaire. Most participants would have liked time for more face-to-face meetings, but the busyness of the practice did not allow for this.

"We don't have a system here where there is protected time for us to sit down with the practitioner and be able to communicate the concerns and that sort of thing. It sort of ends up being something in the hallway: 'Oh by the way, I saw that person and this and that'" (MP).

Conversations were more sporadic at three sites where the NP and MP were not on site together on a regular basis suggesting that physical proximity increased the chances of communication and collaboration. At other sites, the lack of a communal room and facilities impeded opportunities for communication, a defining principle of collaboration. *NP has lunch, standing. There are no chairs to sit. Some admin staff are in the kitchen. There is not much time for conversation. Everyone is standing while eating* (Observation).

Interview data highlighted differing perceptions about the importance of face-to-face meetings. At one site a NP was scheduling her time in between home visits according to the availability of the MPs at the practice. She said: *"I'll catch them informally again, I hover (laughs), make myself available, when I know they have a break"* (NP). One MP also valued this time of direct exchange but noted: *"It just seems to happen that we meet there"* (MP). The MP seemed unaware of the significance of this meeting to the NP, not realising that the NP had actively tried to be around to meet her. For the MP the meetings seemed a convenience, for the NP a priority when working together.

Integrating NPs into existing infrastructure posed a challenge. Due to a shortage of rooms some NPs and MPs frequently changed offices and some NPs used MP consulting rooms. Nurse practitioners stored materials and utensils in a box or movable storage trolley to adjust to this situation. One NP had no consulting room allocated within the practice because she worked mainly in nursing homes or visited patients at home. The lack of designated workspace caused uncertainty about her availability amongst the collaborating MPs because she only returned to the practice sporadically and used different locations within the practice to complete administrative work. I observed her working with a laptop on her knees, surrounded by other staff.

9.30 am – Communal area: In a corner is a 1 m²small desk with computer and printer. The NP wanted to print something there, but it is occupied by someone [...] Standing, she is going through her papers, makes phone calls, operating in the middle of the room. There is no privacy (Observation).

In addition to physical integration, interview statements and observations revealed that NPs experienced pressure to find and assert their position within the existing system. Some MPs were sceptical as to whether NP care differed from care provided by MPs. *"[Is it] just another way [...] of doing something that GPs are already doing?"* (MP). Difficulties with integrating a new health professional were also reflected in the NPs' negative experiences with dismissive MPs, including those not participating in this study or external to the practice setting. Consequently, NPs wanted to prove their worth, for example, one NP reported a patient satisfaction survey she initiated and in which she received very good feedback. That was important for her because *"that was something I could demonstrate to the practice manager and the board that what I am doing is worthwhile"* (NP). This pressure to physically and professionally integrate was not observed for MPs given their long-standing history as PHC professionals.

Influence and consequences of individual role enactment
The second theme reflects on the team roles of NPs and MPs and how NPs and MPs operationalised their work arrangements with complementary roles. For clarity of reading, this theme is divided into three sub-themes.

Influence of NP autonomy
Role enactment refers to the process of participants familiarising themselves with their roles as collaborating colleagues and performing their specific roles within the team. The NPs' level of autonomy led to an expansion of their scope of practice and in some cases caused an overlap with the scope of practice of MPs, which led to blurred professional roles. *"I know that she does some of the work that I would otherwise be doing"* (MP). The lack of differentiation of the NP role from the MP role in practice occurred despite clear statements about the NP's role in practice documents. Understanding the new role of NPs was complicated because NPs had previously been in practice nurse roles with the same MPs and still retained some practice nurse functions. In Australia, practice nurses are enrolled or registered nurses who can autonomously see patients but commonly under the supervision of a general practitioner [55]. In comparison to the NP, a practice nurse participates in many procedures in an assisting capacity and cannot access the Medicare subsidy schemes.

The difficulty to clearly define the NP role may have contributed to some MPs' ambivalence about NP autonomy. Some MPs expressed a general concern about fragmentation of care and appropriate decision-making by NPs. *"I always worry, if there was something missed"* (MP). On the other side, some MPs strongly supported an autonomous NP role and some MPs expected NPs to take more responsibility by making autonomous decisions about patient care. *"I would expect [NP name] to make the actual [patient] management decisions"* (MP).

Nurse practitioners also valued their autonomy but applying it in practice was shaped by two factors; their level of confidence to make autonomous decisions and policy restrictions that required the MPs' involvement as outlined in the first theme. A MP commented on the questionnaire: *Some NPs can't or don't want to make a full decision on her/his scope* (MP).

The ways that NPs exercised and MPs accepted NP autonomy influenced referral and consultation patterns between NPs and MPs. Researcher observations showed that MPs mostly *referred* patients to the NP, that is they passed on the patient for an additional consultation with the NP; while NPs in addition to referrals *consulted* MPs, that is they sought advice from MPs while the patient was with them. While patient referrals to the NP were perceived as an alleviation of workload for MPs, one-sided consultation patterns of NPs caused interruptions to the work of both practitioners. We observed waiting times between 1 and 25 min until a MP was free to assist the NP who was waiting with the patient in her office. Medical practitioners also had to interrupt their workflow and sometimes added an additional patient from the NP to their already full schedule. *"I was really busy and then sometimes, you know, extra referrals from the nurse practitioner can be a little bit too much because it is an extra appointment"* (MP).

Perceptions on reimbursement and legal liability

The joint involvement of practitioners for some patients highlighted that autonomous and collaborative roles of NPs and MPs co-existed. The co-existence of roles affected perceptions of who should be reimbursed and who was legally liable for shared patient care. In regard to reimbursement, NPs consulting the MP for less than a minute to ask a question was a common occurrence but one MP emphasised: *"We don't have a way to bill that"* (MP). Some NPs were concerned that MPs were not reimbursed for these times. Other NPs considered it inappropriate for the MP to bill the patient for a short consultation, which was possible when the MP had joined the NP's session with the patient, because these NPs believed discussing patient issues was a courtesy among colleagues.

"The billing thing is, I think, is the biggest issue. I am troubled with that sometimes and the fact that I don't think somebody walking in the room for two seconds saying 'hello' warrants an item number. And I think some doctors here would dispute that, because they have seen the patient. [...] But I don't think that's fair on Medicare or the patient" (NP).

Despite Medicare policies on what constitutes a consultation [56] there was room for interpretation, depending on whether the MP considered herself as the reimbursable practitioner or an advice-giving colleague. For both NPs and MPs, reimbursement claims relied on an interpretation of their role; that is which of the practitioners considered themselves reimbursable for a joint patient consultation.

Professional guidelines issued by medical and nursing boards in Australia clearly state that each health professional is responsible for his or her own actions and decisions [3, 57]. Practice experience showed that medico-legal liability was less clear when patient care was shared between NP and MP. Contrasting perceptions on liability were identified in interviews.

The majority of MPs but none of the NPs considered MPs as *"ultimately responsible"* (MP), even for those patients cared for by the NP alone. Some MPs thought that the collaborative arrangements served to establish legal liability within the collaborative practice, assigning ultimate responsibility to MPs. One MP stated that collaborative arrangements *"made us, the GPs, much happier about our risk"*, reflecting the assumption of some MPs that the legal determination addressed professional liability. However, the determination does not stipulate the assignment of liability, which is supported by the fact that it can be a verbal agreement.

Nurse practitioners and some MPs considered responsibility lay with the practitioner primarily caring for a patient. *"If I write the order then I would be responsible totally for my actions and if the GP writes the order then they would be totally responsible"* (NP). However, system requirements for NPs to obtain a signature from the MP for certain procedures destabilised the concept of being accountable for one's own practice. For example, it was the NP's decision to refer a patient to mental health services, but the MP became the person responsible because she had to sign the referral form. Without Medicare restrictions the NP could have placed the order and lines of liability would not have been blurred.

Some practitioners agreed that they shared legal liability. Shared responsibility came into effect when a practitioner gave advice to another practitioner and this was recorded in the patient notes and incorporated in the patient's care. However, for MPs it was difficult to know if the "quick" advice in the corridor would be used and regarded as MP involvement in patient care and consequently if it made them legally liable for this patient. Therefore, MPs preferred to be either fully involved in patient care and see the patient or not be included at all. *"If she doesn't refer [to] me I don't want to know anything about her patient [...]. If she refers a patient to me, then I want to know everything. I want to take over"* (MP).

Working in complementary roles

The blurring of roles and responsibilities was not observed to negatively affect direct patient care because the NP and MP worked either in separate autonomous patient consultations or worked with complementary skills for shared patient consultations. For most patient consultations, interview and observation data clearly showed NPs and MPs providing complete episodes of care without collaborative interaction. *"It's a separate process. I usually make my decisions and if she sees a patient she makes her decisions"* (MP). For these autonomous consultations NPs applied what has traditionally been seen as nursing and medical skills whereas for shared episodes of care NPs tended to focus on nursing care and MPs on medical care so that roles complemented each other. Medical practitioners perceived that working in this complementary manner enhanced collaborative practice: *"It just adds another dimension to your understanding of the patient"* (MP). In particular the educational role of NPs, who must also be registered nurses in Australia, complemented MP consultations that focused on diagnostics and medication.

> *"So I think, that [diagnosing] is the cardiologists' role and from then on they can come to me for all the management issues, you know, education, the lifestyle, the action plans, all the other issues that revolve around chronic illness"* (NP).

The complementarity of roles was also evident when NPs and MPs returned to traditional role patterns, with MPs as the dominant care provider and NPs functioning in a subordinate role as practice nurses. Self-perpetuating traditions of MPs "owning" patients and making final decisions were evident in statements of participants: *"But there still is a hierarchy where... In general practice, I feel like the patients still belong to one of the doctors"* (NP). This attitude was also expressed by a practice manager who explained that the MPs could decide if they wanted to squeeze in an acute patient or if the patient should be booked with the NP instead. It implied that MPs had the primary choice of patients.

Language used by MPs also revealed the existence of historical ways of thinking. Some MPs considered themselves as *"supervisor"*, describing the NPs as their *"right hand"* or talking about the NPs, who were all female in this sample, as *"girls"*. Often these statements were explicit acknowledgements of the NPs' importance to patients and the additional value to the practice, particularly evident in the following statement. *"But these girls are helping out enormously in terms of patient load"* (MP). Therefore, this behaviour could be interpreted as a form of subconscious paternalism. The presence of traditional role patterns in day-to-day practice appeared to be accepted by NPs and MPs. This suggests that going back and forth between old and new roles, was part of the process of finding matching roles within the collaborative practice models.

Making it work: adjustment to new routines

Practitioners developed strategies and abilities to successfully work together. Planning and preparation were required to arrange practicalities. At a practice level, these included developing a concept for the collaborative practice model and holding initial meetings to inform staff, clarify questions and dispel concerns. Preparations also needed to address space and equipment. *"So we had to put in a sink, change the curtain; change it into a clinical room. So it wasn't just a matter of slotting someone in. We had to kind of make it happen"* (PM). Practice managers were identified as a resource for adjustments of practice infrastructure. They were involved in the organisation of team meetings, acted as moderator in case of conflicting interests and facilitated information flow between NPs and MPs.

At the interpersonal level, preparatory discussions about the collaborative relationship were held to establish clarity around roles and the scope of practice. Some practices formulated their collaboration in a written collaborative agreement, which NPs thought to be a *"source of clarity"* (NP). Medical practitioners with a good understanding of the role stated that the role had been well explained to them in advance, either by the NP or their medical association, which provided NP job descriptions. Following these preparatory measures, regular communication measures developed for the day-to-day running of the collaborative practice models.

Various communication methods were used to make up for the lack of direct interactions between NP and MP including an internal messaging system and informal face-to-face conversations, described as 'talk in the corridors' or a 'chat over coffee'. Nurse practitioners and MPs considered regular meetings as ideal, but in their absence, the spontaneous conversations were considered satisfactory. *"It feels informal because it is here in the tea room and in between. But it's sufficient"* (NP). Two of the five sites held planned team meetings on a weekly or fortnightly basis. To enable team meetings and manage the busyness of clinicians, one practice introduced a rule that no patients would be booked over lunchtime and all staff could meet during lunch. *"So if you have somewhere where people can sit down and have that meal together or morning tea together or somewhere to sit, that enhances collaboration" (NP)*. Observations confirmed that communication and lunch breaks were significantly longer and more common where participants had the opportunity to sit down together.

Besides working around practical challenges, individual attitudes towards collaboration were found to have a significant impact on the success of collaboration. Nurse practitioners knew that they had to integrate themselves in a *"non-threatening way" (MP)*. A nurse practitioner stated: *"You don't try to take over. That would be a bad thing. And that would make us very unpopular"*. Accordingly NPs developed a strategy of careful negotiation within the MP's domain of patient care. A NP described that she approached the MP in the practice whose idea of patient care was most consistent with hers in a particular case. Thus she found a way of getting approval for care without offending any of the MPs. *"I think, there is a little bit of ... I don't want to say manipulation... umm...a bit of selective choosing (laughs)" (NP)*. It seemed NPs found a strategy of cautious confidence, which allowed them to make autonomous decisions and appear confident but not over-confident in their behaviour.

Nurse practitioners and MPs agreed that collaboration worked because of their trustful and respectful relationship. Developing trust through positive experiences contributed to diminished MP concerns. *"I'm just one of these older GPs who have gone from being totally opposed to the idea of nurse practitioner to being a complete convert" (MP)*. Nurse practitioners reported that after some time MPs transferred tasks to the NP as a sign of increased trust. *"They [MPs] have expanded what they are happy for me to do" (NP)*.

Commitment of individuals was important. Collaborative practice models in this sample worked because most MPs were willing to take a financial risk by working in collaboration with NPs for the advantage of better patient care. *"It is an important part of our practice, so I think, we should do it, even if it's not a money making thing" (MP)*. Considering the restrictions through Medicare policy and legislation, MPs as well as NPs were well aware that the collaboration models in the private sector existed because of the willingness of MPs. *"Collaboration between nurse practitioners and doctors depends on [...] whether the owner of the practice is willing to do that or not" (MP)*.

Findings in comparison with existing models of collaboration

A majority of dimensions of the two theoretical models overlapped with the findings in this study (Table 2). Strong evidence of the importance of mutual trust and respect, compatible role perceptions, communicative behaviour and infrastructure for information exchange, shared goals and decision-making for collaboration were identified in both theoretical models [42, 43] and at sites in this study. Likewise formalisation tools such as policies, protocols and agreements, understood as structural factors affecting collaboration, were found in this study and in the earlier models.

Aspects of role enactment were mostly addressed in Corser's model of nurse-physician interaction [42]. Personality, willingness and personal values as well as traditional role patterns and power symmetry were identified as having a strong influence on the functioning of collaboration in the current study. However, conditions of power symmetry were largely impeded by system structures and to a smaller extent by traditions of professionalisation and traditional gender or role norms as described by Corser [42].

Three dimensions developed by D'Amour et al. were only marginally present at the five sites in our study [43]. First, D'Amour et al. defined connectivity as a connection between individuals and the organisation based on feedback systems, meetings and committees to allow rapid coordination and adjustment of practice [43]. Practice adjustments and opportunities for meetings appeared to be easier to establish at smaller sites where meetings occurred frequently compared to larger sites. However, some participants at large sites and the community centre stated that support from the management level was important for the establishment of the collaborative practice model.

Second, centrality, described as authorities that provide clear directions [43] including professional boards, associations or government institutions, were only of marginal impact in our study. A nurse practitioner expressed her frustration with vague directions by authorities. *"I asked the nurses' board about that [access to PBS] and they weren't clear" (NP)*. It is important to note that D'Amour's Structuration Model was developed in Canada, where 'health authorities' govern the provision of healthcare in designated areas [43]. In Australia, a similar approach with local support for PHC institutions, Medicare Locals, were established in 2011 but a review in 2014 stated low functionality of these authorities [58]. In addition, centrality might play a larger role in inter-organisational collaboration, a focus of the Structuration Model but not of our study.

The third dimension, for which only limited evidence was found, is the influence on collaboration through the presence of a leader of collaboration. None of the participants identified a team member with such a position or role. However, as outlined in theme three, the practice manager played an important coordinating and organisational role in some of the collaborative practice models.

Our study identified two additional factors influencing collaboration not included in the two theoretical models. First, the consequences of NP autonomy on role enactment might be a particular problem for NPs and MPs but were not found to be a problem between other professions or organisations [43] or between general nurses and MPs [42], where lines of authority might be clearer. Corser [42] touched on the issue of autonomy with the dimension of power dynamics. Second, fiscal systems influenced the functioning of collaboration. Corser [42] as well as D'Amour and colleagues in their publications [43, 59] acknowledged that economic constraints and resources influence processes of collaboration but did not consider them as an extra dimension in their models.

Discussion

This study investigated the experiences and perceptions of NPs and MPs in relation to collaborative practice in five PHC settings in Australia following amendments of policies regarding collaborative arrangements and NP access to healthcare services subsidy schemes. Although system structures were the main impediment to establish sustainable collaborative practice models, the willingness of practitioners and their individual relationships partially overcame the effect of system restrictions. Practitioners were able to establish, adjust and accept new routines, noticeable in their moving back and forth between new and traditional roles. While questionnaire results indicated that NPs and MPs experienced both high levels of collaboration and satisfaction with the collaborative relationship, and held strong beliefs in the benefits of collaboration the qualitative results revealed a more ambivalent picture of NPs' and MPs' experiences of collaboration. Financial issues as well as NP autonomy and have an impact on collaboration and expand existing theoretical models.

Collaborative working within policy frameworks and existing infrastructure

Financial issues are a significant influence on collaboration in Australia by disadvantaging NPs in collaborative practice. Nurse practitioners receive lower rates of reimbursement than MPs for patient consultations, and only a limited number of Medicare items are available to them [60]. Differences in reimbursements rates for NPs and MPs reported from an economic case study of an Australian general practice corroborate our findings [61]. However, practitioners both in our study and in the USA highly valued NP access to a health insurance scheme as an enabler of collaborative practice models [27, 62, 63].

Study participants critiqued the fee-for-service model as negatively influencing collaborative practice. North American research supports our finding. A survey of 20,710 Canadian MPs showed that MPs working in a fee-for-service model were significantly less likely to collaborate with NPs [64]. An ethnographic study of three PHC teams in the USA identified fee-for-service models as a disincentive for health professionals to discuss mutual patient cases in the absence of a patient because it solely reimburses practitioners for face-to-face consultation time with patients [65]. The insecurity over financial benefits from collaborative practice inhibits supportive MPs from collaborating with a NP. Australian health care reformers missed a chance to learn from countries where NPs operate on a more sustainable level through targeted government initiatives to support team care approaches [27, 66]. For example, initiatives in Canada and the USA included incentive payments for MPs to join healthcare teams and government funded NP positions [67–69]. Such initiatives foster shared care of patients.

The Australian determination underpinning collaborative arrangements added to the power imbalance between NPs and MPs in collaborative practice models. Nurse practitioners in our sample valued the consultation availability of MPs but questioned the legal determination for two reasons. NPs considered it self-evident that they would consult another health professional if necessary and their choice of work location relied on the agreement of a collaborating MP. Consequently, NPs were in a dependent relationship [70] and disadvantaged in negotiating business terms such as income, leave regulations or payment for administrative support [71]. A literature review about collaborative arrangements in the USA concluded that mandatory collaborative arrangements hindered NP practice in areas of need or remote areas where no MPs are available or willing to enter a collaborative arrangement [72]. A cross-sectional analysis from 2001 to 2008 of 41 USA states showed that restrictive collaborative practice arrangements limited growth of NP numbers by 25 % [73]. Where system-level policies restrict NPs in their choice of practice and force them to practice below their potential, care resources are underutilised [74, 75].

Legal liability can be unclear in team structures [76]. Australian legislation underpinning collaborative arrangements appears to have added to the confusion about such liability [77, 78]. Study participants held diverse views about their accountability for patients who were jointly looked after by an NP and a MP reflecting lack of clarity about such liability. The current determination of Australian collaborative arrangements draws MPs into a commitment of "collaborative" working with a NP with poorly understood implications for practice. Medical practitioners may carry vicarious liability, where they are employers or in some cases practice owners, that is, they may be held accountable for the NP's negligent action [79]. Thus MPs may be wary about entering collaborative arrangements and providing support for patients they have not seen.

Legal liability may be clearer without the legal requirement of collaborative arrangements [78]. Battaglia proposed complete practice independence for NPs so that "a practicing NP would generally bear the full liability for instances of malpractice arising from care provided by that NP" ([78], p. 1151). Resnick and Bronner emphasise the importance of outlining the scope of practice of NP and MP, communication and referral mechanisms in writing [80]. However, such agreements do not have to be linked to legislation and the current Australian determination fails to clarify legal liability.

Organisational structures contributed to the lack of equality between NPs and MPs in this study. The lack of space for NPs in PHC settings has been identified as a problem in a case study of three PHC sites in Canada [81] and in interviews with 16 NPs practicing in PHC settings in the USA [82]. It appeared MPs were given priority for offices and resources, which researchers described as "structural discounting" ([83], p. 90) of NPs.

Disruptions to existing routines, identified in this study in the form of interruptions to patient consultations and communication flow, were highlighted by Greenhalgh as a challenge for collaborative working [84]. Our findings support those from a Canadian ethnographic study of three multiprofessional PHC teams in which a lack of communal space and clinician time constraints impeded frequent meetings [85]. However, face-to-face meetings have been consistently reported as one of the most important features of collaboration because they guarantee exchange of ideas and information with immediate feedback when needed [65, 86, 87]. Consequently, the *"corridor conversations" (NP)* and a *"chat over a cup of coffee" (MP)* became significant routines for information exchange.

Working collaboratively with co-existing roles
The addition of NPs to PHC sites required changes to existing role hierarchies, resulting in the co-existence and blurring of professional roles. A systematic review of studies across all types of healthcare settings reported that the combination of task delegation, substitution and complementarity in NP-MP teams added to the complexity of blurred role boundaries between NPs and MPs [76]. We found that NPs and MPs operationalised collaborative practice with overlapping and complementary roles. Roles overlapped when the NP adopted medical skills in her autonomous patient consultation and they complemented each other in joint patient consultations. The blurring of roles only emerged as a problem when legal and fiscal policies were difficult to apply in clinical practice.

Role theory can help to explain the traditional behaviour of some NPs and MPs. It is assumed that "persons are members of *social positions* and hold *expectations* for their own behaviors and those of other persons" ([88], p. 67). In our study, NPs and MPs worked in distinct nursing and medical roles because these were in line with their identity of nursing and medical care, based on "internalized role expectations" ([89], p. 286). Consequently, the identity of MPs can be linked to their socialisation as silo-workers [90]. Canadian researchers also found that MPs rarely consulted with NPs, even after an intervention addressing collaborative working of NP-MP teams in PHC [75]. We assume that one-sided consultation patterns from NPs to MPs in our study can be partially explained by the fact that MPs had not needed communication or collaboration with other health professionals in the past.

For NPs in our study, a strong influence on their role and identity adjustment was based in the way they used their autonomy. Feminist researchers developed the term 'relational autonomy', claiming that autonomy is hardly ever absolute but context bound and linked with given structures [91]. Nurse practitioners in our study possessed relational autonomy in the sense that they were entitled to work as autonomous health practitioners *within* a framework of professional structures, policy restrictions and their individual level of confidence to make autonomous decisions. An example of NPs practicing with relational autonomy relates to those NPs who adopted a level of assertiveness that did not undermine the MPs' position. Assertiveness and confidence of NPs have been reported as facilitators of collaborative working in a mixed methods study of NPs and MPs in long-term care homes in Canada [47]. In our study, unassertive behaviour, including MP involvement where not strictly required, by otherwise very confident and highly competent NPs, was used as a purposeful strategy by all six NPs to enter existing MP-dominated structures.

Successful collaboration relies on the commitment of individuals
Considering the barriers for collaborative practice from existing systems, organisational structures and neglect from government agendas, collaboration between NPs and MPs in our sample appeared to exist through individual relationships and personal experiences. This accords with other studies that identified relationships and the personality of practitioners as significant factors for successful collaboration [82, 87, 92].

Collaborative practice models in the Australian PHC context would not exist without the personal commitment of NPs and MPs. Their willingness and ability to work around system barriers was based on the value they ascribed to their relationship. This was reflected in largely positive perceptions of the collaborative relationship in interviews and the questionnaire. Furthermore, in contrast to the Canadian Structuration model of collaboration [43] Australian PHC collaboration models were a bottom-up approach, driven by individuals who received limited support and governance through government and healthcare system structures as identified in the deductive analysis.

Strengths and limitations

The inclusion of five different sites spread across four Australian states generated a broad perspective on collaboration based on a multi-method dataset. The similarity with other research and theoretical models strengthened the credibility of findings and suggests their transferability within the Australian context of PHC, whilst noting that findings from case study research cannot be directly generalised to the general population of NPs and MPs.

Participating sites had well-established patterns of working together and recruitment of a negative or disconfirming case [36, 44] would have been a valuable addition to the sample. However, while we attempted to include sites with obvious inter-professional challenges, none were willing to participate. The recruitment of well-functioning teams was partly balanced out by participant statements about negative experiences in previous practices.

Recommendations for practice, policy and research

While this study was conducted in the Australian setting, similarity with international experience suggests that recommendations coming from this study are relevant to health professionals in other countries where NP roles are being implemented.

The influence of existing policies on the success of collaborative practice models needs consideration. Reimbursement structures for NPs have to ensure financial viability of NPs in PHC to increase the motivation for MPs to work in collaboration. For example, NPs should be granted access to a similar range of MBS items currently available for MPs, including procedure-based items (e.g. conducting and interpreting electrocardiography and spirometry, ordering female pelvic ultrasounds and suturing wounds) in addition to time-based consultation items. Further funding for collaborative practice models may come from private health funds if they reimburse patients who use NP care services. In line with trends in the USA, mandatory collaborative arrangements for NPs should be removed from legislation to facilitate autonomous NP practice and to minimise blurring of legal liability.

Improvements in infrastructure and practice level arrangements are recommended to facilitate NP-MP

interaction within practice settings. Opportunities for face-to-face meetings should be enhanced because face-to-face conversations were the most valued mode for information exchange. Regular meetings can serve as an occasion to address practical issues between participants, to foster information exchange about mutual patients and increase mutual learning. Where scheduled meetings are not possible, opportunities for informal conversations can be enhanced through communal areas and facilities where this is possible. Practice managers should be utilised for their potential leadership role in fostering collaboration. Nurse practitioners should be given access to space and resources that equal the MP's access to infrastructure, including office space. Preparatory clarification of scope of practice, consultation and referral mechanisms as well as roles and responsibilities is recommended. It appeared useful for practitioners to put this agreement in writing (on a voluntary basis and not based on legislative requirements) and to address liability of practitioners for different scenarios such as 1) patients seen together; 2) patients seen by only one practitioner but advice was given by another practitioner (by phone, email, face-to-face conversation); and 3) NPs working under vicarious liability, when the employer (MP) may hold some responsibility for the employee (NP).

Most patient consultations occurred in separate sessions affirming that NPs are autonomous healthcare providers. Future research could investigate frameworks within which NPs are able to establish their own businesses. This study showed that the dependence on MPs and low reimbursement rates made it difficult for NPs to establish their own clinics in Australia.

Conclusions

These findings represent the experiences and perceptions of NPs and MPs in collaborative practice models following the introduction of new policies in the Australian setting regarding NP access to the public health insurance scheme and collaborative arrangements. Numerous challenges posed by system structures at policy and practice level and differing perceptions of role enactment were identified. Findings provided an understanding about the difficulty of NPs to enter existing healthcare systems and help to understand some reservations of MPs towards collaboration with NPs. Nevertheless with their willingness and ability to modify routines and roles and accept existing structural frameworks, NPs and MPs were able to establish well-functioning models of collaboration. The individual determination of practitioners to make it work was crucial for the implementation of these models of care because their establishment was challenging at those sites where external support by government agencies was lacking. The evidence-base from this study on collaborative practice models in Australian PHC settings will facilitate new discussions with policy makers, healthcare funds, medical and nursing associations, politicians and key stakeholders who influence healthcare reform.

Abbreviations

ACNP, Australian College of Nurse Practitioners; AHPRA, Australian Health Practitioner Regulation Agency; FFS, fee-for-service; GP, general practitioner; MBS, medicare benefit schedule; MMR, mixed methods research; MP, medical practitioner; NP, nurse practitioner; PBS, pharmaceutical benefit scheme; PHC, primary healthcare; PM, practice manager; UK, United Kingdom; USA, United States of America; WHO, World Health Organisation

Acknowledgements

We wish to thank the nurse practitioners, medical practitioners and practice managers who provided their valuable time for study participation.

Funding

Verena Schadewaldt was funded with a Victorian International Research Scholarship by the Victorian Department of Economic Development, Jobs, Transport and Resources (formerly Department of State Development, Business and Innovation) and the Australian Catholic University. The funding sources had no role in the study and no influence on data collection and analyses, interpretation of results or writing of publications.

Authors' contributions

VS contributed to the study design, data collection, analysis and data interpretation, and drafted the first version of the manuscript. EM contributed to the study design and data interpretation. JEH contributed to the study design. AG was the principal supervisor and contributed to study design, data analysis and interpretation. All authors critically reviewed and approved the final version of the manuscript.

Authors' information

None provided.

Competing interests

All authors declare that they have no competing interests.

Author details

[1]Faculty of Health Sciences, School of Nursing Midwifery and Paramedicine, Australian Catholic University, Melbourne, Australia. [2]Nursing Research Institute, St Vincent's Health Australia/Australian Catholic University, Sydney, Australia. [3]School of Health Sciences, Faculty of Health, Arts and Design, Swinburne University of Technology, Melbourne, Australia. [4]School of Public Health, University of Adelaide, Adelaide, Australia. [5]Faculty of Health Sciences, School of Nursing, Midwifery and Paramedicine, Australian Catholic University, Canberra, Australia. [6]James Cook University, Townsville, Australia.

References

1. Australian college of nurse practitioners history [http://acnp.org.au/history]. Accessed 04 May 2014.
2. Statistics [http://www.nursingmidwiferyboard.gov.au/About/Statistics.aspx]. Accessed 05 May 2014.
3. Nursing and Midwifery Board of Australia. Nurse practitioner standards of practice. Melbourne, Australia: ANMB; 2014. p. 1–5.
4. Nursing and Midwifery Board of Australia. Guidelines on endorsement as a nurse practitioner. Melbourne, Australia: Nursing and Midwifery Board of Australia; 2011.
5. Stanik-Hutt J, Newhouse RP, White KM, Johantgen M, Bass EB, Zangaro G, Wilson R, Fountain L, Steinwachs DM, Heindel L, et al. The quality and effectiveness of care provided by nurse practitioners. J Nurse Pract. 2013;9(8):492–500. e413.
6. Parkinson AM, Parker R. Addressing chronic and complex conditions: What evidence is there regarding the role primary healthcare nurses can play? Aust Health Rev. 2013;37(5):588–93.
7. Australian Government. A national health and hospitals network for australia's future. Canberra: Commonwealth of Australia; 2010.
8. World Health Organisation. A universal truth: No health without a workforce. Geneva: WHO; 2013.
9. McInnes L. Review of processes for the implementation of the role of nurse practitioners in south australia. Report for SA Health; unpublished report 2008. p. 1–42
10. Primary health care in australia [http://www.aihw.gov.au/australias-health/2014/preventing-ill-health/]. Accessed 25 Jul 2016.
11. Australia's health system [http://www.aihw.gov.au/australias-health/2014/health-system/]. Accessed 06 Nov 2014.
12. The pharmaceutical benefits scheme - nurse practitioner pbs prescribing [http://www.pbs.gov.au/browse/nurse]. Accessed 08 Nov 2014.
13. Health insurance (midwife and nurse practitioner) determination. In. Edited by Australian Government ComLaw; 2011.
14. Phillips SJ. 26th annual legislative update: Progress for aprn authority to practice. Nurse Pract. 2014;39(1):29–52.
15. National health (collaborative arrangements for nurse practitioners) determination. In. Edited by Australian Government ComLaw; 2010.
16. Lowe G, Plummer V, Boyd L. Nurse practitioner roles in australian healthcare settings. Nurs Manag (Harrow). 2013;20(2):28–35.
17. Burgess J, Purkis ME. The power and politics of collaboration in nurse practitioner role development. Nurs Inq. 2010;17(4):297–308.
18. Offredy M, Townsend J. Nurse practitioners in primary care. Fam Pract. 2000; 17(6):564–9.
19. Government of Western Australia. Nurse practitioner business models and arrangements - final report. Perth, Australia: Government of Western Australia, Department of Health, Nursing and Midwifery Office; 2011
20. Schadewaldt V, McInnes E, Hiller JE, Gardner A. Views and experiences of nurse practitioners and medical practitioners with collaborative practice in primary health care – an integrative review. BMC Fam Pract. 2013;14(132):1–11.
21. San Martín-Rodríguez L, Beaulieu MD, D'Amour D, Ferrada-Videla M. The determinants of successful collaboration: A review of theoretical and empirical studies. J Interprof Care. 2005;19 Suppl 1:132–47.
22. Christensen CM, Bohmer R, Kenagy J. Will disruptive innovations cure health care? Harv Bus Rev. 2000;78(5):102–12. 199.
23. Christensen CM, Baumann H, Ruggles R, Sadtler TM. Disruptive innovation for social change. Harv Bus Rev. 2006;84(12):94–101. 163.
24. Barton TD. Clinical mentoring of nurse practitioners: The doctors' experience. Br J Nurs. 2006;15(15):820–4.
25. Stein LI. The doctor-nurse game. Arch Gen Psychiatry. 1967;16(6):699–703.
26. Willis E. Medical dominance: The division of labour in australian health care. Sydney: Allen & Unwin; 1983.
27. Bourgeault IL, Mulvale G. Collaborative health care teams in canada and the USA: Confronting the structural embeddedness of medical dominance. Health Sociol Rev. 2006;15(5):481–95.
28. McMurray R. The struggle to professionalize: An ethnographic account of the occupational position of advanced nurse practitioners. Human Relations. 2011;64(6):801–22.
29. Willis E. Introduction: Taking stock of medical dominance. Health Sociol Rev. 2006;15(5):421–31.
30. Carrigan C. Collaborative arrangements. Are expanded roles for nurses and midwives being stifled? Aust Nurs J. 2011;18(10):24–7.
31. Defining the nurse practitioner role [https://www.mja.com.au/insight/2011/2/claire-jackson-defining-nurse-practitioner-role]. Accessed 05 Jan 2015.
32. Collaborative agreements spark litigation fears [https://www.mja.com.au/insight/2011/18/collaborative-agreements-spark-litigation-fears]. Accessed 05 Jan 2015.
33. Cashin A. Collaborative arrangements for australian nurse practitioners: A policy analysis. J Am Assoc Nurse Pract. 2014;26(10):550–4.
34. Stake RE. The art of case study research. Thousand Oaks: Sage; 1995.
35. Simons H. Case study research in practice. SAGE: Los Angeles, London; 2009.

36. Yin RK. Case study research - design and methods. 4th ed. Los Angeles: Sage; 2009.

37. Eisenhardt KM, Graebner ME. Theory building from cases: Opportunities and challenges. Acad Manag J Arch. 2007;50(1):25–32.

38. Yin RK. Case study research - design and methods. 5th ed. Thousand Oaks: SAGE Publications; 2014.

39. Creswell JW. Research design - qualitative, quantitative, and mixed methods approaches. 4th ed. London: Sage; 2014.

40. Johnson RB, Onwuegbuzie AJ, Turner LA. Toward a definition of mixed methods research. J Mix Methods Res. 2007;1(2):112–33.

41. Morse JM, Niehaus L. Mixed method design - principles and procedures. Walnut Creek: Left Coast Press; 2009.

42. Corser WD. A conceptual model of collaborative nurse-physician interactions: The management of traditional influences and personal tendencies. Sch Inq Nurs Pract. 1998;12(4):325–41.

43. D'Amour D, Goulet L, Labadie JF, Martin-Rodriguez LS, Pineault R. A model and typology of collaboration between professionals in healthcare organizations. BMC Health Serv Res. 2008;8:188–202.

44. Patton MQ. Qualitative research & evaluation methods, vol. 3rd. Thousand Oaks: Sage; 2002.

45. Schadewaldt V, McInnes E, Hiller JE, Gardner A. Investigating characteristics of collaboration between nurse practitioners and medical practitioners in primary healthcare: A mixed methods multiple case study protocol. J Adv Nurs. 2013;70(5):1184–93.

46. Way D, Jones L, Baskerville NB. Improving the effectiveness of primary health care through nurse practitioner/family physician structured collaborative practice - final report to the health transition fund. Ottawa: University of Ottawa; 2001. p. 1–158.

47. Donald F. Collaborative practice by nurse practitioners and physicians in long-term care homes: A mixed methods study. Hamilton: McMaster University; 2007.

48. Sicotte C, D'Amour D, Moreault M-P. Interdisciplinary collaboration within quebec community health care centres. Soc Sci Med. 2002;55(6):991–1003.

49. Braun V, Clarke V. Using thematic analysis in psychology. Qual Res Psychol. 2006;3(2):77–101.

50. Fetters MD, Curry LA, Creswell JW. Achieving integration in mixed methods designs - principles and practices. Health Serv Res. 2013;48(6pt2):2134–56.

51. Kitto SC, Chesters J, Grbich C. Quality in qualitative research. Med J Aust. 2008;188(4):243–6.

52. J, Corter A, Brewerton R, Watts I. Nurse practitioners in primary care: Benefits for your practice. Julian King & Associates Limited; Kinnect Group; Australian General Practice Network, Auckland, New Zealand 2012.

53. Bosque E. A model of collaboration and efficiency between neonatal nurse practitioner and neonatologist: Application of collaboration theory. Adv Neonatal Care. 2011;11(2):108–13.

54. D'Amour D, Ferrada-Videla M, San Martin Rodriguez L, Beaulieu MD. The conceptual basis for interprofessional collaboration: Core concepts and theoretical frameworks. J Interprof Care. 2005;19 Suppl 1:116–31.

55. About general practice nursing [http://www.apna.asn.au/scripts/cgiip.exe/WService=APNA/ccms.r?PageId=11137]. Accessed 18 Sept 2014.

56. Medicare benefits schedule - item 3 [http://www9.health.gov.au/mbs/fullDisplay.cfm?type=item&qt=ItemID&q=3]. Accessed 09 Nov 2014.

57. Medical Board of Australia. Good medical practice: A code of conduct for doctors in australia. Melbourne, Australia: Medical Board of Australia; 2014. p. 1–25.

58. Horavath J. Review of medicare locals. Canberra, Australia: Australian Government - Department of Health; 2014.

59. D'Amour D, Goulet L, Pineault R, Labadie J-F, Remondin M. Comparative study of interorganizational collaboration in four health regions and its effects: The case of perinatal services. Montreal: University of Montreal; 2004.

60. Australian Government - Department of Health. Mbs online - medicare benefits schedule. Canberra, Australia: Australian Government - Department of Health; 2014.

61. Helms C, Crookes J, Bailey D. A case study examining financial viability, benefits and challenges of employing a nurse practitioner in general practice. Aust Health Rev. 2014. in print.

62. Phillips S. Nps face challenges in the u.S. And the uk. Nurse Pract. 2007; 32(7):25–9.

63. Brooten D, Youngblut JM, Hannan J, Guido-Sanz F. The impact of interprofessional collaboration on the effectiveness, significance, and future of advanced practice registered nurses. Nurs Clin North Am. 2012;47(2):283–94. vii.

64. Sarma S, Devlin RA, Thind A, Chu M-K. Canadian family physicians' decision to collaborate: Age, period and cohort effects. Soc Sci Med. 2012;75(10):1811–9.

65. Chesluk BJ, Holmboe ES. How teams work - or don't - in primary care: A field study on internal medicine practices. Health Affairs (Millwood). 2010; 29(5):874–9.

66. Naccarella L, Southern D, Furler J, Scott A, Prosser L, Young D. Siren project: Systems innovation and reviews of evidence in primary health care narrative review of innovative models for comprehensive primary health care delivery. Australia: Australian Primary Health Care Research Institute (APHCRI), Australian National University; The Department of General Practice & Melbourne Institute of Applied Economics and Social Research, The University of Melbourne; 2006. p. 1–179.

67. The ontario family care enrolment example [http://aphcri.anu.edu.au/news-events/communique-unlocking-potential-general-practice]. Accessed 20 May 2014.

68. Mable AL, Marriott J, Mable ME. Canadian primary healthcare policy - the evolving status of reform. Ottawa: Canadian Health Services Research Foundation; 2012. p. 1–45.

69. Roots AC. Outcomes associated with family nurse practitioner practice in fee-for-service community-based primary care. Doctoral thesis. British Columbia: University of Victoria; 2012.

70. Currie J, Chiarella M, Buckley T. An investigation of the international literature on nurse practitioner private practice models. Int Nurs Rev. 2013; 60(4):435–47.

71. Minarik PA, Zeh MA, Johnston L. Collaboration with psychiatrists in connecticut. Clin Nurse Spec. 2001;15(3):105–7.

72. Iglehart JK. Expanding the role of advanced nurse practitioners - risks and rewards. N Engl J Med. 2013;368(20):1935–41.

73. Reagan PB, Salsberry PJ. The effects of state-level scope-of-practice regulations on the number and growth of nurse practitioners. Nurs Outlook. 2013;61(6):392–9.

74. Bauer JC. Nurse practitioners as an underutilized resource for health reform: Evidence-based demonstrations of cost-effectiveness. J Am Acad Nurse Pract. 2010;22(4):228–31.

75. Bailey P, Jones L, Way D. Family physician/nurse practitioner: Stories of collaboration. J Adv Nurs. 2006;53(4):381–91.

76. Niezen MGH, Mathijssen JJP. Reframing professional boundaries in healthcare: A systematic review of facilitators and barriers to task reallocation from the domain of medicine to the nursing domain. Health Policy. 2014;117(2):151–69.

77. Cashin A, Carey M, Watson N, Clark G, Newman C, Waters CD. Ultimate doctor liability: A myth of ignorance or myth of control? Collegian. 2009;16(3):125–9.

78. Battaglia LE. Supervision and collaboration requirements: The vulnerability of nurse practitioners and its implications for retail health. Wash Univ Law Rev. 2010;87(5):1127–61.

79. Staunton P, Chiarella M. Law for nurses and midwives. 7th ed. Sydney: Elsevier; 2013.

80. Resnick B, Bonner A. Collaboration: Foundation for a successful practice. Review. 2003;4(6):344–9.

81. Sangster-Gormley E, Martin-Misener R, Burge F. A case study of nurse practitioner role implementation in primary care: What happens when new roles are introduced? BMC Nurs. 2013;12:1.

82. Poghosyan L, Nannini A, Stone PW, Smaldone A. Nurse practitioner organizational climate in primary care settings: Implications for professional practice. J Prof Nurs. 2013;29(6):338–49.

83. Martin PD, Hutchinson SA. Negotiating symbolic space: Strategies to increase np status and value. Nurse Pract. 1997;22(1):89–91. 94–86, 101–102.

84. Greenhalgh T. Role of routines in collaborative work in healthcare organisations. BMJ. 2008;337(7681):1269–71.

85. Oandasan IF, Gotlib Conn L, Lingard L, Karim A, Jakubovicz D, Whitehead C, Miller K-L, Kennie N, Reeves S. The impact of space and time on interprofessional teamwork in canadian primary health care settings: Implications for health care reform. Prim Health Care Res Dev. 2009;10(02):151.

6

Process evaluation of a stepped-care program to prevent depression in primary care: patients' and practice nurses' experiences

Alide D. Pols[1,2] (iD), Karen Schipper[3], Debbie Overkamp[2], Susan E. van Dijk[1], Judith E. Bosmans[1], Harm W. J. van Marwijk[2,4], Marcel C. Adriaanse[1*] and Maurits W. van Tulder[1]

Abstract

Background: Depression is common in patients with diabetes type 2 (DM2) and/or coronary heart disease (CHD), with high personal and societal burden and may even be preventable. Recently, a cluster randomized trial of stepped care to prevent depression among patients with DM2 and/or CHD and subthreshold depression in Dutch primary care (Step-Dep) versus usual care showed no effectiveness. This paper presents its process evaluation, exploring in-depth experiences from a patient and practice nurse perspective to further understand the results.

Methods: A qualitative study was conducted. Using a purposive sampling strategy, data were collected through semi-structured interviews with 24 participants (15 patients and nine practice nurses). All interviews were audiotaped and transcribed verbatim. Atlas.ti 5.7.1 software was used for coding and structuring of themes. A thematic analysis of the data was performed.

Results: The process evaluation showed, even through a negative trial, that Step-Dep was perceived as valuable by both patients and practice nurses; perceived effectiveness on improving depressive symptoms varied greatly, but most felt that it had been beneficial for patients' well-being. Facilitators were: increased awareness of mental health problems in chronic disease management and improved accessibility and decreased experienced stigma of receiving mental health care. The Patient Health Questionnaire 9 (PHQ-9), used to determine depression severity, functioned as a useful starting point for the conversation on mental health and patients gained more insight into their mental health by regularly filling out the PHQ-9. However, patients and practice nurses did not widely support its use for monitoring depressive symptoms or making treatment decisions. Monitoring mental health was deemed important in chronically ill patients by both patients and practice nurses and was suggested to start at the time of diagnosis of a chronic disease. Appointed barriers were that patients were primarily motivated to participate in scientific research rather than their intrinsic need to improve depressive symptoms. Additionally, various practice nurses preferred offering individually based therapy over pre-determined interventions in a protocolled sequence and somatic practice nurses expressed a lack of competence to recognise and treat mental health problems. (Continued on next page)

* Correspondence: marcel.adriaanse@vu.nl
[1]Department of Health Sciences and the EMGO Institute for Health and Care
Research, Vrije Universiteit, Amsterdam, De Boelelaan 1085, 1081 HV
Amsterdam, The Netherlands
Full list of author information is available at the end of the article

(Continued from previous page)

Conclusion: This study demonstrates both the benefits and unique demands of programs such as Step-Dep. The appointed facilitators and barriers could guide the development of future studies aiming to prevent depression in similar patient groups.

Keywords: Qualitative study, Process evaluation, Major depressive disorder, Subthreshold depression, Stepped care, Diabetes mellitus type 2, Coronary heart disease

Background

Major depression is estimated to currently affect 350 million people around the world. Depression is the leading cause of disability worldwide and is a major contributor to the overall global burden of disease [1]. People with chronic physical health problems, like type 2 diabetes mellitus (DM2) and coronary heart disease (CHD), are approximately twice as likely to suffer from major depression as compared to the general adult population. Furthermore, when co-occurring, major depression is significantly associated with greater reductions in health status compared with depression alone, or with single or multiple chronic physical conditions alone [2]. It is furthermore increasingly conceptualized as a chronic condition [3].

One approach to reduce the burden of major depression could be to prevent the influx of new cases. Recent meta-analyses have shown that psychological interventions can reduce the incidence of depression, which in high-risk populations can be as high as 25% annually [4, 5]. Offering these in a stepped care format could be an efficient and cost-effective approach to prevent depression, but the evidence is not unequivocal [6]. In stepped care, patients start with minimally intensive evidence-based treatments. Progress is monitored systematically and those patients who do not improve adequately step up to a treatment of higher intensity, thereby making the best use of available resources [7], although the steps perhaps do not make the best use of available clinical expertise [8]. Current evidence on the effectiveness of prevention of depression using stepped care is conflicting. While effective in reducing the incidence of major depressive disorder in some elderly or visually impaired populations [9–11], it was not superior to usual care in other elderly, diabetic or primary care populations [12–15].

We recently performed a randomized controlled trial evaluating a nurse-led stepped-care program to prevent depression among patients with DM2 and/or CHD and subthreshold depression (indicated prevention) in primary care (Step-Dep) in several regions in the Netherlands. Patients with subthreshold depression were identified via screening which is not common practice in Dutch primary care. Our first finding was that both arms had a surprisingly low overall annual incidence of depression (11%). This pragmatic intervention was also not effective

in comparison with usual care in our quantitative analyses (Pols AD, Van Dijk, Bosmans SEM, Hoekstra JET, Van Marwijk HWJ, Van Tulder MW, Adriaanse M. Effectiveness of a stepped-care intervention to prevent major depression in patients with type 2 diabetes mellitus and/or coronary heart disease and subthreshold depression: apragmatic cluster randomized controlled trial, submitted). To gain more insight into the facilitators and barriers of the Step-Dep program and to better understand the effects of the intervention in daily life, a qualitative process evaluation study was performed alongside the trial. Qualitative studies can complement the quantitative outcomes by gaining deeper understanding of interventions and this can yield valuable input for the development and implementation of the next generation of care models in the management of mental-physical multimorbidity and frailty, and can inform the policy debate [16]. This paper reports the results of this process evaluation exploring experiences with the Step-Dep program from a patient and practice nurse perspective.

Methods
Step-Dep study

The process evaluation entailed semi-structured face-to-face interviews with both patients and practice nurses in the intervention arm of the Step-Dep study. The methods and design have been described previously [17]. In short, we screened all patients with DM2 and/or CHD in 27 participating General Practitioner (GP) practices for subthreshold depression, defined as a Patient Health Questionnaire 9 (PHQ-9; range 0–27) score of six or more [18, 19], and no major depressive disorder according to the Mini International Neuropsychiatric Interview (MINI) [20, 21]. Patients in the intervention arm were offered a stepped care preventive program, and patients in the control arm received care as usual. The stepped care intervention consisted of four sequential but flexible treatment steps, each lasting 3 months; 1) watchful waiting, 2) guided self-help, 3) problem solving treatment (PST) and 4) referral to the general practitioner. After each step, patients with a persisting PHQ-9 score of six or more were offered the next treatment step of the intervention. Due to the pragmatic nature of the Step-Dep trial, treatment steps could be personalized or skipped if deemed necessary. A trained practice nurse delivered the stepped care program. This training focused on how to implement the stepped-care program, how to provide guidance with the self-help course using motivational interviewing techniques and how to provide the PST (see Appendix 1 for a detailed description of patient an practice nurse roles during Step-Dep). The training was developed and provided by a qualified trainer in collaboration with research team members. During the trial, all practice nurses were regularly supervised by the training staff and could contact them to discuss any questions or problems.

Participant selection and recruitment

We used purposeful sampling in order to include patients with as many perspectives on the pre-specified topics as possible [22]. Based on a literature review of factors influencing depression incidence and outcome, we selected patients on: gender, age, presence of DM2 and/or CHD, self-reported history of depression, self-reported current depression, level of education, baseline depression severity (PHQ-9), baseline anxiety severity (HADS-a), baseline quality of life score (EQ5D), baseline social support scores, and locus of control scores. We also selected patients who had received different elements of the stepped care program as well as a patient that had dropped-out of the program. We included patients from all different GP practices.

All nine practice nurses involved in the actual implementation of the Step-Dep program were interviewed. Amongst them were both somatic practice nurses, whose primary task is the physical health management of primary care patients with diabetes and/or cardiovascular disease, and psychological practice nurses, whose primary task is to provide low-intensity mental health care for primary care patients. In the Netherlands, the educational programs for these two types of practice nurses are separate and generally take 1 year after an appropriate pre-registration education of 4 years at an University of Applied Sciences. Patients are not charged for practice nurse consultations in primary care; this type of care is reimbursed within public health insurance. At the start of the intervention in 2013, per standard practice size of 2350 registered patients, 0.33FTE somatic practice nurse and 0.25FTE psychological practice nurse were available.

Patients and practice nurses were asked by an investigator (ADP or DO) to participate in the evaluation of the Step-Dep study by phone. All selected participants agreed to be interviewed, except for three patients due to terminal illness of themselves or their partners.

Data collection

To structure the interviews and maintain conformity in the different interviews, a topic guide was used (Appendix 2), which was developed based on study aims and patients' and practice nurses' feedback during the Step-Dep study.

Additionally, to systematically evaluate the experiences with the Step-Dep program, we added questions based on the RE-AIM model [23]. RE-AIM assesses five dimensions of an intervention: reach, efficacy, adoption, implementation, and maintenance. Reach explores characteristics of study participants compared to the target population; efficacy refers to whether the targeted outcome was achieved; adoption assesses variables of the staff and settings executing the intervention; implementation refers to intervention fidelity and resources (i.e. time); maintenance evaluates both individual-level and organizational/setting-level intervention sustainability. Based on the topic guide, semi-structured open-ended questions were formulated (Appendix 3 and 4). The process of data collection and analysis was iterative, meaning that the researchers started data analysis after the first interviews to further explore and validate emerging themes in the next interviews. This process evaluation was summative and retrospective; the results were not used to adjust the program along the way.

All interviews were conducted between September and November 2015 by ADP and DO. Interviews with individual participants were held at home (patients $n = 11$), at the GP practice (practice nurses $n = 8$) or at the Vrije Universiteit Amsterdam (patients $n = 4$, practice nurses $n = 1$). The interviews lasted about 45 min each. The interviews were audio-recorded and transcribed verbatim with the permission of the participants. To check the validity of the transcription, participants received a summary of their interview and were asked if they recognized the main themes (member check) [22]. All participants but one (a patient who could not be reached despite multiple attempts) confirmed the content of the summary by mail to be representative for the interview.

Data analysis

The transcriptions of the interviews were analysed by two researchers (AP and DO) and emerging themes and subthemes were identified individually. First, using Atlas.ti 5.7.1 software codes and labels were attached to citations related to specific topics (open coding), leading to a set of descriptive topics per transcript. Then, all labels of all transcripts were compared and redefined, and clustered into themes and subthemes (axial coding). Eventually, overarching themes were formulated (selective coding), and similarities and differences between cases were identified (cross case analysis of constant comparison) to provide further insight into the research questions. Furthermore, 'check coding' was used, meaning that three different researchers (AP, DO and KS) were involved in the process of data analysis, in order to enhance the reliability [22]. Relevant themes were agreed upon and for each theme the most illustrating quotes were selected and only adjusted if necessary for readability for the final report.

Data saturation

In qualitative research, the process of data collection and analysis ends when 'saturation' is reached [22]. This is the point where no new information is added and data replication occurs. From the patient perspective, we reached this point after interviewing 11 patients. We have subsequently interviewed four more patients to confirm this.

Results

Description of participants

Of the participating patients, eight were female and seven male. The age range was from 48 to 84 years. PHQ-9 levels at baseline varied from 2 to 16. Additional data regarding the chronic condition, education level,

self-reported depression at baseline, self-reported history of depression, and number of program steps terminated can be found in Table 1. Of the interviewed practice nurses, six were psychological practice nurses and three were somatic practice nurses. One of the three somatic practice nurses had been a psychological practice nurse before. The number of Step-Dep patients per practice nurse varied from 3 to 24. To ensure anonymity, age and gender are not mentioned.

Themes

The results from this study can be understood using five overarching themes; 1) motivation to participate, 2) the Step-Dep program, 3) patient care, 4) patient wellbeing and 5) recommendations for future care. They illuminate

Table 1 Participant characteristics

Patients

Interview nr	Age	Sex	DM2/CHD	Educational level	Self-reported depression at baseline	Self-reported history of depression	PHQ-9 score at inclusion	PHQ-9 score at baseline[a]	Number of program steps terminated
P1	66	f	CHD	high	no	yes	7	5	2
P2	61	f	CHD	high	no	yes	7	4	1
P3	63	f	Both	intermediate	yes	yes	9	16	referred
P4	84	f	CHD	low	yes	no	10	11	3
P5	53	f	DM2	high	no	yes	16	14	2
P6	72	m	CHD	intermediate	no	yes	10	2	1
P7	56	m	DM2	high	no	yes	10	10	3
P8	73	f	Both	low	no	no	11	6	1
P9	55	m	Both	intermediate	no	yes	14	12	4
P10	48	m	DM2	intermediate	yes	yes	12	12	1
P11	61	m	DM2	low	yes	yes	8	4	Drop-out
P12	56	f	Both	high	yes	yes	14	12	3
P13	66	m	CHD	high	no	yes	7	5	referred
P14	57	m	DM2	intermediate	no	no	14	7	3
P15	55	f	CHD	low	no	no	15	8	4

Practice nurses

Interview nr	Practice nurse type	Number of Step-Dep patients treated
N1	Psychological practice nurse	24
N2	Psychological practice nurse	15
N3	Psychological practice nurse	13
N4	Psychological practice nurse	10
N5	Somatic practice nurse	3
N6	Somatic practice nurse	6
N7	Psychological practice nurse	15
N8	Currently somatic practice nurse, previously psychological practice nurse	3
N9	Psychological practice nurse	7

Abbreviations: F female, M male, CHD Coronary Heart Disease, DM2 Diabetes Mellitus type 2, PHQ-9 Patients Health Questionnaire 9 score
[a]Scores do not equal inclusion PHQ-9 scores due to time between inclusion and baseline

the main experienced facilitators and barriers of Step-Dep. The term facilitator used in this paper translates to what interviewees named as experienced successful, useful, effective or strong elements of the program. The term barriers is used to express the opposite. An overview of the main results per theme can be found in Table 2.

Theme: motivation to participate

Patients reported widely different reasons to participate. Interestingly, less than half named the desire to improve their mood as a primary motivation. A few wanted to use the study to analyse their mood, whereas others were curious about the possible interaction of their depressive symptoms with their chronic disease or felt that the study acknowledged this link. Another reason mentioned, was the GP's advice to enrol.

All interviewed patients stressed the importance of contributing to scientific research, and named this as (one of) their main motivator(s) to participate.

Table 2 Overview of main results by theme

Motivation to participate

- Patients were primarily motivated to participate in Step-Dep to contribute to scientific research rather than having a desire to improve their depressive symptoms
- Practice nurses perceived this as a barrier to motivate patients for the different treatment steps, especially the self-help course

The Step-Dep program

Role and competences of the practice nurse:

- In order to discuss their mental health problems, patients needed to feel a connection to the practice nurse
- Somatic practice nurses expressed a lack of competence to recognise and treat mental health problems

Treatment steps and stepped care protocol:

- The offered treatments were viewed to be only suitable for specific patients
- Practice nurses preferred flexibility in the choice of therapy over pre-determined interventions in a one-size fits all protocol

Using the PHQ-9:

- The PHQ functioned as a useful starting point for the conversation on mental health, but was not widely supported as monitoring instrument or to base treatment decisions on

Patient care

- Interviewees experienced improved accessibility and decreased experienced stigma of receiving mental health care
- The increased awareness and attention for mental aspects in chronic disease management were experienced as very valuable
- Monitoring mental health is deemed important

Patient wellbeing

- Patients gained more insight into their mental health status by regularly filling out the PHQ-9

Recommendations for future care

- Monitoring of mental health in chronically ill patients should start from the time of diagnosis of the chronic disease

"In my opinion, if you can get certain results from a research program like this, that could help other people, you should collaborate." (P14)

Practice nurses picked up on this issue when treating Step-Dep participants and perceived it as a barrier to motivate some patients for the different treatment steps. Especially with the self-help module, a treatment which requires a relatively large input from patients, this lack of intrinsic motivation was perceived as problematic.

"By many, this wasn't actively requested. They were asked: 'Would you like to participate in a research program?' It did not come from within, like: 'I am stumbling upon problems, I am stuck, I want help.' It's a different story if it would originate from intrinsic motivation." (N1)

This phenomenon might explain some of the lack of effectiveness and the relatively low uptake of the Step-Dep intervention. Around 30% of patients who were offered one of the treatment steps, declined this step (Pols AD, Van Dijk, Bosmans SEM, Hoekstra JET, Van Marwijk HWJ, Van Tulder MW, Adriaanse M. Effectiveness of a stepped-care intervention to prevent major depression in patients with type 2 diabetes mellitus and/or coronary heart disease and subthreshold depression: a pragmatic cluster randomized controlled trial, submitted). Possibly, the research setting created an artificial situation, motivating patients to participate without much need for care.

Theme: the step-Dep program

The role and competences of the practice nurse The patient interviews illuminated that a good personal connection with the practice nurse determined whether they felt they could discuss their mental health problems. For several patients, the contact with the practice nurse itself even was the most important facilitator of the program, whereas for two others the lack of a good connection was the most important barrier.

"The best element...that (name practice nurse) listened to me so carefully [...] He made me feel calm [...] we just got along well." (P4)

"If I am with someone, with whom I can easily talk and I feel like he understands me and we click, I can open up more. I did not feel like I was really able to do that now." (P10)

Reflecting on their role and competences as mental health caregivers, the somatic practice nurses who lacked mental health work experience, cited that they lacked education, skills and experience to recognise and treat mental health problems in general, despite the Step-Dep training. They pointed this out as the main barrier to participate and function in the Step-Dep program.

"That (mental health care for chronic illnesses) is not something you learn during the practice nurse educational program. [...] Purely somatic health." (N5)

"As a somatic practice nurse, I felt like I utterly failed these people in certain aspects. They clearly indicated that they were dealing with problems and that they were struggling [...] I felt like I wasn't really able to help out." (N6)

They did want to master these competences, since in their experience, various mental health problems often interfere with somatic problems and they found these skills essential for a holistic treatment.

"I have often noticed that the insulin dependent patients are very afraid of injections or hypoglycaemia. There is a lot of anxiety involved. There are lots of people who just don't want to exercise. That is partly lifestyle, but also often psychological. People who are severely overweight are better off being referred to a psychologist than to a dietician. I feel that one of the most imperative things to do then is to offer psychological help, but as a somatic practice nurse, you need more education on how to do that and how to recognise such cases." (N5)

All practice nurses felt that the PST training was very useful and informative. Even so, the delivery of the PST was frequently experienced as difficult. Two somatic practice nurses referred their patients to the psychological practice nurse for this step *"Because I did not feel competent, I reckoned it required more know-how." (N5)*

Even psychological practice nurses said that in order to work with PST with every possible patient, they would require more practice. Since they only had a few patients that required PST within Step-Dep, these skills could not be extensively trained.

"I had that training and found it very useful; I learned a lot from it. Before I would be able to fully use it in daily practice at work, I would like some extra training." (N2)

The treatment steps and protocol Practice nurses found it easy to work with the simple and straightforward

Step-Dep protocol and deviations were hardly deemed necessary. However, ideally, they would prefer more room for their own choice of therapy, based on the estimated needs of a patient, instead of pre-determined steps in a protocolled sequence. Some practice nurses did not find the watchful waiting step fitting for patients they considered in need of care and would have preferred to skip this step. Also the self-help and PST were viewed as suitable for specific patients only.

"I would like to have a little more freedom of choice though." (N3)

"You should always keep in mind if it matches one's individual level and learning style and consider carefully if it will be of use to someone." (N9)

In line with the findings from the practice nurses' interviews, the experienced usefulness for patients was mixed for both the self-help and PST. Half of the interviewed patients that were offered the self-help course considered it one of the best elements of the Step-Dep program, whereas the other half did not find it helpful. Commonly mentioned benefits were the practical advices it offers, the accessible and understandable writing style, the insight it provided into their symptoms, and the advantage of being able to look up information at their own convenience later on. Barriers were how the course confronted them with their negative current mental state and the seemingly overwhelming amount of information.

"It is difficult to face at times. [...] To admit that you have a problem and then pick up that book." (P9)

Patients figured that more intensive guidance from the practice nurse was helpful to comply with the course *"...in order to be forced to actually go through that book..." (P9)* and to reduce the amount of information by recommending specific chapters applicable to them.

"(Name practice nurse) would say: 'Let's go to chapter 9; it is precisely what you have been through. Why don't you read that so we can go from there.' That helps." (P7)

Most practice nurses also experienced that their guidance, especially in combination with using motivational interviewing techniques, did improve patients' motivation, which could be a barrier as mentioned in the previous theme.

Three of the interviewed patients had received PST and their experiences were again quite personal. One patient felt it was too similar to his work approach and this therapy therefore did not work for him.

"[...] that is how you approach a project. It gets on my nerves if you analyse your own health in that same, simplistic manner." (P7)

The other two patients felt it did help to deal with their problems, although it was sometimes hard to face them.

"To look at it differently, from another perspective. It made me face my problems. It did help me, but not all the time, because I can't just change like that." (P12)

The PHQ-9 questionnaire

During the Step-Dep study, the PHQ-9 questionnaire was used for screening and monitoring of depressive symptoms and treatment decisions were based on its scores. A positive side-effect was that the majority of both patients and practice nurses felt that filling out the PHQ-9 together was an easy starting point to talk about patients' mental state.

"Filling out the questionnaire is convenient, because it is a natural way to start conversation." (P5)

Two patients, however, felt that their 3-monthly sessions were limited to this purpose, which was dissatisfying for them.

When investigating patients' experiences with how accurately their scores on the PHQ-9 questionnaire reflected their depressive symptom severity, all but two interviewed patients recognized themselves in the (sub-threshold) depressed profile at the start of Step-Dep. However, four patients felt that the scores during the 1-year follow-up did not measure the change in their mood accurately.

"When she would say: 'Your score has improved since last time,' I would feel like: 'Ok, if you say so.' It did not feel like it had improved." (P14)

In concordance with these patients, most of the practice nurses did not feel that the PHQ-9 measured changes in depressive symptoms during the year of follow-up accurately and making treatment decisions solely based on the PHQ-9 was not considered sufficient; clinical judgement was deemed necessary.

"You should always look at the PHQ as a whole. [...] I don't think you should ever use an instrument like that to make a stand-alone decision or base that on a certain score." (N3)

Theme: patient care

Due to the preventive approach, meaning that care was pro-actively offered as standard care, many patients and practice nurses experienced improved accessibility of mental health care. Especially the advantage of receiving care without a stigma was expressed.

"I had been depressed, but I was doing a bit better. I thought: 'If I participate and get this help, it won't be so hard to deal with.' You won't say: 'Ring the alarm, I need help because I am not well mentally.'" (P7)

"A low threshold. An easy access without a stigma. [...] Like this, it is offered as 'This is standard care for this group.' This way you are not crazy, it is not all in your head, it is just standard care." (N4)

Many patients said that during the care for their chronic condition, no or very little attention is ever paid to mental health.

"I have had that chronic disease for a long time now. No attention was ever paid to it, mentally. It was just like: 'Well, you have diabetes. You can't do this, but you can do that. Take some pills and that's it.'" (P14)

Participation in the Step-Dep study also made somatic practice nurses realise that normally, they put all emphasis on physical and none on mental health.

"What I liked, was that every 3 months you would ask: 'How are you? How are you feeling mentally?' That actually never comes up during diabetes treatment." (N8)

The psychological practice nurses considered this increased awareness and attention on mental health an important improvement of current chronic disease management.

"Just paying that explicit attention; 'How did things evolve for you, ever since you knew you had diabetes or heart failure?' That was received positively by many, and had been missing as well. Many people had to cope with it on their own, where an intervention might have been necessary. A project like this makes us health care providers more aware of the fact that we should monitor closely what the effect of our bad news will be." (N1)

One other highly valued aspect of the Step-Dep intervention was that the practice nurse visits were every 3 months. Both patients and practice nurses felt that this monitoring of depressive symptoms was beneficial; it felt like a safety net.

"What worked for me was that because of the consultations with (name practice nurse), someone was keeping an eye on me." (P5)

"Especially those who weren't doing all too well and who were struggling a bit, which doesn't necessarily lead to a depression, but is quite difficult, those were pleased to be monitored so closely." (N3)

However, a few patients felt it was an extra burden to come to the GP practice every 3 months during a year, but at the same time said it was necessary to adequately monitor their mental health state.

"It is indeed strenuous and a year seems like a lot at the beginning, but I do think you actually need that." (P7)

Part of this burden might have been caused by the research setting, since patients also had to fill out 3-monthly online questionnaires containing the HADS, PHQ-9, EQ5D, TIC-P, locus of control and perceived recovery questionnaires.

Theme: patient wellbeing
Remarkably, almost all patients indicated that they gained more insight into their mental state just by regularly filling out the PHQ, which they pointed out as one of the most important benefits of the program. Taking the time to analyse their mental state and depressive symptoms served as a form of self-reflection.

"The real eye-opener for me was that I became aware of my own behaviour. As I filled out the questionnaires again and again, I realised: 'This is how people see me.' Whereas I hadn't really noticed my negativity or that I was feeling a bit down myself. That was the biggest plus for me." (P10)

The majority of interviewed patients and practice nurses felt that Step-Dep had been beneficial for patients' wellbeing somehow, however sometimes in other ways than improving depressive symptoms per se.

"Just talking about depression or stress, that by itself is so useful. Not to make it go away, but to keep it under control, to be heard or to feel supported." (P1)

"They mainly benefitted from being more aware of and having more insight into how a chronic disease like diabetes or heart-failure can affect how we function and feel. And the acknowledgment; somebody is really taking it seriously and listening carefully." (N1)

Almost all patients would therefore recommend others to participate in a program like Step.

"With very little investment, it might become clearer to you what your problem is and be of help." (P11)

When evaluating the perceived effectiveness on improving depressive symptoms of the program, it became apparent that this varied greatly between patients. Several felt that their depressive symptoms had evidently improved because of Step-Dep, whereas a few said that the program had made no difference at all.

Practice nurses viewed this in a similar way, saying that "... some really benefitted from it and others did not." (N4)

Almost all practice nurses had several examples of patients where they felt that Step-Dep had really improved depressive symptoms.

"I definitely see positive results. I see, and that is also how they describe it, that they have more tools, a big repertoire of possible solutions to try out when they are not doing well. They have more control over their problems." (N9)

When investigating why for some the program had not been useful, explanations were diverse. For some patients, the fact that they were participating in a scientific research lowered the expectations of possible benefits from the program, which seems to have formed a barrier for effective care for these patients.

"Because the program is called 'research', you don't expect it to offer help. [...] I've just always looked at it as research." (P13)

Others did not get practical advices on how to improve their mood, the treatment they wanted or enough treatment sessions. One patient disengaged from the program because it did not help him, whereas a work re-integration project he was simultaneously engaged in did, because of the purpose of and link to coming back to work.

When questioning why the practice nurses felt that the program had not been useful for some patients, explanations were just as diverse. One said the program had been offered too late. Another said that it was hard to really measure the experienced benefits.

"I think that most people benefitted from it in some way, but that is very so hard to measure." (N2)

Two practice nurses concluded that the program sometimes did not work because many patients said they did not have any depressive symptoms.

"Almost everybody said that they had no depressive symptoms. So you can ask yourself whether you've reached the target population you were aiming for." (N2)

A program like Step-Dep was felt not to be suitable for patients with psychiatric comorbidity, which was indeed an exclusion criterion. Nonetheless, two practice nurses did have such patients in their Step-Dep treatment and reckoned that to be the reason why these patients did not improve during the program.

"If people have a lot of mental baggage, this doesn't work sufficiently. [...] If you would exclude these vulnerable individuals, I think it would work very well." (N4)

Theme: recommendations for future care

When discussing future prevention of depression, both patients and practice nurses agreed that this should take place in the GP practice. Patients prefer having chronic disease management clustered in one facility and enjoy the familiarity with the caregivers present in a primary care practice. Both a patient and a practice nurse suggested offering a prevention program like Step-Dep at the time of a new diagnosis of a chronic disease.

"Caring for people who are confronted with this for the first time, by their general practitioner, could be a good idea." (P2)

"We were too late for a very large part of the target population. Because some had already been through a phase of excessive sadness, which made me think: 'We might have been able to avoid this by offering a program like Step-Dep earlier on.'" (N1)

When testing this idea with others patients and practice nurses, most viewed it as an improvement of current chronic care. A few practice nurses added that one should avoid unnecessary medicalization of patients. In their opinion, patients should be made aware of the possibilities of mental health care, but only start therapy when experiencing problems.

Discussion

This qualitative study reports the results of a process evaluation exploring experiences with the Step-Dep program from a patient and practice nurse perspective. Our findings show that the main facilitators were: increased awareness of and insight into mental health in chronic disease management and improved accessibility and decreased experienced stigma of receiving mental health care. Main barriers were that patients were primarily motivated to participate to contribute to scientific research rather than their intrinsic need to improve depressive symptoms. Additionally, the PHQ-9 was not widely supported to monitor depressive symptoms or base treatment decisions on. Furthermore, somatic practice nurses expressed a lack of competence to recognise and treat mental health problems.

This process analysis has several strengths. Interviewing both patients and practice nurses enabled an evaluation from two essential perspectives; caregiver and care receiver. These perspectives were assessed within the context of a pragmatic trial, approximating a routine setting as much as possible. Additionally, the use of the theoretical RE-AIM framework in this evaluation ensured a thorough investigation of barriers and facilitators. Other strengths are the utilisation of two independent analysts, the systematic development of codes and code definitions, the use of a qualitative computer program, and complete data saturation of information after coding the interviews.

Limitations of this study are that one of the researchers conducting the interviews was also one of the main researchers of the Step-Dep program, possibly influencing interviewees' answers. However, before starting the interviews, strong emphasis was put on the importance of all feedback to improve future depression care. Our findings may not generalise to contexts where chronic disease management relies on different professionals than the GP and the somatic practice nurse, or where psychological practice nurses are not co-located or available in primary care. Furthermore, due to the aim of this process evaluation, we only interviewed patients from the intervention arm. Information from the control arm patients, on for example their own 'self-help' strategies and experiences with filling out the PHQ-9, could have been of added value. Considering the strengths and limitations of this study, our findings give important input for future research. We will discuss the principal findings in the light of current literature.

Firstly, the improved accessibility of care and the perception of a less stigmatising way in which care was delivered are in line with findings from another qualitative interview study among patients, GPs and practice nurses performed alongside a comparable randomised clinical trial on depression care [24]. Such benefits are important to patients, but hard to measure and usually not evaluated in effectiveness studies.

Secondly, it seemed of added value to standardly use the PHQ-9 in chronic disease management to offer patients a form of self-reflection on their mental state and facilitate the conversation on this topic. In another study, patients also saw it as an efficient and structured supplement to medical judgment, and as evidence that general practitioners were taking their problems seriously [25]. Even though the PHQ-9 has been shown to be a valid instrument to both screen for [18, 19] and monitor depressive symptoms [26], many patients and practice nurses in our study did not find this instrument appropriate for the latter. The preference of caregivers to rely on clinical judgment rather than depression severity scales has been described before [25]. Possibly, the most acceptable use of the PHQ-9 for caregivers would be as an instrument of self-reflection and as an 'ice-breaker', but not to base treatment decisions on.

Thirdly, our data revealed that somatic practice nurses experience a lack of competence in recognizing and handling depressive symptoms in chronically ill patients. Other qualitative studies have observed the same [24, 27, 28]. While for both somatic and psychological practice nurses the competence with the delivery of PST seemed dependent on the number of patients treated in Step-Dep, this general lack of confidence for the somatic practice nurses did not. The 2-day Step-Dep training appeared insufficient to compensate for experienced educational shortcomings. Despite the small number of somatic practice nurses in this study, this is an important finding given the prevalence of depressive symptoms in chronically ill patients and the increasing lead of the somatic practice nurse in chronic disease management. Therefore, we consider it important to educate somatic practice nurses better in recognizing and handling mental health problems. The interviewed somatic practice nurses in this study felt this need and were willing to do so. In contrast to our findings, the study by Barley et al. [29] showed that practice nurses do not see mental healthcare as part of what they do. In addition, a recent qualitative study on integrated care from the UK indicated that patients might prefer not to discuss mental health problems with their somatic health caregiver [24]. However, this was not in line with our study outcomes, where this preference was not expressed by patients. To explain these differences and to determine potential improvements in the somatic practice nurse education on mental health and how to best offer future integrated care, these views and preferences should be evaluated further.

Finally, most interviewed patients said to have been motivated to participate in order to contribute to scientific research, which practice nurses perceived as a barrier to deliver optimal care. It is possible that patients were not sufficiently aware of the possible benefits of the intervention for their depressive symptoms. However, both this potential benefit and the positive screening result on subthreshold depression were explicitly mentioned in two separate letters and in the final phone call during the consenting process, and during the first practice nurse visit both the rationale of Step-Dep and the depressive symptoms were discussed as well. It seems more plausible that the extent to which patients experienced a need for the offered mental health care played a role. Having a need for care is an essential motivator to take up offered care, especially in view of the self-activating nature of the offered psychological interventions within the Step-Dep study. Since prevention is often offered to people in an early or mild stage of their mood disorder, implicating less distress or suffering of the patient and therefore a limited need for care [30], this barrier may be challenging to overcome. The depression guidelines of the Dutch College of General Practitioners stress the importance of the existence of the need for care to increase the probability of treatment success, and plead against pro-actively offering depression care to patients having depressive symptoms as indicated by screening [31].

Further research should focus on approaches within chronic disease management to identify and proactively treat only those who are likely to benefit from preventive depression care but also experience a need for such care. Finding optimal strategies to routinely assess and monitor mental health issues while supporting resilience is perhaps required for the rest.

Conclusion

Although Step-Dep was not superior to care as usual in the prevention of major depression, it was perceived as valuable by the interviewed patients and practice nurses. The perceived effectiveness on improving depressive symptoms varied greatly among interviewees, but most felt that the program had been beneficial for patients' well-being. Main facilitators, such as increased awareness and understanding of mental health problems, improved accessibility and decreased experienced stigma of mental health care in chronic disease management are difficult to capture in conventional quantitative outcomes. These difficulties in combination with the appointed barriers may have contributed to the non-significant difference in effects of the Step-Dep intervention compared to usual care. Notwithstanding, both the facilitators and barriers described in this process evaluation might guide the development of future studies aiming to reduce the burden of depression among patients with a chronic physical disorder.

Appendix 1

Table 3 Practice nurse and patient roles per step in the Step-Dep program

Step	Role of practice nurse	Role of patient
1. Watchful waiting	Introductory consultation with patient. Explains stepped-care program and its rationale. If applicable, gives information and/or brochure about mild depression with simple advices on how to cope with mild depressive symptoms. Is available for patient, if needed	Gets acquainted with practice nurse. Receives information on stepped-care program and its rationale. Contacts practice nurse if needed
2. Guided self-help	Explains self-help course, hands out materials. Contacts patient every other week by phone to monitor progress. Uses motivational interviewing techniques to activate the patient, if needed. If needed, invites patient to discuss current depressive symptoms; if needed offers early progress to step 3	Starts self-help and works through course at own convenience. Discusses progress every other week. If needed, visits practice nurse and starts step 3
3. Problem Solving Treatment	Offers brief cognitive behavioral intervention focusing on practical skill building in 7 sessions. Explains stages of problem solving and applies to problems encountered in daily life, helping to regain control of life	Visits practice nurse for 7 PST sessions, working through problems together, learning practical skill building
4. Referral to GP	Refers patients to GP for further assessment of depressive symptoms. Provides a summary of the offered treatment	Visits GP to discuss provided treatment and following treatment for depressive symptoms

Appendix 2

Table 4 Topic list

RE-AIM	Topic
Reach	Appropriateness Step-Dep patients (target population)
	Depression: recognition, severity, causes, improving factors
	Need for care
	Motivation to participate
	Access mental health care
Efficacy	Perceived effectiveness
	Perceived usefulness
Adoption	Information practices, caregivers
Implementation	Barriers & facilitators
	Deviations from protocol
	Reasons for dropout
	Prerequisites for implementation
Maintenance	Satisfaction
	Feasibility for future

Appendix 3

Table 5 Patients interview

Topic	Question
General	How was your experience participating in Step-Dep/the program in your general practitioner practice?
	What was the best part for you?
	What was the weakest part for you?
Motivation	Why did you decide to participate in Step-Dep?
Mental state	How would you describe your mental state before starting Step-Dep? If not depressed: please tell more about it?
	If depressed: please tell more about it? Did it influence your life? What do you think caused it? Is there a relationship with your chronic disease? How? How is your mental state now? If improved: what are the reasons for that improvement?
	Did you feel the PHQ-9 reflected your mental state correctly? Why? Why not?
Need for care	Were you in need of care/a preventive program to improve depressive symptoms?
	How would it have been, if you had not received an invitation for Step-Dep?
	What were your expectations/hopes from the program?
	Did the program match your needs?
	What would your care of choice have been like? And to improve depressive symptoms?
	How would it have been for you to be offered a program at the time of diagnosis of your chronic disease?
Perceived effectiveness	Was the offered program useful to improve your depressive symptoms? Why? Why not? What was most useful to you? How do you see that in the long-term?
	How were/was the consultations with the practice nurse/self-help/problem solving treatment/referral to general practitioner for you?
Suggestions for future care	Would you recommend this program to others? Why? Why not? To whom?
	What would your suggestions be to improve Step-Dep?
	Is there anything you would like to add to the interview?

Appendix 4

Table 6 Practice nurse interview

Topic	Question
General	How did you experience executing Step-Dep?
	What is your opinion on the Step-Dep program?
	What were the main facilitators?
	What were the main barriers?
Reach	Were the selected patients appropriate for this prevention program? Why? Why not?
	How did you view their mental state/depressive symptoms? Did patients recognize themselves in the depressed profile? What are causes for depressive symptoms? How do you view the relationship with the chronic disease? What coping strategies do patients have with a chronic disease?
	Were the patients in need for care for depression? Other need for care? Why? Why not?
Efficacy	Did the program match their need for care?
	Was Step-Dep effective in your opinion on preventing depression/improving depressive symptoms for these patients? Why? Why not? How?
	What is your view on the program elements: consultations, self-help, problem solving treatment, referral to general practitioner?
	If the depressive symptoms improved in your patients; what was the reason for this improvement? Did the program play a part?
Implementation	Why did you decide to participate in Step-Dep?
	How do you view your competences to execute the program?
	Was it necessary to deviate from the protocol? Why? Why not?
	How was using the PHQ-9 for you? And as a screening/monitoring/decision tool?
	How much time would you need for the consultations/self-help/problem solving treatment?
Maintenance	Is this program (or elements) useful in daily practice for this group? Why? Why not?
	Would you use this program (or elements) in the future? Why? Why not?
	What would be necessary to implement this in your practice?
	How would you ideally see depression prevention?
	What is your opinion on offering a program like that at the time of diagnosis of the chronic disease?

Abbreviations

CHD: Coronary heart disease; DM2: Diabetes mellitus type 2; GP: General practitioner; PHQ-9: Patients health questionnaire 9; PST: Problem solving treatment

Acknowledgements

The authors would like to thank Lotte Bakker for the transcriptions of the interviews. We also would like to thank all the participating general practices and the research networks of general practitioners (ANH, THOON and LEON) for their participation and collaboration in the implementation and execution of the Step-Dep study. Furthermore, this study has been possible thanks to all interviewed participants. We would like to extend our gratitude to all Step-Dep participants.

Funding

This study is funded by ZonMw, the Netherlands Organisation for Health Research and Development (project number 80-82310-97-12110). The sponsor had no role in the design and conduct of the present study or in the writing of the manuscript.

Authors' contributions

LP constructed the design of the study and drafted the manuscript. LP and DO performed all interviews and analyses. KS collaborated in constructing the design, supervised the analyses and revised the manuscript. MA, JB, SvD, MvT and HvM collaborated in constructing the design and revised the manuscript. The final manuscript was read and approved by all authors.

Competing interests

The authors declare that they have no competing interests.

Consent for publication

Not applicable.

Author details

[1]Department of Health Sciences and the EMGO Institute for Health and Care Research, Vrije Universiteit, Amsterdam, De Boelelaan 1085, 1081 HV Amsterdam, The Netherlands. [2]Department of General Practice & Elderly Care Medicine and EMGO Institute for Health and Care Research, VU University Medical Centre, Amsterdam, The Netherlands. [3]Department of Medical Humanities, EMGO+ Institute, VU Medical Centre (VUmc), Amsterdam, The Netherlands. [4]CLAHRC Greater Manchester and NIHR School for Primary Care Research, the University of Manchester, Manchester, UK.

References

1. World Health Organization. Depression fact sheet [Internet]. 2016. Available from: http://www.who.int/mediacentre/factsheets/fs369/en/.
2. Moussavi S, Chatterji S, Verdes E, Tandon A, Patel V, Ustun B. Depression, chronic diseases, and decrements in health: results from the world health surveys. Lancet. 2007;370:851–8.
3. Vos T, Haby MM, Barendregt JJ, Kruijshaar M, Corry J, Andrews G. The burden of major depression avoidable by longer-term treatment strategies. Arch Gen Psychiatry. 2004;61:1097–103.
4. van Zoonen K, Buntrock C, Ebert DD, Smit F, Reynolds CF, Beekman ATF, et al. Preventing the onset of major depressive disorder: a meta-analytic review of psychological interventions. Int J Epidemiol. 2014;43:318–29.
5. Cuijpers P, van Straten A, Smit F, Mihalopoulos C, Beekman A. Preventing the onset of depressive disorders: a meta-analytic review of psychological interventions. Am J Psychiatry. 2008;165:1272–80.
6. Muñoz RF, Cuijpers P, Smit F, Barrera AZ, Leykin Y. Prevention of major depression. Annu Rev Clin Psychol. 2010;6:181–212.
7. Bower P, Gilbody S. Stepped care in psychological therapies: access, effectiveness and efficiency. Narrative literature review. Br J Psychiatry. 2005;186:11–7.
8. van Straten A, Hill J, Richards DA, Cuijpers P. Stepped care treatment delivery for depression: a systematic review and meta-analysis. Psychol Med. 2015;45:231–46.
9. van't Veer-Tazelaar PJ, van Marwijk HWJ, van Oppen P, van Hout HPJ, van der Horst HE, Cuijpers P, et al. Stepped-care prevention of anxiety and depression in late life: a randomized controlled trial. Arch Gen Psychiatry. 2009;66:297–304.
10. Dozeman E, van Marwijk HWJ, van Schaik DJF, Smit F, Stek ML, van der Horst HE, et al. Contradictory effects for prevention of depression and anxiety in residents in homes for the elderly: a pragmatic randomized controlled trial. Int. Psychogeriatrics. 2012;24(08):1242–51.
11. van der Aa HP, van Rens GH, Comijs HC, Margrain TH, Gallindo-Garre F, Twisk JW, et al. Stepped care for depression and anxiety in visually impaired older adults: multicentre randomised controlled trial. BMJ. 2015;351:h6127. doi:10.1136/bmj.h6127.
12. Zhang DX, Lewis G, Araya R, Tang WK, Mak WWS, Cheung FMC, et al. Prevention of anxiety and depression in Chinese: a randomized clinical trial testing the effectiveness of a stepped care program in primary care. J Affect Disord. 2014;169:212–20.
13. Van der Weele GM, De Waal MWM, Van den Hout WB, De Craen AJM, Spinhoven P, Stijnen T, et al. Effects of a stepped-care intervention programme among older subjects who screened positive for depressive symptoms in general practice: the PROMODE randomised controlled trial. Age Ageing. 2012;41:482–8.
14. van Beljouw IM, van Exel E, van de Ven PM, Joling KJ, Dhondt TD, Stek ML, et al. Does an outreaching stepped care program reduce depressive symptoms in community-dwelling older adults? a randomized implementation trial. Am J Geriatr Psychiatry. 2014;23:807–17.
15. Bot M, Pouwer F, Ormel J, Slaets JPJ, de Jonge P. Predictors of incident major depression in diabetic outpatients with subthreshold depression. Diabet Med. 2010;27:1295–301.
16. Craig P, Dieppe P, Macintyre S, Michie S, Nazareth I, Petticrew M. Developing and evaluating complex interventions: the new medical research council guidance. Br Med J. 2008;337:979–83.
17. van Dijk SEM, Pols AD, Adriaanse MC, Bosmans JE, Elders PJM, van Marwijk HWJ, et al. Cost-effectiveness of a stepped-care intervention to prevent major depression in patients with type 2 diabetes mellitus and/or coronary heart disease and subthreshold depression: design of a cluster-randomized controlled trial. BMC Psychiatry. 2013;13:128.
18. Kroenke KSR. The PHQ-9: a new depression diagnostic and severity measure. Psychiatr Ann. 2002;32:509–15.
19. Lamers F, Jonkers CCM, Bosma H, Penninx BWJH, Knottnerus JA, van Eijk JTM. Summed score of the patient health questionnaire-9 was a reliable and valid method for depression screening in chronically ill elderly patients. J Clin Epidemiol. 2008;61:679–87.
20. Sheehan DV, Lecrubier YSK. The mini-international neuropsychiatric interview (MINI): the development and validation of a structured diagnostic psychiatric interview for DSM-IV and ICD-10. J Clin Psychiatr. 1998;59:22–33.
21. Van Vliet I, De Beurs E. Het Mini Internationaal Neuropsychiatrisch Interview (MINI). Een kort gestructureerd diagnostisch psychiatrisch interview voor DSM-IV en ICD-10-stoornissen [The Mini International Neuropsychiatric Interview (MINI). A short structured diagnostic psychiatric interview for DSM-IV and ICD-10 disorders]. Tijdschrift voor Psychiatrie. 2007;49(6):393–7.
22. Meadows LM, Morse JM. Constructing evidence within the qualitative project. In Morse JM, Swanson JM, Kuzel AJ, editors. The nature of qualitative evidence. Thousand Oaks: Sage. 2001:187–200.
23. Glasgow RE, Vogt TM, Boles SM. Evaluating the public health impact of health promotion interventions: the RE-AIM framework. Am J Public Health. 1999;89:1322–7.
24. Knowles SE, Chew-Graham C, Adeyemi I, Coupe N, Coventry PA. Managing depression in people with multimorbidity: a qualitative evaluation of an integrated collaborative care model. BMC Fam Pract. 2015;16:32.

25. Dowrick C, Leydon GM, McBride A, Howe A, Burgess H, Clarke P, et al. Patients' and doctors' views on depression severity questionnaires incentivised in UK quality and outcomes framework: qualitative study. BMJ. 2009;338:b663.

26. Lowe B, Unutzer J, Callahan CM, Perkins AJ, Kroenke K. Monitoring depression treatment outcomes with the patient health questionnaire-9. Med Care. 2004;42:1194–201.

27. Murphy R, Ekers D, Webster L. An update to depression case management by practice nurses in primary care: a service evaluation. J Psychiatr Ment Health Nurs. 2014;21:827–33.

28. Peters S, Wearden A, Morriss R, Dowrick CF, Lovell K, Brooks J, et al. Challenges of nurse delivery of psychological interventions for long-term conditions in primary care: a qualitative exploration of the case of chronic fatigue syndrome/myalgic encephalitis. Implement Sci. 2011;6:132.

29. Barley EA, Walters P, Tylee A, Murray J. General practitioners' and practice nurses' views and experience of managing depression in coronary heart disease: a qualitative interview study. BMC Fam Pract. 2012;13:1–10.

30. Freud S. Verdere adviezen over de psychoanalytische techniek I: Over het inleiden van de behandeling. Werken 6. 1913c;184:186–205.

31. Van Weel-Baumgarten E, Grundmeijer H, LichtStrunk E, van Marwijk H, van Rijswijk H, Tjaden B, et al. The NHG guideline Depression (second revision of the NHG guideline Depressive disorder). Huisarts & Wetenschap. 2012;55:25–9.

7

The impact of substituting general practitioners with nurse practitioners on resource use, production and health-care costs during out-of-hours

Mieke Van Der Biezen[1][*] (iD), Eddy Adang[2], Regi Van Der Burgt[3], Michel Wensing[1,4] and Miranda Laurant[1,5]

Abstract

Background: The pressure in out-of-hours primary care is high due to an increasing demand for care and rising health-care costs. During the daytime, substituting general practitioners (GPs) with nurse practitioners (NPs) shows positive results to contribute to these challenges. However, there is a lack of knowledge about the impact during out-of-hours. The current study aims to provide an insight into the impact of substitution on resource use, production and direct health-care costs during out-of-hours.

Methods: At a general practitioner cooperative (GPC) in the south-east of the Netherlands, experimental teams with four GPs and one NP were compared with control teams with five GPs. In a secondary analysis, GP care versus NP care was also examined. During a 15-month period all patients visiting the GPC on weekend days were included. The primary outcome was resource use including X-rays, drug prescriptions and referrals to the Emergency Department (ED). We used logistic regression to adjust for potential confounders. Secondary outcomes were production per hour and direct health-care costs using a cost-minimization analysis.

Results: We analysed 6,040 patients in the experimental team (NPs: 987, GPs: 5,053) and 6,052 patients in the control team. There were no significant differences in outcomes between the teams. In the secondary analysis, in the experimental team NP care was associated with fewer drug prescriptions (NPs 37.1 %, GPs 43 %, $p < .001$) and fewer referrals to the ED (NPs 5.1 %, GPs 11.3 %, $p = .001$) than GP care. The mean production per hour was 3.0 consultations for GPs and 2.4 consultations for NPs ($p < .001$). The cost of a consultation with an NP was €3.34 less than a consultation with a GP ($p = .02$).

Conclusions: These results indicated no overall differences between the teams. Nonetheless, a comparison of type of provider showed that NP care resulted in lower resource use and cost savings than GP care.
To find the optimal balance between GPs and NPs in out-of-hours primary care, more research is needed on the impact of increasing the ratio of NPs in a team with GPs on resource use and health-care costs.

Keywords: Substitution, Skill mix, General practitioner, Nurse practitioner, Out-of-hours care, Resource use, Costs

* Correspondence: mieke.vanderbiezen@radboudumc.nl
[1]Radboud Institute for Health Sciences, Scientific Center for Quality of Healthcare, Radboud University Medical Center, P.O. Box 91016500 HB Nijmegen, The Netherlands
Full list of author information is available at the end of the article

Background

In many Western countries primary healthcare is under pressure due to a rising demand on primary care and rising health-care costs [1–3]. These developments fuel the need for innovative models for organizing health-care delivery more efficiently. Substituting general practitioners (GPs) with nurse practitioners (NPs) is considered worldwide a promising health-care delivery model [4–6]. Substitution of care is feasible since NPs have the ability to treat a large proportion of the complaints presented in primary care autonomously [7–9]. The deployment of NPs has the potential to reduce GPs' workload, improve efficiency, increase service capacity and improve quality of care [5, 10].

Nurses as GPs' substitutes in primary daytime practices can provide good quality and safe care, with patient outcomes at least similar to those of GPs [11–14]. Nurse-led care is associated with longer consultation times and lower productivity, an equal number of prescriptions, and equal or more referrals to other services [10, 11, 14]. This would imply that nurse-led care does not necessarily save costs, and might potentially increase costs. Therefore, monitoring the impact of substituting GPs with NPs on resource use and health-care costs is an essential part in the evaluation of skill mix changes [10]. However, only a few studies have investigated the effect of NPs in primary care on health-care costs and the results of the available studies are inconclusive [4, 6, 12, 14]. Outcomes of substitution, resource use and health-care costs in particular are likely to depend on the particular context of care and outcome measures.

Just like in daytime practice, the debate is rising over whether NPs are capable of substituting for GPs in out-of-hours care, where patients present themselves with acute problems. In the Netherlands, GPs provide care for their patients 24/7 and are the gatekeepers to hospital care. As in the UK and Denmark, out-of-hours primary care is most often organized in large-scale general practitioner cooperatives (GPCs). This means GPs take turns in being on duty to take care of all patients within a region outside office hours [15, 16]. Although the deployment of NPs in general practices during daytime is increasing, it is relatively new in the GPCs and there is a lack of evidence about the efficiency of substituting GPs with NPs in those services. Results from daytime are not generalizable to out-of-hours care due to the potentially acute character of the presented symptoms and complaints [17, 18]. As far as we know, there hasn't been a study conducted on the impact of nurses substituting in out-of-hours primary care on resource use and health-care costs.

Methods

Aim

To evaluate the effect of substituting GPs with NPs in out-of-hours care on resource use, production and health-care costs.

Design

Pragmatic quasi-experimental trial comparing two types of teams providing out-of-hours primary care. In the experimental arm, care is provided by a team of four GPs and one NP, from 10 a.m. – 5 p.m. on a weekend day. In the control arm, care is provided by a team of five GPs on the other weekend day from 10 a.m. – 5 p.m. In addition, care provided by the NPs is compared to that of GPs in the experimental arm.

Study setting

The evaluation was part of a quasi-experimental study, which was conducted at a general practitioner cooperative (GPC) situated within a hospital next to the Emergency Department (ED) in the south-east of the Netherlands. In this GPC, GPs work in shifts from 5 p.m. – 8 a.m. on weekdays and the entire weekend to take care of a population of approximately 304,000 people. All patients in need of acute care during out-of-hours contact the GPC via a single, regional telephone number where triage nurses decide whether patients receive telephonic advice, a consultation at the GPC, a home visit or referral to the ED. Patients who receive a consultation at the GPC are scheduled in a common presentation list. GPs and NPs choose attending patients from this presentation list [16].

Study population

General practitioners and nurse practitioners

A sample of five NPs and 138 GPs participated in this study. GPs' mean age was 49.3 years (SD 9); 60 % were male and on average the GPs had been associated with the GPC for 7.3 years (SD 3.7).

All NPs had at least five years of experience working as a licensed NP in primary care or elderly care. None of the NPs had experience working at the GPC prior to the study. Therefore, they received three half days of additional training in commonly presented complaints during out-of-hours [16]. In the Netherlands, the title 'Nurse Practitioner' is protected by law and exclusively reserved for those who have completed a Master Advanced Nursing Practice (NLQF/EQF level 7; accredited by the NVAO), and are registered in the specialist register. All NPs have previous experience in nursing at Bachelor of Nursing level. NPs have the authority to independently indicate and perform reserved procedures (including prescribing medicines) in his/her area of expertise using the same guidelines as GPs [19, 20]. This is a major difference from the widely implemented practice in the Netherlands whereby practice nurses take care of patients with chronic complaints following evidence based protocols. These practice nurses are usually operating at a Bachelor of Nursing level (NLQF/EQ Level 6) and are, in contrast to NPs, always working under supervision of a GP and not authorised to diagnose and prescribe medicine autonomously [21].

Based on the educational training of the NPs, the GPC in this study excluded the following patients from NP care: those younger than one year and those with psychiatric complaints, abdominal pain, chest pain, a neck ailment, headache or dizziness. Based on the information of the triage nurse, NPs decided which patients from the common presentation list they would call in for consultation. Patients excluded from NP care would receive consultation from a GP. In cases where the complaint of the patient during the triage was different from the complaint during the consultation, NPs were allowed to decide autonomously whether they felt competent or not to complete the consultation themselves, whether they consulted the GP about the patient or whether to refer the patient to the GP.

Patients

All patients who visited the GPC during the data collection were included in the study. Due to the explorative character of the study a statistical power calculation could not be done reliably. In order to get reasonably accurate estimates, a 15-month follow-up was chosen to get a sufficiently large sample.

Randomization

The experimental and control days were rotated systematically between Saturday and Sunday. The five-week rotation scheme was determined in advance. Days were randomized between Saturday and Sunday to avoid bias due to possible differences in patient presentations on those weekend days. Patients were unaware of experimental or control days when they contacted the GPC. The GPs were randomly assigned to the weekend days; they did not know whether they would work with an NP at the time of scheduling.

Measures and data collection

The primary outcome was resource use following a consultation at the GPC. Resource use included X-rays, drug prescriptions and referrals to the ED. Other imaging tests or laboratory samples than X-rays could not be ordered by the providers. If such diagnostic tests were necessary patients were referred to the ED or to their own GP the next day. Data related to resource use were measured as dichotomous outcome variables.

Secondary outcomes were production per hour (indicated as the mean number of patients per care provider per hour) and direct health-care costs. Direct health-care costs were based on personnel costs (based on production per hour and salary) and costs per unit of resources used for each consultation (X-rays, drug prescriptions and referrals to the ED). Here volumes are combined by unit prices that constitute costs.

Data abstracted to compare baseline characteristics included potential confounders for the comparison: age (in four categories), urgency (in five categories), gender, and type of complaint (indicated as an International Classification Primary Care [ICPC] code). All data were abstracted from the electronic medical patient records at the GPC and coded by the care providers as part of their routine during the consultation.

Data were collected from April 2011 to July 2012.

Analysis
Baseline characteristics
Baseline characteristics of the study population are presented as a proportion (%) since all measures (age, gender, urgency level and type of complaint (ICPC)) were measured in categorical variables. Differences between the experimental arm and control arm were tested using a Chi^2 test. The same analysis was performed in secondary analysis comparing baseline characteristics between patients treated by the NP and patients treated by the GP in the experimental arm.

Resource use
Resource use (i.e., X-rays, drug prescriptions and referrals to the ED) was evaluated by analysing differences in volumes between groups. Logistic regression analysis for dichotomous outcomes was conducted to compare the two study arms. To adjust for potential confounders a second logistic regression model was used that corrected for age, gender, urgency level and ICPC group. The same analysis was performed in the secondary analysis to compare the NPs and GPs in the experimental arm.

Production per hour
Production per hour was calculated by dividing the total number of patients per care provider by the exact number of hours per care provider. This resulted in a mean number of patients treated per hour per care provider. A linear mixed model was used to test the differences in production per hour between the teams. Results were corrected for holidays, weekend days, number of professionals and the total number of patients per day. The same analysis was performed in the secondary analysis to compare the NPs and GPs in the experimental arm.

Direct health-care costs

The economic evaluation was designed as a cost-minimization analysis, considering direct health-care costs of the consultation only. In this analysis, based on previous study reviews, patient outcomes of the two study conditions are assumed to be equal [22]. Direct costs were calculated for each consultation separately including costs for care provider, X-rays, drug prescriptions and referral to the ED.

Costs for the GP and NP time per consultation were calculated by dividing the tariff per hour by the mean production per hour. For NPs the tariff was based on their salary from the GPC, including social security contributions (approximately 40 %) and premium pay (50 %). For GPs the tariff was based on the payment agreements with health insurance companies. This tariff is calculated on the basis of a total tariff per GPs' patients for providing 24/7 care.

The tariff valid for the GPC per care provider per hour was €77 for GPs, and €65,46 and €66,38 for NPs (see Table 1). Next, following the guidelines of the Dutch Manual for Costing, the cost for each referral to the ED was set at €151 and €43,98 and €45,37 for an X-ray [23]. As a result of the differences between the minimum and maximum price for medicine, two separate costs were calculated per drug prescription. All the direct health-care costs were calculated using the tariffs that were valid for the intervention period (see Table 1).

To provide further insight into the cost differences, a *t*-test was performed to compare the unadjusted estimates between the experimental and control arm. Second, to adjust for potential confounders a linear regression model was used that corrected for case mix (i.e., age, gender, urgency level, ICPC group). For the cost of drug prescriptions the minimum price per medicine was used in the primary analysis. Deterministic uncertainty was explored by one-way sensitivity on costs of drug prescriptions by including the maximum price per medicine. The same analysis was used in the secondary analysis to compare NPs and GPs in the experimental arm.

Finally, we applied a bootstrapping procedure (with 1,000 replications) to manage the highly skewed costs across patients. The statistical analysis, including the bootstrapping, was carried out using SPSS software version 22 (SPSS Inc, Chicago, IL, USA).

Results

The experimental arm included 34 Saturdays and 29 Sundays (63 intervention days), and the control arm included 29 Saturdays and 34 Sundays (63 control days). In total, 12,092 patients had a consultation during the study period. In the experimental arm, 987 patients visited an NP and 5,053 patients visited one of four GPs. In the control arm, 6,052 patients visited one of five GPs. A total of 3,101 cases (10.0 % with an NP, 27.0 % with a GP) could not be analysed due to a missing ICPC code (a flow diagram of the study is shown in Fig. 1).

Baseline characteristics

There were no significant differences in patient characteristics between the experimental and the control arm (Table 2 shows the 10 most presented complaints). However, as expected given the exclusion criteria, significant differences were found between GPs and NPs for patients' age ($p = .002$), urgency level ($p < .001$) and type of complaint ($p < .001$) [18]. GPs saw more patients aged >64 years, with an urgency level of U2, and suffering digestive, cardiovascular and neurological complaints. NPs saw more patients suffering skin and respiratory complaints and with an urgency level of U4.

Resource use

Experimental arm vs control arm

Table 3 shows both the unadjusted and adjusted differences in X-rays, drug prescriptions and referrals to the ED. Across the overall sample, the team in the experimental arm compared to the control arm less often ordered an X-ray (4.4 % vs. 5.3 %; $p = .017$), less often prescribed drugs (42.0 % vs. 44.1 %; $p = .022$) and less often referred patients to the ED (10.2 % vs. 11.6 %; $p = .02$). However, none of these differences remained significant after

Table 1 Prices per unit in 2011-2012

Resource	Unit	Costs (€)	Data source
Salary costs GP	Hour	€77	GPC (based on agreements with health insurance companies)
Salary costs NP	Hour	€65,46 (as per 1-4-2011)	GPC
		€66,38 (as per 1-4-2012)	
Drug prescription	Consultation	Variable (minimum and maximum prices)	http://www.medicijnkosten.nl/ (indicated by Dutch Manual for Costing [23])
X-ray	Consultation	2011: €43,98	The Dutch Healthcare Authority (NZa) (indicated by Dutch Manual for Costing [23])
		2012: €45,37	
Referral to the Emergency Department	Consultation	€151	Dutch Manual for Costing [23]

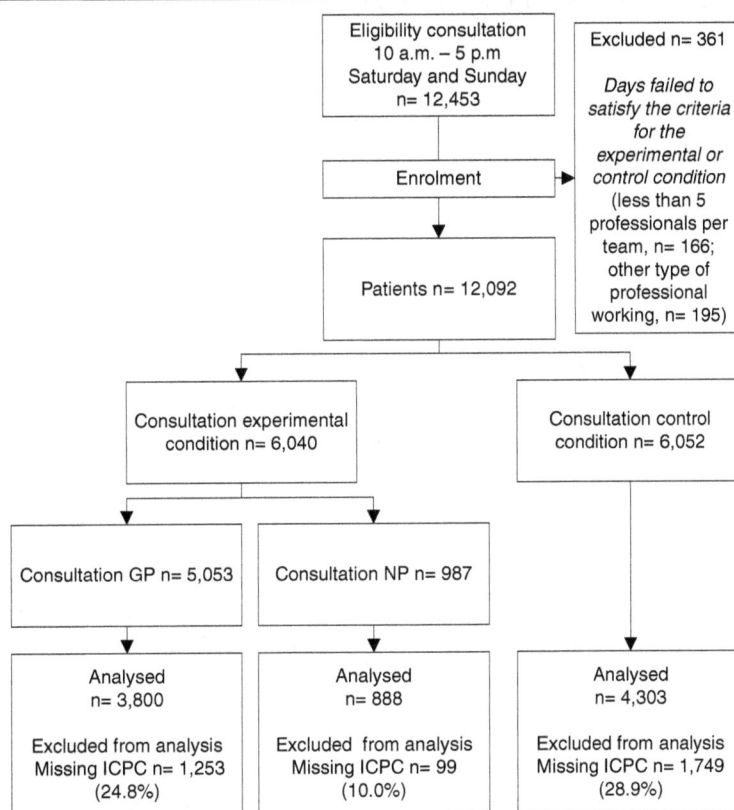

Fig.1 Flow diagram of the study

Table 2 Baseline characteristics, top 10 ICPC groups

	Control arm	Experimental arm	GP Experimental arm	NP Experimental arm
Complaints (%)[a]				
Skin	21.7	22.7	20.7	31.2
Musculoskeletal	20.5	20.1	19.6	22.2
Respiratory	15.2	14.2	13.7	16.3
Digestive	10.5	9.9	11.4	3.0
Eye	6.0	6.1	6.5	4.4
General and unspecified	5.9	6.5	6.6	6.0
Ear	5.7	5.8	5.6	6.8
Urological	5.5	5.7	5.7	5.6
Cardiovascular	2.5	2.5	2.9	0.7
Neurological	2.3	2.3	2.8	0.3
Other	4.2	4.2	4.5	3.5

Tested using a Chi[2] test
[a]significant difference between the GP and NP in the experimental arm

Table 3 Rate differences of resource use following a visit to the GPC

	Experimental vs control arm				Experimental arm GP vs NP			
		95 % CI for exp *b*				95 % CI for exp *b*		
	B (SE)	Lower	Exp *b*	Upper	B (SE)	Lower	Exp *b*	Upper
Unadjusted estimates								
X-ray	-.202* (.09)	.692	.817	.965	-.303 (.156)	.544	.738	1.002
Drug prescription	-.084* (.037)	.855	.919	.988	.246 *** (.072)	1.111	1.279	1.472
Referral ED	-.136* (.058)	.779	.873	.979	.866 *** (.152)	1.766	2.378	3.202
Adjusted estimates								
X-ray	-.203 (.11)	.682	.816	1.006	-.168 (.19)	.588	.846	1.115
Drug prescription	-.09 (.05)	.838	.916	1.001	.317 *** (.077)	1.167	1.373	1.616
Referral ED	-.13 (.07)	.759	.877	1.014	.60** (.179)	1.277	1.814	2.576

Tested within a logistic regression model. Adjusted estimates are adjusted for age, gender, urgency level and ICPC group
* $p < .05$
** $p < .01$
*** $p < .001$

adjusting for case mix (i.e., age, gender, urgency level, ICPC group).

NPs vs GPs in the experimental arm
NP care was associated with fewer drug prescriptions (37.1 % vs. 43 %; $p < .001$) and fewer referrals to the ED (5.1 % vs 11.3 %; $p < .001$) than GP care. These differences remained significant after adjusting for case mix. There was no statistical significant difference between NPs and GPs with regard to ordering X-rays (NPs 5.6 % vs. GPs 4.2 %).

Production per hour
The mean production per professional was 2.9 consultations per hour in both the experimental arm and the control arm. In the experimental arm the mean number of consultations per hour was 3.0 for GPs and 2.3 for NPs ($p < .001$).

Direct health-care costs
Based on the tariff per hour and the production per hour, the mean costs per GP consultation were

calculated at €25,67 and the costs per NP consultation were calculated at €27,28 (as per April 2011) and €27,66 (as per April 2012).

Experimental arm vs control arm
Table 4 presents the unadjusted and adjusted cost differences between the experimental and the control arm. The mean costs of a consultation in the experimental arm were €2,05 less than a consultation in the control arm (95 % CI: €-3,79; €-0,29; $p = .02$). However, this difference did not remain significant after correcting for case mix (i.e., age, gender, urgency level, ICPC group). In the sensitivity analysis with the maximum cost per medication the adjusted difference remained non-significant (95 % CI: €-3,65; €0,15).

GPs and NPs in the experimental arm
The mean cost per consultation on the experimental day was €7,58 less for a consultation with an NP than for a consultation with a GP (95 % CI: €-10,82; €-4,34; $p < .001$) (see Table 4). After correction for case mix a significant difference of €-3,34 remained in favour of the

Table 4 Unadjusted and adjusted differences in direct health-care costs following a consultation at the GPC

	Experimental vs control arm			
	experimental arm	control arm	Mean difference	95 % CI
Unadjusted mean cost per consultation (minimal medication costs)	€44,93	€46,98	€-2,04*	€-3,79; €-0,29
Adjusted mean cost per consultation (minimal medication costs)			€-1,53	€-3,36; €0,46
	Experimental arm GP vs NP			
	GP	NP	Mean difference	95 % CI
Unadjusted mean cost per consultation (minimal medication costs)	€46,17	€38,59	€-7,58**	€-10,82; €-4,34
Adjusted mean cost per consultation (minimal medication costs)			€-3,34*	€-5,97; €-0,65

Tested within a linear regression model. Adjusted estimates are adjusted for age, gender, urgency level and ICPC group
* $p < .05$
** $p < .001$

NP (95 % CI: €-5,97; €-0,65; p = .02). The main influence on the difference in costs was the number of patients referred to the ED. In the sensitivity analysis with the maximum costs per medication the adjusted difference between the experimental and control arm increased to €-3,51 (95 % CI: €-6,77; € -0,24; p = .04).

Discussion
Statement of principal findings
This study did not find a significant difference between teams with an NP and teams with only GPs with regard to X-rays, drug prescriptions and referrals to the ED. Moreover, the production per hour and the cost per consultation for the team with an NP were not different from teams with only GPs.

In the experimental team, NP care was found to be associated with significantly fewer drug prescriptions and fewer ED referrals than care delivered by GPs. NPs were shown to have a lower production per hour than GPs. The cost per consultation with an NP was lower than with a GP.

Strengths and weaknesses
A strength of the current study is its large patient sample and a long follow-up period, but limitations include the single-centre character of the study and the low number of nurse practitioners involved. Moreover, we had a relatively large number of missing ICPC codes. There appeared to be only a few GPs who repeatedly did not report ICPC codes, which means the bias is related to the GP and not the ICPC diagnosis or day. This is supported by the fact that the ICPC codes in our study are comparable to those of other out-of-hours services in Western countries [18]. Therefore, we don't suspect that the missing ICPC codes will cause any bias to our outcomes.

It should be noted that the current study shows the effect of NPs within a GPC. Although many countries have organized out-of-hours care in large-scale organizations in previous years, the various types of health-care systems influence the generalizability of the research findings [15]. Moreover, the education and deployment of NPs differs between, and even within, countries and health-care systems. In the Netherlands, as in most countries, NPs providing care are always working as part of primary care teams alongside GPs [21, 24]. Our results can therefore not be generalized to other models of care in which NPs are working in teams without GPs [25]. Moreover, in the current study the NPs were primarily responsible for treating minor ailments. The complexity of tasks can differ between regions and countries.

In the current study, NPs with no experience working at the GPC at the start of the study were compared with GPs who had on average 7.3 years of experience at the GPC. This may have influenced resource use or production per hour. A strength of the current study is the fact that researchers did not change patient allocation, which gives an accurate representation of the daily practice and related cost estimates.

We only included costs relevant from the GPCs' viewpoint (tariff per hour, production per hour) and direct health-care costs relevant from health insurance companies' viewpoint (X-rays, drug prescriptions and referrals to the ED). This implies that it is not possible to draw conclusions on whether the deployment of NPs is cost saving from a societal viewpoint. Therefore, other factors, such as the difference in costs of training, rates of sick leave, patient follow-up after a GPC visit or after ED referral, et cetera, should have been included [23, 26].

Comparisons with other studies
Meta-analyses based on research conducted in daytime primary care did not show differences between nurses and GPs in terms of prescriptions, diagnostic test orders and referrals [10]. Although, in line with these meta-analyses, we did not find differences at team level, our secondary analysis in the experimental team showed a difference between GPs and NPs in terms of drug prescriptions and referrals to the ED. We cannot determine whether this difference in resource use is an overuse of medication or referrals by GPs, or an underuse by NPs. There is no capacity to examine how clinical outcomes would differ from the likely outcomes if patient care was provided by the other care provider [27]. Inappropriate referrals and prescriptions may further increase health-care costs and unnecessary treatments in the hospital. Based on reviews of research, we do not expect an underuse by NPs since patient outcomes in primary care were found to be at least equivalent for NPs and GPs [12, 14]. Moreover, research on the ED and hospital care shows that the diagnostic accuracy of NPs is comparable to that of doctors [28, 29].

We found a lower production per hour for NPs than for GPs. However, it was not possible to adjust this outcome for case mix. This makes comparison between GPs and NPs difficult since they treat different patients. However, we expect the number of consultations per hour to be a reliable measure. This is supported by the fact that our outcomes are comparable to results from meta-analyses on consultation times [10]. Besides treating different patients, lower production per hour can also be associated with less experience [30]. Although NPs had at least five years of experience in primary or elderly care, none of them had any experience in out-of-hours primary care at the start of the study. Other possible explanations for longer consultations include a higher use of protocols [10], and a more holistic approach and greater provision of information by NPs than by GPs [31]. In addition, the provision of more health education and information by NPs may result in fewer prescriptions [32].

Based on previous research, we expected NP care to be cost saving due to a lower salary for NPs than for GPs [33]. However, in line with another study, lower production per hour appeared to lessen the influence of salary differences on consultation costs [34]. Another reason for the small influence of salary costs on overall costs is the small difference in tariff between the GPs and NPs during out-of-hours care. This is because the GPs receive financial compensation for out-of-hours care based on the total tariff for providing care to their patients 24/7. This means that the GPs receive a fixed tariff, whereas the tariff per hour for NPs was based on their gross salary including social security contributions and premium pay. The differences in tariff per hour would have been bigger in cases where the care providers were employed by the GPC in the same way. For example, the difference in gross salary of a GP employed by another GP and the NPs in our study is approximately 60 % [35]. In another Dutch study in daytime primary care, the salary of an NP appeared to be less than half of that of a GP. As a consequence, in that study, cost differences were mainly caused by the difference in salary [36]. It is expected that bigger differences in salary will result in more cost savings when GPs are substituted with NPs.

The current study shows that the differences in referral rates to the ED strongly influenced consultation costs. The fewer referrals by NPs resulted therefore in lower mean costs of care provided by NPs than by GPs. It is difficult to compare these findings with previous research due to conflicting results on the effect of substituting GPs with NPs in primary care on the cost of health care. Moreover, due to heterogeneous outcome reporting and the small number of studies they are hard to interpret. However, in general, NP care seems to be associated with lower or equal health-care costs per consultation [6, 12]. Only one study found increased costs associated with NP care. These results were based on two factors that we did not measure: time spent by GPs on supervising and number of return visits [34]. The time spent on supervising in the current study was, however, relatively low. The NPs consulted a GP in only 7.1 % of all consultations. Only 0.2 % of the patients were taken over by the GP; the other consultations were completed by the NP. Consultations between the NP and GP are considered part of daily practice and comparable to consultations GPs have with other GPs Therefore, we do not expect this to bias our outcomes.

Study implications

The current study shows no differences in resource use and direct health-care costs between teams with an NP and teams with GPs only. Therefore we conclude that during out-of-hours, involvement of NPs in multidisciplinary teams can increase capacity without increasing resource utilization.

Our results show that using NPs as substitutes for GPs in out-of-hours care is a feasible solution for decreasing GPs' workload or increasing service capacity. It should be noted that tasks at GPCs are limited to providing acute care and do not use NPs' competences to the full. Tasks such as preventive projects, psycho-social home visits, providing ongoing training for staff and developing protocols are only performed during the daytime. In countries where GPs deliver 24/7 care, the implementation of NPs in primary care will only succeed when they (just like GPs) provide care 24/7.

With the need for extra workforce in primary care, our data suggests that substitution by NPs can be considered an solution economical equal to the care delivered by GPs. However, because we only included one GPC, and only measured direct costs, results should be interpreted with caution. Economic evidence on which to make judgments on future out-of-hours care is far more complicated [37]. Other costs from a societal perspective such as training cost and unemployment rates of physicians in hospital care have to be taken into account. This implies that decisions on the substitution of GPs by NPs in out-of-hours primary care should not only depend on costs, but on other factors such as a view on professional roles, responsibilities, and quality and safety of care [34].

As this study showed a significant difference in cost per consultation in favour of NPs, it may be possible that deploying more NPs in a team with GPs is more cost saving. Future research is needed to indicate an optimal balance in which teams with NPs and GPs provide the most efficient care for patients in out-of-hours primary care.

Conclusion

The current study indicated no differences between teams with an NP and teams with only GPs with regard to resource use, production per hour and direct health-care costs. However, in teams with an NP, the NP appeared to make fewer drug prescriptions and fewer referrals to the ED than the GPs. Due to lower resource use, the cost of a consultation with an NP was less than that of a consultation with a GP. The current study shows that involvement of NPs in teams with GPs can increase capacity without increasing resource utilization during out-of-hours. More research is needed to find the optimal balance between GPs and NPs to cover all

The impact of substituting general practitioners with nurse practitioners on resource use, production...

77

patient care in out-of-hours primary care efficiently. Obviously, decisions on substituting GPs with NPs should be based on the full range of considerations, including a view on the professional roles and responsibilities of NPs in of out-of-hours care, rather than just arguments related to resource use and costs.

Abbreviations

ED: Emergency Department; GP: General practitioner; GPC: General practitioner cooperative; ICPC: International Classification Primary Care; NP: Nurse practitioner

Acknowledgement

We thank the Centrale Huisartsenposten Zuidoost Brabant for making this study possible. They agreed to act as an experimental site and carried out some organizational changes in order to implement the nurse practitioners. We also thank them for facilitating the collection of data on health-care utilization. Finally, we thank the nurse practitioners and general practitioners for acting as 'pioneers' during this study.

The views expressed in this paper are those of the authors and not necessarily those of the funding organizations or the Centrale Huisartsenposten Zuidoost Brabant.

Funding

This study was funded by The Netherlands Organisation for Health Research and Development (ZonMw) (project number: 8271.1010), Vereniging Huisartsenposten Nederland (VHN) and Brabant Medical School (BMS).

Authors' contributions

ML, RB and MB conceived and designed the study. MB, EA and ML performed the data analysis. MB, RB, MW and ML interpreted the results. MB wrote the first draft of the manuscript. EA, RB, MW and ML revised the manuscript with important intellectual contributions. All authors read and approved the final manuscript.

Authors' information

MB, MSc, PhD student; EA, PhD associate professor cost-effectiveness analysis; RB, MSc, project coordinator; MW, PhD professor of health services research and implementation science; ML, PhD, professor organisation of healthcare and services.

Competing interests

The authors declare that they have no competing interests.

Consent for publication

Not applicable.

Author details

¹Radboud Institute for Health Sciences, Scientific Center for Quality of Healthcare, Radboud University Medical Center, P.O. Box 91016500 HB Nijmegen, The Netherlands. ²Department for Health Evidence, Radboud Institute for Health Sciences, Radboud University Medical Center, P.O. Box 91016500 HB Nijmegen, The Netherlands. ³Foundation for Development of Quality Care in General Practice, Tilburgseweg-West 100, 5652 NP Eindhoven, The Netherlands. ⁴Department of General Practice and Health Services Research, Heidelberg University, INF Marsilius Arkaden, Heidelberg, Germany. ⁵Faculty of Health and Social Studies, HAN University of Applied Sciences, P.O. Box 69606503 GL Nijmegen, The Netherlands.

References

1. Bodenheimer T, Pham HH. Primary care: current problems and proposed solutions. Health Aff (Millwood). 2010;29(5):799–805. doi:10.1377/hlthaff.2010.0026.
2. Huibers LA, Moth G, Bondevik GT, Kersnik J, Huber CA, Christensen MB, Leutgeb R, Casado AM, Remmen R, Wensing M. Diagnostic scope in out-of-hours primary care services in eight European countries: an observational study. BMC Fam Pract. 2011; doi:10.1186/1471-2296-12-30
3. Porter ME, Pabo EA, Lee TH. Redesigning primary care: a strategic vision to improve value by organizing around patients' needs. Health Aff (Millwood). 2013;doi:10.1377/hlthaff.2012.0961.
4. Goryakin Y, Griffiths P, Maben J. Economic evaluation of nurse staffing and nurse substitution in health care: a scoping review. Int J Nurs Stud. 2011; doi:10.1016/j.ijnurstu.2010.07.018
5. Laurant M, Harmsen M, Wollersheim H, Grol R, Faber M, Sibbald B. The impact of nonphysician clinicians: do they improve the quality and cost-effectiveness of health care services? Med Care Res Rev. 2009; doi:10.1177/1077558709346277.
6. Martinez-Gonzalez NA, Djalali S, Tandjung R, Huber-Geismann F, Markun S, Wensing M, Rosemann T. Substitution of physicians by nurses in primary care: a systematic review and meta-analysis. BMC Health Serv Res. 2014; doi:10.1186/1472-6963-14-214.
7. Bruijn-Geraets D, Daisy P, Eijk-Hustings V, Yvonne J, Vrijhoef HJ. Evaluating newly acquired authority of nurse practitioners and physician assistants for reserved medical procedures in the Netherlands: a study protocol. J Adv Nurs. 2014;70(11):2673–82.
8. Vrijhoef HJ. Nurse Practitioners. In: Cockerham WC, Dingwall R, Quah SR, editors. The Wiley Blackwell Encyclopedia of Health, Illness, Behavior, and Society. 1st ed. Oxford: Wiley; 2014.
9. Everett CM, Schumacher JR, Wright A, Smith MA. Physician assistants and nurse practitioners as a usual source of care. J Rural Health. 2009; 25(4):407–14.
10. Martinez-Gonzalez NA, Rosemann T, Djalali S, Huber-Geismann F, Tandjung R. Task-shifting from physicians to nurses in primary care and its impact on resource utilization: a systematic review and meta-analysis of randomized controlled trials. Med Care Res Rev. 2015; doi:10.1177/1077558715586297
11. Laurant M, Reeves D, Hermens R, Braspenning J, Grol R, Sibbald B. Substitution of doctors by nurses in primary care. Cochrane Database Syst Rev. 2005; doi:.10.1002/14651858.CD001271.pub2
12. Martin-Misener R, Harbman P, Donald F, Reid K, Kilpatrick K, Carter N, Bryant-Lukosius D, Kaasalainen S, Marshall DA, Charbonneau-Smith R et al. Cost-effectiveness of nurse practitioners in primary and specialised ambulatory care: systematic review. BMJ Open. 2015;doi:10.1136/bmjopen-2014-007167.
13. Martinez-Gonzalez NA, Tandjung R, Djalali S, Huber-Geismann F, Markun S, Rosemann T. Effects of physician-nurse substitution on clinical parameters: a systematic review and meta-analysis. PLoS One. 2014; doi:10.1371/journal.pone.0089181
14. Swan M, Ferguson S, Chang A, Larson E, Smaldone A. Quality of primary care by advanced practice nurses: a systematic review. Int J Qual Health Care. 2015;doi:10.1093/intqhc/mzv054.
15. Huibers L, Giesen P, Wensing M, Grol R. Out-of-hours care in western countries: assessment of different organizational models. BMC Health Serv Res. 2009; doi:10.1186/1472-6963-9-105
16. Wijers N, Schoonhoven L, Giesen P, Vrijhoef H, van der Burgt R, Mintjes J, Wensing M, Laurant M. The effectiveness of Nurse Practitioners working at a GP cooperative: a study protocol. BMC Fam Pract. 2012;doi:10.1186/1471-2296-13-75.
17. Giesen P, Braspenning J. Out-of-hours GP care compared with office GP care: common complaints with an urgent character. Huisarts Wet. 2004; 47(4):177.
18. van der Biezen M, Schoonhoven L, Wijers N, van der Burgt R, Wensing M, Laurant M. Substitution of general practitioners by nurse practitioners in out-of-hours primary care: a quasi-experimental study. J Adv Nurs. 2016; doi:10.1111/jan.12954
19. De Bruijn-Geraets DP, Van Eijk-Hustings YJ, Vrijhoef HJ. Evaluating newly acquired authority of nurse practitioners and physician assistants for reserved medical procedures in the Netherlands: a study protocol. J Adv Nurs. 2014; doi:10.1111/jan.12396
20. Dutch Professional Nurse Practitioner Organisation (V&VN VS). The nurse practitioner in the Netherlands. http://venvnvs.nl/wp-content/uploads/sites/164/2015/08/2015-10-30-Factsheet-Nurse-Practitioner-Netherlands-2015.pdf: Accessed 5 July 2016.

21. Freund T, Everett C, Griffiths P, Hudon C, Naccarella L, Laurant M. Skill mix, roles and remuneration in the primary care workforce: who are the healthcare professionals in the primary care teams across the world? Int J Nurs Stud. 2015; doi:.10.1016/j.ijnurstu.2014.11.014

22. Drummond MF, Sculpher MJ, Torrance GW, O'Brien BJ, Stoddart GL. Methods for the economic evaluation of health care programmes. Vol. 3. Revised edition. Oxford: Oxford University Press; 2005.

23. Hakkaaer van Roijen L, Tan S, Bouwmans CAM. Handleiding voor Kostenonderzoek. In: Methoden en standaard kostprijzen voor economische evaluaties in de gezondheidszorg. Rotterdam: Health care Insurance Council; 2010.

24. Iglehart JK. Expanding the role of advanced nurse practitioners—risks and rewards. N Engl J Med. 2013;368(20):1935–41.

25. Venning P, Durie A, Roland M, Roberts C, Leese B. Randomised controlled trial comparing cost effectiveness of general practitioners and nurse practitioners in primary care. BMJ. 2000;320(7241):1048–53.

26. Curtis L, Netten A. The costs of training a nurse practitioner in primary care: the importance of allowing for the cost of education and training when making decisions about changing the professional-mix. J Nurs Manag. 2007; doi:10.1111/j.1365-2834.2007.00668.x

27. Parker R, Forrest L, Desborough J, McRae I, Boyland T. Independent evaluation of the nurse-led ACT Health Walk-in Centre. Acton: The Australian National University; 2011.

28. Pirret AM, Neville SJ, La Grow SJ. Nurse practitioners versus doctors diagnostic reasoning in a complex case presentation to an acute tertiary hospital: a comparative study. Int J Nurs Stud. 2015; doi:10.1016/j.ijnurstu. 2014.08.009

29. van der Linden C, Reijnen R, de Vos R. Diagnostic accuracy of emergency nurse practitioners versus physicians related to minor illnesses and injuries. J Emerg Nurs. 2010;doi:10.1016/j.jen.2009.08.012

30. Laurant M, Reeves D, Hermens R, Braspenning J, Grol R, Sibbald B. Substitution of doctors by nurses in primary care. Cochrane Database of Systematic Reviews. 2004; doi:10.1002/14651858.CD001271.pub2.

31. Seale C, Anderson E, Kinnersley P. Treatment advice in primary care: a comparative study of nurse practitioners and general practitioners. J Adv Nurs. 2006;doi:10.1111/j.1365-2648.2006.03865.x.

32. Weiss MC, Deave T, Peters TJ, Salisbury C. Perceptions of patient expectation for an antibiotic: a comparison of walk-in centre nurses and GPs. Fam Pract. 2004;doi:10.1093/fampra/cmh504.

33. Dierick-van Daele AT, Metsemakers JF, Derckx EW, Spreeuwenberg C, Vrijhoef HJ. Nurse practitioners substituting for general practitioners: randomized controlled trial. J Adv Nurs. 2009; doi:10.1111/j.1365-2648.2008. 04888.x

34. Hollinghurst S, Horrocks S, Anderson E, Salisbury C. Comparing the cost of nurse practitioners and GPs in primary care: modelling economic data from randomised trials. Br J Gen Pract. 2006;56(528):530–5.

35. LHV/VHN. CAO Huisartsenzorg. 1 April 2011 – 31 December 2012. Utrecht: Landelijke Huisartsen Vereniging & Vereniging Huisartsenposten Nederland; 2011.

36. Dierick-van Daele ATM, Steuten LMG, Metsemakers JFM, Derckx EWCC, Spreeuwenberg C, Vrijhoef HJM. Economic evaluation of nurse practitioners versus GPs in treating common conditions. Br J Gen Pract. 2010; doi: 10. 3399/bjgp10X482077

37. McClellan CM, Cramp F, Powell J, Benger JR. A randomised trial comparing the cost effectiveness of different emergency department healthcare professionals in soft tissue injury management. BMJ Open. 2013;doi:10.1136/ bmjopen-2012-001116.

38. Laurant M, Wijers N, Van der Biezen M. Nurse practitioners in out-of-hours primary care. *DANS*. 2012; doi:http://dx.doi.org/10.17026/dans-xgr-v4u3.

8

Nurse-led home visitation programme to improve health-related quality of life and reduce disability among potentially frail community-dwelling older people in general practice: a theory-based process evaluation

Mandy M N Stijnen[1*], Maria W J Jansen[2,3], Inge G P Duimel-Peeters[1,4] and Hubertus J M Vrijhoef[5,6]

Abstract

Background: Population ageing fosters new models of care delivery for older people that are increasingly integrated into existing care systems. In the Netherlands, a primary-care based preventive home visitation programme has been developed for potentially frail community-dwelling older people (aged ≥75 years), consisting of a comprehensive geriatric assessment during a home visit by a practice nurse followed by targeted interdisciplinary care and follow-up over time. A theory-based process evaluation was designed to examine (1) the extent to which the home visitation programme was implemented as planned and (2) the extent to which general practices successfully redesigned their care delivery.

Methods: Using a mixed-methods approach, the focus was on fidelity (quality of implementation), dose delivered (completeness), dose received (exposure and satisfaction), reach (participation rate), recruitment, and context. Twenty-four general practices participated, of which 13 implemented the home visitation programme and 11 delivered usual care to older people. Data collection consisted of semi-structured interviews with practice nurses (PNs), general practitioners (GPs), and older people; feedback meetings with PNs; structured registration forms filled-out by PNs; and narrative descriptions of the recruitment procedures and registration of inclusion and drop-outs by members of the research team.

Results: Fidelity of implementation was acceptable, but time constraints and inadequate reach (i.e., the relatively healthy older people participated) negatively influenced complete delivery of protocol elements, such as interdisciplinary cooperation and follow-up of older people over time. The home visitation programme was judged positively by PNs, GPs, and older people. Useful tools were offered to general practices for organising proactive geriatric care.

Conclusions: The home visitation programme did not have major shortcomings in itself, but the delivery offered room for improvement. General practices received useful tools to redesign their care delivery from reactive towards proactive care, but perceived barriers require attention to allow for sustainability of the home visitation programme over time.

Keywords: Frail elderly, General practice, Geriatric assessment, Home visit, Mixed-methods, Practice nurse, Primary care, Process evaluation, Program implementation

* Correspondence: mandy.stijnen@maastrichtuniversity.nl
[1]Department of Family Medicine, School for Public Health and Primary Care (CAPHRI), Faculty of Health, Medicine and Life Sciences, Maastricht University, P.O. Box 616, 6200 MD Maastricht, The Netherlands
Full list of author information is available at the end of the article

Background

Healthcare professionals worldwide are increasingly called upon to organise and deliver care to a growing number of older people. This stimulated the development of various multifactorial interventions and care models aimed at maintaining independent living and the prevention of disability and other adverse outcomes in community-dwelling older people [1-3]. Especially primary care has been considered ideally suited to address the needs of older people, and more specifically frail older people who are at risk of functional decline and hospitalisation, predominantly due to their patient-oriented focus [4,5]. In several countries with a strongly developed primary healthcare system, such as the UK, Denmark and the Netherlands, interventions comprising comprehensive geriatric assessment (CGA) exist in which the general practitioner (GP) acts as the central care provider [6-8]. However, primary care based models for care for older people also pose challenges to GPs. These relate to difficulties in dealing with multiple and often co-occurring medical conditions, (inter)personal challenges (e.g., communication barriers, time pressure), and the burden of administrative work [9].

There is a growing recognition that the primary care setting, and particularly general practices, have the potential to deliver patient-centred, coherent, and proactive care to older people [4,10]. Therefore, in the south of the Netherlands, the [G]OLD ('Getting OLD the healthy way') preventive home visitation programme has been developed aimed at improving health-related quality of life and reducing disability among potentially frail community-dwelling older people in general practice [11]. Care delivery within general practices is redesigned by applying components of the Chronic Care Model (CCM), a model developed to improve chronic illness management in primary care [12,13]. In addition, the Guided Care Model informed the development of the intervention protocol of the [G]OLD home visitation programme. So far, Guided Care seems to be the only evidenced-based model that translated components of the CCM in a stepwise intervention model in an effort to transform care for vulnerable older people with multiple chronic conditions and complex care needs [14]. As a result, the [G]OLD home visitation programme consists of a CGA of older people's health and well-being during a home visit by the practice nurse (PN), a tailored care and treatment plan, multidisciplinary care management, and targeted intervention and follow-up over time.

Due to its multi-component nature and integration in the dynamic primary care setting, the [G]OLD home visitation programme can be characterised as a complex intervention. Besides investigating the effects on patient outcomes in a large-scale controlled trial, it is equally important to obtain a profound understanding of how complex interventions function in their intended context [15-17]. Therefore, we prospectively designed a process evaluation to follow the implementation of the [G]OLD home visitation programme from its initial use until continued use [18]. Such pre-planned process evaluations performed alongside the effect evaluation allow for in-depth information to differentiate between interventions that have shortcomings in itself (intervention failure) and those that are badly delivered (implementation failure) [19,20]. Instead of merely implementing, the present home visitation programme required general practices to redesign their care delivery for potentially frail older people from reactive, disease-oriented care towards proactive, patient-oriented care. As a result, the objectives of the process evaluation are to examine (1) the extent to which the [G]OLD home visitation programme was implemented as planned in general practices, and (2) the extent to which general practices successfully redesigned their care delivery.

Methods

Process evaluation design

The process evaluation plan was designed according to seven theoretical elements proposed by Saunders and colleagues [21], as adapted from Baranowski and Stables [22] and Linnan and Steckler [23]: fidelity (quality of implementation), dose delivered (completeness), dose received (exposure; satisfaction), reach (participation rate), recruitment, and context. The element 'context' was explored into more detail using the Normalisation Process Model [24] to identify factors that affect the success or failure of delivering and implementing the intervention in a dynamic and complex primary care setting. The process evaluation questions per component of the process evaluation are summarised in Table 1. Further details concerning the design of the process evaluation plan are discussed elsewhere [18].

The Medical Ethical Committee (MEC) of Maastricht University Medical Centre (MUMC+) judged the protocol of the [G]OLD-study and the accompanying process evaluation as not needing formal ethical approval (METC 10-4-015). Nonetheless, the MEC approved the study protocol and related documents. Written informed consent was obtained from participants at recruitment and additional verbal informed consent was obtained for the interviews on behalf of the process evaluation.

Setting and participants

The process evaluation was conducted parallel to a longitudinal, quasi-experimental trial investigating the effects of the [G]OLD home visitation programme on health-related quality of life and disability [11]. Twenty-four general practices from three regions in the south of the Netherlands ('Maastricht-Heuvelland', 'Parkstad', and

Table 1 Process evaluation questions and data collection tools per component of the process evaluation plan

Component	Process evaluation questions	Data collection tools
Fidelity (quality of implement-tation)	1) To what extent were all elements of the home visitation programme implemented as planned?	Semi-structured interviews GP/PN; structured registration forms
	2) Is care delivery for older people within general practices successfully redesigned?	
	a. Did GPs and PNs change their mindset from delivering reactive care to proactive care?	
	b. To what extent were linkages established with other professionals or organisations?	
	c. Did general practices receive useful decision-aids to support decision-making?	
	d. Is a registration system realised that is (practically) useful for general practices?	
Dose delivered (completeness)	3) To what extent did PNs follow all steps of the intervention protocol (see Figure 1)?	Semi-structured interviews GP/PN and older people; structured registration forms
Dose received (exposure)	4) To what extent were older people compliant with follow-up actions formulated in the care and treatment plan?	Structured registration forms
Dose received (satisfaction)	5) To what extent were GPs and PNs satisfied with organising care according to the home visitation programme?	Semi-structured interviews GP/PN
	6) To what extent were older people satisfied with the home visit?	Semi-structured interviews older people
	7) To what extent did older people benefit from the home visit and, if necessary, subsequent follow-up actions?	Structured registration forms
Reach (participation rate)	8) What proportion of the intended target population participated?	Registration trial database
	9) What were the reasons for non-participation of older people?	Reminder non-responders and notes in trial database
	10) Was the right target population reached according to GPs/PNs?	Semi-structured interviews GP/PN
	11) What proportion of older people completed all steps of the intervention protocol?	Registration trial database
	12) What were the reasons for drop-out of older people enrolled?	Notes in trial database
Recruitment	13) What procedures were used to recruit general practices and older people for participation?	Narrative report by project team
Context	14) What barriers and facilitators influenced implementation of the home visitation programme within general practices?	Semi-structured interviews GP/PN
	15) To what extent did the control group receive the intervention or similar types of proactive care (contamination)?	Short semi-structured interview GP by phone
Interactional workability	16) To what extent was congruence accomplished between PNs and older people and GPs and PNs regarding detected (health) problems and/or follow-up actions?	Semi-structured interviews GP/PN and older people
Relational integration	17) Did PNs have sufficient knowledge, expertise and skills to perform the activities as part of the home visitation programme?	Semi-structured interviews GP/PN and older people; evaluation form during training session
	18) To what extent did PNs feel confident that they could assess and address older people's health problems?	
Skill-set workability	19) Was the division of work between GP and PN acceptable?	Semi-structured interviews GP/PN
Contextual integration	20) Did the home visitation programme fit within the range of health care services offered by general practices?	Semi-structured interviews GP/PN
	21) Were sufficient resources (e.g., time, staff, and money) available for the adequate performance of the home visitation programme by general practices?	

'Midden-Limburg') were involved in the trial and all participated in the accompanying process evaluation. Thirteen general practices were instructed to redesign their care delivery from reactive to proactive care by implementing the [G]OLD preventive home visitation programme between July 2010 and September 2011 (intervention group), whereas 11 general practices offered usual care to older people (i.e., reactive care when older people present themselves with health problems or complaints) (control group). GPs and PNs from the intervention group were the key actors within the home visitation programme and therefore the main sources from which process data were gathered. Mean age of the 14 GPs from the intervention group participating in the process evaluation was 46.8 years (SD = 7.9; range: 31–60), 64.3% was male, and their average working experience as GP was 17.6 years SD = 8.5; range: 4–30). Thirteen PNs (one PN worked in two participating general practices; one general practice had two PNs) were responsible for implementing the home visitation programme. In several countries, including the Netherlands, PNs increasingly substitute the GP in chronic disease management and in care for older people now as well [25-27]. PNs had a mean age of 38.0 years (SD = 10.8; range: 22.6-57.3) and were predominantly female (91.7%). Their mean working experience as PN was 2.6 years (SD = 1.8; range: 0.5-6.5). Finally, the experiences of older people were incorporated. The target population were all community-dwelling older people aged 75 years and older who had been selected by general practices from their GP Information System. Older people not living independently, those on a waiting list for admission to a nursing home or home for older people, those under close medical supervision (chemotherapy, chronic haemodialysis or other therapies posing a high burden on the older person), and the terminally ill were excluded. The remaining older people eligible to participate were referred to as potentially frail older people whose frailty status would be judged by the CGA during a home visit.

[G]OLD home visitation programme

Figure 1 illustrates the steps of the [G]OLD home visitation programme that need to be undertaken by PNs, in collaboration with the GP, to ensure optimal delivery of the intervention to older people. The active ingredients of the [G]OLD home visitation programme for it to reach the intended effects were a home visit for conducting a CGA, a tailored care and treatment plan, multidisciplinary care management, and targeted intervention and follow-up. Although PNs could adapt certain steps (i.e., how to arrange follow-up of older people over time) to older person's needs and their own working routine, no steps were allowed to be omitted. PNs used the [G]OLD-instrument, which is a CGA to obtain a complete overview of older people's physical, psychological, mental, and social functioning, as well as lifestyle and medication use. This instrument was specifically developed for application by PNs in general practices [28]. If required, PNs could administer part

two of the [G]OLD-instrument consisting of more elaborate tests concerning cognition, depression, and personality disorders.

Besides these steps, care delivery to older people within general practices could only be successfully redesigned if four additional aspects from the Chronic Care Model [12] were realised. In line with the underlying philosophy of the intervention, general practices had to change their mindset from delivering reactive care towards offering proactive care ('delivery system design'). In order to achieve this, PNs were required to perform proactive home visits for the early identification of health and well-being problems among older people, followed by the other steps of the [G]OLD home visitation programme as depicted in Figure 1. In addition, to offer individually appropriate care to older people, PNs were instructed to achieve interdisciplinary collaboration by establishing linkages (e.g., multidisciplinary meetings) with (local) professionals or organisations offering care and/or well-being services to older people ('community resources'). Further, the project team delivered decision-aids and tools to assist general practices in deciding about the presence or absence of problems detected through the CGA, as well as a service map of where to refer older people with specific problems to within the available range of health and well-being services ('decision support'). Finally, the local primary care organisations were instructed to realise an ICT-based clinical information system within existing systems in general practices to register the findings from the CGA and the results of monitoring and follow-up of older people over time ('clinical information systems').

Before the start of the intervention period in July 2010, all PNs participated in a two-day training session that focused on gaining knowledge and skills to carry out the different steps of the home visitation programme. PNs received background information on the [G]OLD-instrument, they practiced applying the [G]OLD-instrument among older people, and they were brought into contact with several professionals or organisations offering care and/or well-being services to older people.

Data collection

Mixed-methods research was conducted in which quantitative and qualitative data complemented one another to yield an enriched understanding of the implementation process and of the extent to which general practices redesigned their care delivery. Using a convergent-parallel approach, quantitative and qualitative methods were given equal priority, data were gathered concurrently, and integration took place at the interpretation or conclusion stage of the research. This resulted in a so-called parallel-databases design [29] or also called a triangulation design model, which is frequently applied in primary care research

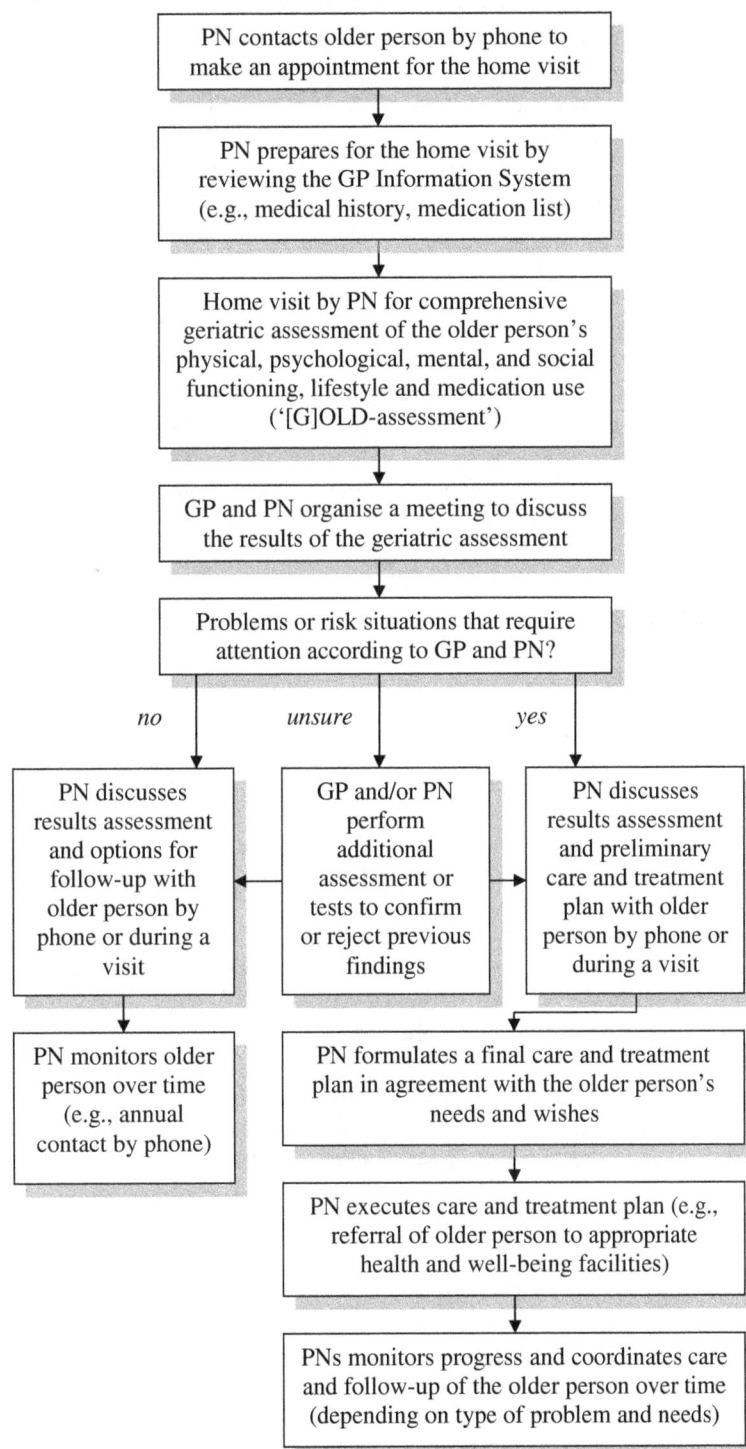

Figure 1 Steps of the [G]OLD home visitation programme (intervention protocol).

[30]. Apart from the use of quotes, the qualitative components of our study adhered to RATS guidelines [31]. An overview of the data collection tools per research question guiding the process evaluation is presented in Table 1.

Semi-structured interviews

Individual semi-structured interviews were conducted with PNs and GPs in the general practice and with older people in their homes. Semi-structured interviews are well suited to explore people's opinions and perceptions with flexibility and at the same time cover fixed elements as a part of the process evaluation. The process evaluation questions guided the topic lists for the interviews. All 13 participating PNs were interviewed three times (i.e., after three months, six months, and at the end of the intervention period) to gain a detailed overview of their experiences in various phases of the implementation process. For example, their experiences with conducting the home visits and the extent to which general practices redesigned their care delivery from reactive to proactive care were among the topics being discussed. The interviews lasted approximately 30 to 60 minutes each.

At the end of the intervention period, one GP from each general practice participated in a 30-minute interview. In general practices with several GPs, the one who was most closely involved in implementing the home visitation programme was approached. As a result, 13 interviews were conducted with 14 GPs (in one general practice both GPs participated in the interview). Examples of topics discussed were the involvement of the GP in the home visitation programme, the extent to which a transition from reactive to proactive care was achieved, as well as intended continuation of the home visitation programme over time within the general practice. At the end of the follow-up period of the trial (18 months after baseline), one GP per control practice was interviewed shortly by phone to determine the extent to which the general practice had been involved in proactive care similar to the intervention group (contamination).

After the home visit, older people were invited to share their experiences and views regarding the home visitation programme. Interviews lasted approximately 30 minutes and took place three to five weeks after the home visit. This gave PNs sufficient time to communicate the care and treatment plan to the older person, while the risk that the older person would not remember details of the home visit anymore was not yet too high. Initially, one older person (or a couple, if both received a CGA) per general practice/PN was purposefully selected (total n = 17 older people, including 3 couples) in consultation with the PN based on the principle of maximum variation by taking into account gender, age, household status (living alone vs. living together), and health status (no/few problems detected vs. multiple problems detected). After the initial interview round, data saturation was reached as no new themes or issues arose during the coding process.

Structured registration forms
Several structured registration forms were distributed among PNs to gain insight into complete and acceptable delivery of steps of the home visitation programme. PNs received the [G]OLD-instrument on paper, which also

included a form to register details of the post-discussion with the GP, and the care and treatment plan according to the official format as recommended by the Dutch College of General Practitioners [32]. The care and treatment plan contained details per detected problem of the goal to be achieved, who will undertake action, and when evaluation will take place. Returned forms were checked for completeness and accuracy of reporting by a research assistant, thereby serving as a proxy for complete delivery of elements of the intervention protocol.

At the end of the 18-month follow-up period, PNs were asked to register on a structured form for each older person the number of follow-up contacts, the extent to which this person in general complied with follow-up actions or advice given (5-point scale: 'always', 'most of the time', 'sometimes', 'rarely', 'never', including the options 'I don't know' and 'not applicable, no action/ help needed'), and the extent to which the older person in general benefitted from follow-up actions, referral or advice given (4-point scale: 'very much', 'somewhat', 'a little', 'not at all', including the reason for their judgement).

The two-day training programme for PNs was evaluated using a structured evaluation form to be filled-out at the end of each day. Besides their satisfaction with the training in general (on a scale ranging from 0 (worst score) to 10 (best score)), PNs were asked to what extent the training prepared them for the performance of the home visits and to what extent they felt confident that they could perform a home visit independently (both measured on 7-point scales ranging from 1 ('not at all') to 7 ('very much')).

At baseline, older people received the [G]OLD care diary to register details of their contacts with professionals offering care and/or well-being services during the 18-month follow-up period. This information was intended as an indicator of compliance to follow-up actions besides the judgement of the PN. Unfortunately, only 7.1% of the older people (n = 42 out of 590 older people who had a home visit) filled-out the [G]OLD care diary and returned it at 18-months follow-up. According to some of the older people who gave remarks on the use of the [G]OLD care diary, they did not see the added value of it and/or forgot to fill it out after contacts with professionals. Since we did not obtain a representative sample for estimating compliance, this information was not used for process evaluation purposes.

Continuous registration and notes
The number of participants, non-participants, and dropouts, including reasons for non-participation and dropout were registered by members of the research team in the trial database. Furthermore, members of the research team made notes or narrative descriptions of the recruitment procedures and feedback meetings with all PNs

together. These meetings were organised twice: after approximately six months and at the end of the intervention period. PNs were offered the possibility to exchange experiences and interim results of the individual semi-structured interviews were discussed (member check).

Data analysis

Descriptive statistics (e.g., means, frequencies, and percentages) were computed for quantitative process data using IBM SPSS Statistics for Windows, version 21.0. All individual semi-structured interviews with GPs, PNs, and older people from the intervention group were digitally recorded, after obtaining verbal consent from participants, and transcribed verbatim. The analysis of the interview transcripts was supported by the software package NVivo 7. Two members of the research team (PhD-student, who also performed all interviews, and a research assistant; both with an academic background) independently coded the data to enhance credibility of the findings. One member of the research team coded all transcripts (PhD-student), while a second coder (research assistant) served as a control and coded a random selection of one quarter of the transcripts to reduce workload. A general inductive approach was applied in which the coding process was guided by a coding tree based on the process evaluation objectives. This relatively simple approach allows for deriving findings in the context of focused evaluation questions [33]. Systematic and rigorous reading and coding of the transcripts allowed major themes to emerge, which were compared for overlap. Consensus was reached after discussion and since the most important themes had already emerged, it was not considered necessary for the second coder to analyse the remaining transcripts. Credibility of the qualitative findings was also enhanced using member checks (i.e., preliminary findings were documented and send to PNs for feedback) and method triangulation (i.e., using multiple methods to collect data on a particular process evaluation question). Other qualitative data (i.e., notes of the feedback sessions with PNs) were analysed using conventional content analysis [34]. Direct information is obtained from participants without imposing preconceived ideas on them, which allows categories or new themes to emerge from the data that did not yet emerge from the semi-structured interviews. Descriptions of procedures applied by the research team for recruitment of general practices during the intervention period were summarised in a narrative report.

Results

The results of the process evaluation are described below, structured according to the process evaluation questions as presented in Table 1.

Fidelity (Q1)

All steps of the home visitation programme were largely implemented as planned. Exceptions are PNs who changed or omitted questions in the CGA, no or delayed post-discussion between the GP and PN, and no or inappropriately formulated care and treatment plans. Both PNs and GPs struggled most with how to arrange long-term monitoring of older people considering the limited number of hours PNs could dedicate to care for older people. Besides this, each PN developed his/her own routine in performing the different steps.

Change in mindset (Q2a)

The shift from reactively to proactively approaching older people in a structured and comprehensive way was evident for PNs, as well as for most GPs. One PN mentioned that GPs were not used to approaching older people in a proactive way. They usually offer care and/or treatment upon request, whereas PNs are more familiar with delivering preventive care.

At the end of the intervention period, all general practices intended to continue with the home visitation programme, but the proactive versus a more reactive approach posed a dilemma for half of the practices. Proactively visiting all older people (75+) allows for primary prevention of problems but is a huge time investment for general practices. Purposefully visiting older people who show signs of decline would be more feasible, but this is at the expense of detecting problems which could have been prevented if addressed earlier.

Interdisciplinary collaboration (Q2b)

Due to the home visitation programme, PNs' extended their network of professionals or disciplines involved in care for older people and they used their network to a greater extent. The number of referrals to secondary care was limited and the majority of contacts took place within primary care, for instance with home care organisations, physiotherapists, and occupational therapists. Several PNs indicated that they only had few contacts with other care professionals since not that many problems had been detected. Collaboration with other professionals was facilitated when they were located nearby, preferably in the same building.

In three general practices, multidisciplinary meetings took place on a structural base (e.g., once a month) already before the start of this study, and older people were discussed in these meetings from time to time as well. In other general practices, no structural meetings were organised yet with disciplines outside the general practice, mostly because no or only few complex problems were detected among older people. Three general practices had concrete plans to organise multidisciplinary meetings in the near future. Others were not convinced of their added value compared to existing meetings or contacts with other disciplines on an individual base.

Decision-aids to support decision-making (Q2c)

Half of the PNs used the service map made available by the project team and considered it useful. Others had not encountered any situations in which the service map could have been helpful.

Both PNs and GPs were positive about the [G]OLD-instrument. Its extensiveness offered a comprehensive overview of the older person's health and well-being, yet the instrument was time-consuming to administer. Consequently, several PNs and GPs sought for a balance in restricting the time investment without losing important content (e.g., application to a limited group of older people).

Clinical information system (Q2d)

Only in the region 'Parkstad', the digital system for registering the findings from the CGA and the care and treatment plan was finished at the start of the intervention period, although PNs could not yet register the results of monitoring and follow-up of older people over time. Initially, PNs considered it time-consuming and double work.

Dose delivered (completeness) (Q3)

The dose delivered is illustrated in Figure 2. In total, 590 participants were visited at home by the PN for a CGA between July 2010 and September 2011. An underestimation of the actual number of post-discussions is likely, since not all PNs consistently filled-out the registration form. The percentage of formulated care and treatment plans per PN varied widely from 4.0% to 95.2%. In case PNs did not use the official format, we did not count them as care and treatment plans. Finally, we had no valid details per older person of their follow-up within the chain of care as PNs could not easily differentiate between follow-up contacts on behalf of the home visitation programme and other contacts with the general practice within the 18-month period. Nonetheless, the follow-up process might have been suboptimal in several cases, as some PNs experienced time constraints and/or they did not have a concrete plan for monitoring and follow-up (this was not provided as part of the intervention protocol).

Dose received (exposure) (Q4)

According to the forms filled-out by PNs ($n = 384$, 65.1%), of the 229 older people who received follow-up actions or advice, 67.7% complied 'always' or 'most of the time', while 10.5% complied 'rarely' or 'never'. Six older people admitted during the interview that they did not comply with a specific advice given by the PN.

Half of the PNs noticed that they often came across older people who did not want any follow-up action(s) in the first place. Especially mental problems were difficult to deal with. Often older people agreed to undertake actions when it was already too late. Some PNs struggled with how to deal with these older people and how to find a balance between respecting the older person's wishes and maintaining contact to try to achieve the desired actions over time.

Dose received (satisfaction) (Q5-Q7)
Practice nurses (Q5)

PNs liked the performance of the home visits because of the ability to get to know the older person and to offer help or advice. The home visit lowers the threshold for older people to contact the general practice should problems arise in the future. PNs were in favour of a home visit instead of a consultation in the general practice, as it offered a more objective picture of the older person's functioning. At the general practice level, the home visitation programme resulted in more attention for older people in general and closer collaboration between the GP and PN in organising care for older people. The majority of the PNs did not like the administrative work. Moreover, opinions of PNs diverged regarding the added value of the care and treatment plan over and above the registration of follow-up actions in the GP's Information System. In general, PNs evaluated the preparatory training rather positively (M = 7.64, SD = 0.50 for the first day vs. M = 6.64. SD = 0.92 for the second day).

General practitioners (Q5)

Half of the GPs liked most that they obtained a comprehensive and complete picture of older people's functioning and the social network surrounding older people. As a result, GPs considered the home visits useful, because it offered them additional information which might be valuable for future reference. At the general practice level, the home visitation programme had offered a starting point and useful tools for organising care for older people. Seven GPs mentioned that, against their expectations, no or only few previously unknown problems were detected. Furthermore, the older people that were out of the picture according to the GP and that would therefore particularly benefit from the home visit often did not consent to participate.

Older people (Q6)

Although the majority had no specific expectations about the home visit, three older people were hesitant about the purpose of the home visit at first. All older people were very satisfied with the home visit and afterwards, they had a good feeling about it or they emphasised that it had been interesting. They were very positive about the PN and felt

Figure 2 flowchart contents:

n=1,251 non-participants → Reasons non-participation (n=648):
- Not interested (*n*=168)
- Unwillingness to participate (e.g., feels to old) (*n*=112)
- Home visit considered unnecessary (e.g., is doing fine) (*n*=109)
- Participation inconvenient at the moment (e.g., due to illness) (*n*=91)
- Reasons related to filling-out questionnaires (e.g., too burdensome) (*n*=53)
- Does not want PN to visit him/her (*n*=35)
- Ineligible to participate (*n*=34)
- Does not want to participate in scientific research in general (*n*=19)
- Children decide or disagree with participation (*n*=13)
- Other reasons (*n*= 14)

n= 199 dropouts during 18-month FU → Reasons:
- Does not want to continue participation (*n*=58)
- Death (*n*=36)
- Illness / decline in health status / under close medical supervision (*n*=28)
- Admission to nursing home (*n*=27)
- Moved or switched to other general practice (*n*=16)
- Admission to home for older people (*n*=10)
- Unknown reason (*n*=24)

n=1,972 eligible older people (≥75 years) from 13 general practices approached for participation

n=721 older people (36.6%) consented to participate

Home visit
n=590 older people (81.8%) were visited at home by the PN for a comprehensive geriatric assessment (CGA)

Additional assessment
n=216 older people (36.6%)

Post-discussion
n=465 of the visited older people (78.8%) were discussed by the GP and PN

Care and treatment plan
n=354 of the visited older people (60.0%) had a care and treatment plan according to the official format of the Dutch College of General Practitioners; for *n*=45 of the visited older people (11.3%) the plan for follow-up was registered in GP Information System or otherwise

Follow-up
No details available per older person of their follow-up within the chain of care

Completion steps of the intervention protocol:
- Home visit + post-discussion between the GP and PN + care and treatment plan: *n*=274 participants (38.0%)
- Home visit + post-discussion between the GP and PN: *n*=157 participants (21.8%)
- Home visit + care and treatment plan: *n*=80 participants (11.1%);
- Home visit only: *n*=34 participants (4.7%)
- None of the steps completed: *n*=131 participants (those who had no home visit) (18.2%)

n=45 participants (6.2%): unofficial care and treatment plan formulated by PN

Reasons no home visit (n=131):
- Lack of time PN (*n*=42)
- Older person declined participation (*n*=26)
- Death (*n*=14)
- Home visit inconvenient according to GP due to illness / health problems / under close medical supervision (*n*=14)
- Older person moved or switched to other general practice (*n*=13)
- Admission to nursing home (*n*=7)
- Older person felt no need for home visit (*n*=3)
- Admission to home for older people (*n*=2)
- Unknown reason (*n*=10)

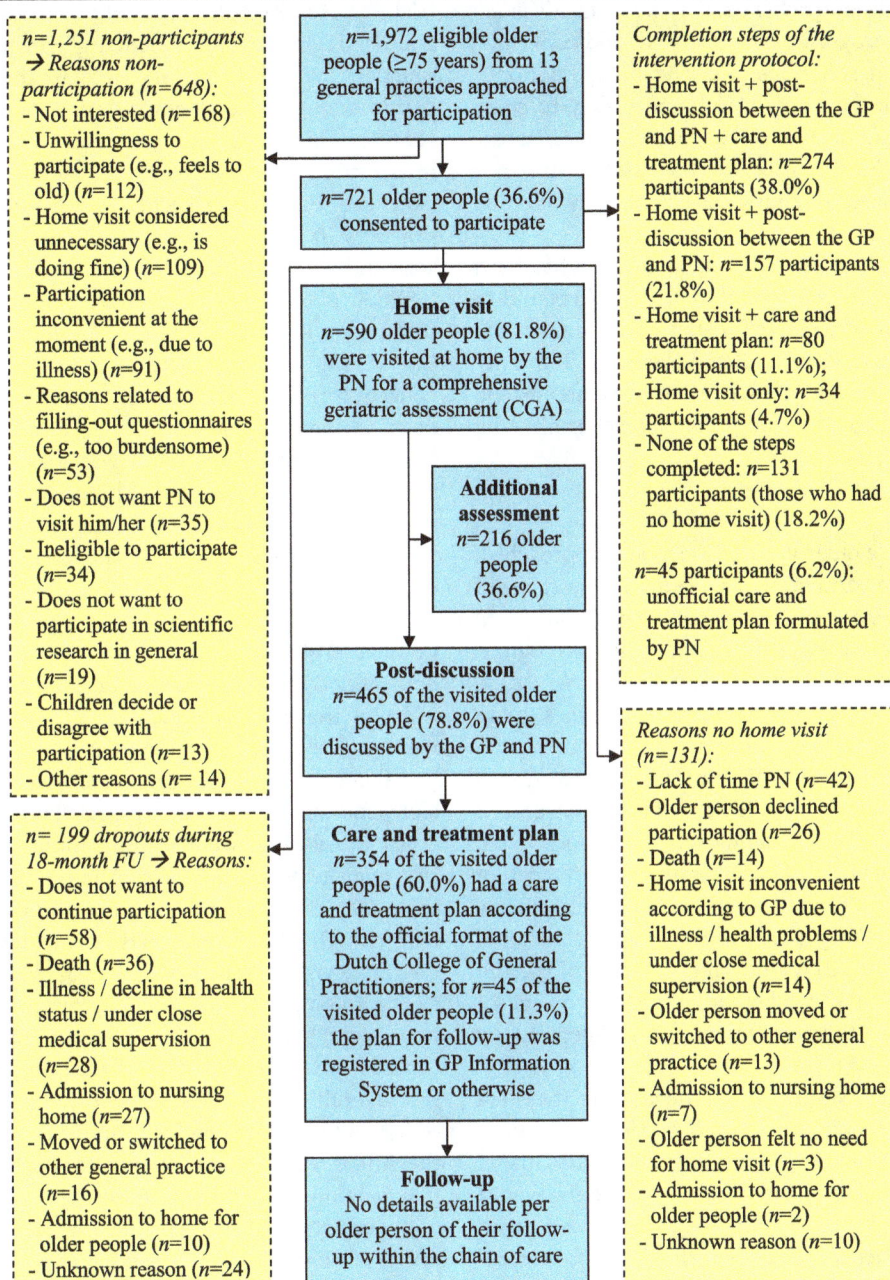

Figure 2 Dose delivered and reach of the [G]OLD home visitation programme.

that they could discuss everything with him/her. The home visit was neither too short nor too long and they felt that everything that they considered to be important was discussed. The questions asked as part of the CGA were not difficult to understand, impolite, awkward, or strange. Older people liked the ability to talk about different things, the unexpected attention from their general practice, and the fact that they now had a familiar face in the general practice. One person indicated that these visits tend to go towards too extensive meddling with other people's affairs, especially among older people who are doing relatively well and do not have a specific request for help.

Benefits to older people (Q7)

According to the forms filled-out by PNs (*n* = 394, 66.8%), for 29.9% of the older people follow-up actions, referral or advice had been 'very much' or 'somewhat' beneficial, while the remaining 70.1% of the older people benefitted 'a little' or 'not at all'. Most PNs indicated that the majority of older people experienced few benefits, because no problems had been detected or only problems that could be addressed easily or problems that had already been taken care of. As recognised by a PN, a GP and confirmed by one older person, sometimes older people did not optimally benefit from the home visit because they to some extent hold a façade of normalcy. Finally, one GP commented that the home visits are less useful for older people without a specific request for help as they often do not want to undertake action.

Six older people mentioned that the home visit had been useful for them, mostly because it lowered a threshold to discuss matters for which they do not easily contact the general practice themselves. Others believed that you are just old and there is nothing that can be done about that, and that certain problems (e.g., loneliness) cannot be solved.

Reach (Q8-Q12)

Of the 1,972 eligible older people (≥75 years) approached, 36.6% consented to participate (see Figure 2). Mean age of participants was 80.6 years (SD = 4.26; range: 74.4-95.4) and 56.0% ($n = 972$) were female. Participants were significantly younger compared to non-participants (M = 81.2, SD = 4.39) ($p = 0.004$) and men were 1.43 times more likely to participate than women. Participants who dropped out (27.6%, $n = 199$) during the 18-month follow-up period (see Figure 2), received usual care if necessary. Drop-outs were significantly older (M = 81.1, SD = 4.76) compared to those who continued participation (M = 80.3, SD = 3.95), ($p =0.027$) and women were equally likely to drop-out as men (OR = 0.99). As Figure 2 shows, for only 38.0% of the 721 participants all steps of the [G]OLD-protocol up to the follow-up process were completed according to the registration forms filled-out by PNs.

Nearly all PNs and several GPs believed that they had missed the older people who would particularly benefit from the home visitation programme, since participants were the relatively healthy older people, those for whom care was already arranged quite well, or the ones who often visit the practice. They felt that due to the informed consent procedure of the trial, people who are not doing well or the more frail older people are suspicious about the consequences of participation.

Recruitment (Q13)

All general practices in the regions 'Maastricht-Heuvelland' and 'Parkstad' were informed about the [G]OLD-project by means of a letter from the primary healthcare organisation of their region, followed by information sessions and practice visits for those interested to participate. Non-responders were contacted by phone to inquire about their willingness to participate in the control group. Since insufficient general practices agreed to participate in the control group, jeopardising the continuation of the

trial, the recruitment of control practices was extended to another region ('Midden-Limburg'). In total, 188 general practices from three regions were approached for participation and 24 general practices consented to participate (12.8%). Thirteen general practices were included in the intervention group (7 from the region 'Parkstad' and 6 from the region 'Maastricht-Heuvelland') and 11 general practices in the control group (2 from the region 'Parkstad' and 9 from the region 'Midden-Limburg').

Older people were approached for participation by means of an information letter and consent form. In the intervention group, those who did not return the signed consent form within two weeks were contacted by phone once to inquire whether they received the information letter. One postal reminder was send to older people who could not be contacted by phone. Due to the substantial time investment of calling older people, non-responders in the control group only received a postal reminder.

Context (Q14-Q21)
Barriers and facilitators for implementation (Q14)

Most of the barriers experienced by PNs during implementation were related to logistical difficulties in planning the different steps of the home visitation programme alongside other daily work. Especially the introduction of a new disease management programme for cardiovascular risk management (CVRM) by the primary care organisations during the intervention period posed challenges to PNs and GPs, causing several PNs to invest less time in the home visitation programme than planned. Finally, barriers for continuing the home visitation programme over time were the lack of an adequate reimbursement by health insurers of the costs of care for older people and the overall time investment of the home visitation programme (total time investment from preparation of the home visit to formulating the care and treatment plan was on average 85 minutes per older person).

A facilitator for implementation according to several PNs was gaining routine in efficiently planning and executing the different steps of the home visitation programme. Moreover, some PNs expressed the need for regular meetings with other PNs to exchange experiences or the ability to consult an expert panel with practical questions. For GPs, having a PN in the general practice who is largely responsible for performing the home visitation programme and who gained experience in it, was a positive development conducive to successful implementation.

Contamination control group (Q15)

None of the participating general practices in the control group had been involved in any form of proactive care for community-dwelling older people during the 18-month study period.

Interactional workability (Q16)

All PNs were satisfied with how they worked together with the GP in deciding about follow-up actions for detected problems. Yet one PN and one GP noticed that sometimes there was incongruence between the two of them: the proactive approach required GPs to address different kinds of problems and/or needs that otherwise might not have received attention at that point in time. Mostly, older people agreed with the suggestions done by the PN for follow-up actions. However, both PNs and GPs observed that quite a few older people were not willing to undertake any follow-up actions or only when problems had progressed substantially (incongruence).

Relational integration (Q17 + Q18)

At the end of the training programme, PNs felt very confident that they could perform a home visit independently (M = 6.27, SD = 0.91). In general, both PNs and GPs thought that the PN's knowledge, expertise or skills regarding care for older people were sufficient and, according to PNs, even increased during the intervention period. Those inexperienced with structural assessments would benefit from feedback, supplementary information, or examples on how to administer certain tests of the CGA and how to assign a score to the answers given by older people. A few PNs did not have that much expertise yet in deciding whether or not to undertake follow-up actions for detected problems and in formulating care and treatment plans correctly. One GP sensed a lack of affinity of the PN regarding care for older people. All older people believed the PN had sufficient knowledge about health, listened to them, took sufficient time for the home visit, and respected their needs and wishes.

Skill-set workability (Q19)

Both PNs and GPs considered the division of work regarding the home visitation programme clear and acceptable. As GPs often cannot attribute as much time to older people as they would like, the expertise gained by PNs in care for older people was very much appreciated. One PN was a little disappointed that the GPs did not use her expertise more often in arranging follow-up actions for older people.

Contextual integration (Q20 + Q21)

Six PNs felt that the home visitation programme was well integrated within the health care services offered by the general practice. According to two GPs, the home visitation programme fits within the health care services offered by general practices, as older people are familiar with the general practice. Furthermore, it enabled GPs to be the central care provider and to collect information that is relevant to them.

According to PNs and GPs, sufficient time for care for older people was an essential resource for adequate performance of the home visitation programme. PNs' available time had to be carefully divided over various patient categories within the general practice. Five GPs thought that the time investment was disproportionate compared to the benefits in terms of detected problems. The other GPs thought the time investment was justifiable, as it yielded a lot more information about the older person.

Opinions of GPs diverged with respect to the importance of the reimbursement policy of health insurers for implementing care for (frail) older people. While some GPs considered it to be of minor importance, others believed its importance will grow over time due to competition between various disease management programmes for the available time of the PN. Finally, some GPs stated that continuation of the home visitation programme would largely depend on it.

Discussion

This paper reports on a pre-planned, theory-based process evaluation into redesigning care delivery by general practices and implementation of a home visitation programme for potentially frail community-dwelling older people (aged ≥75 years). The process evaluation plan was structured using the theoretical elements 'fidelity' (quality of implementation), 'dose delivered' (completeness), 'dose received' (exposure; satisfaction), 'reach' (participation rate), 'recruitment', and 'context' as proposed by Saunders and colleagues [19], as well as the Normalisation Process Model [22] to explore the element 'context' in greater detail. Overall, the home visitation programme was delivered completely according to protocol to only 38.0% of the 721 study participants. This is considerably lower than the completion rate of 78% of a similar intervention [35]. Several threats to complete delivery of the intervention have been identified.

First of all, lack of time emerged as a crucial factor in various elements of the process evaluation and prior research showed that it is an important barrier in providing structured care to older people in general practice [36,37]. Administering the [G]OLD-instrument during the home visit, post-discussion between the PN and GP, administrative work (e.g., registering the findings from the CGA in the digital registration system), and monitoring older people were (initially) judged to be time-consuming activities or were influenced by time constraints of either the PN or GP. The time investment and corresponding available financial reimbursement were considered disproportionate compared to the benefits in terms of detected problems, thereby influencing the intention of general practices to continue using the home visitation programme. Furthermore, the time investment posed logistical challenges for some general practices in dividing the limited time of the PN over various patient categories. Interestingly, solutions to reduce the time investment were not sought in shortening the [G] OLD-instrument or adapting the intervention protocol in general, but in targeting the home visitation programme to a selected group of older people who benefit most from it.

Secondly, few new or complex health and/or well-being problems had been detected, which was the main cause of no post-discussions and no care and treatment plans for specific cases, and limited interdisciplinary cooperation. Both PNs and GPs believed that the relatively healthy older people were visited, suggesting inadequate reach. On the one hand, volunteer bias may have been introduced by the recruitment procedure on behalf of the parallel quasi-experimental trial. Alternatively, the population-based screening approach may have resulted in few (newly) detected problems among older people. While some opt for population-based screening of older people in general practice [6], other studies suggest that general practices benefit most from a more targeted screening approach [38,39].

While coding the transcripts of the semi-structured interviews, we retrieved relevant information regarding fidelity that went beyond mere quality of implementation. In agreement with Hasson and colleagues [40], we found that implementation fidelity was influenced by the care professionals' commitment to the home visitation programme, as well as their ability to execute the intervention protocol with the resources at hand. Both PNs and GPs were satisfied with the home visitation programme. It had resulted in more attention for older people, closer collaboration between the GP and PN, and a comprehensive picture of older people's functioning and social network. This positive attitude made them willing to find solutions for barriers encountered during the implementation (e.g., monitoring older people via other disease management programmes). Such small changes to the intervention protocol were not considered threats to fidelity, but as necessary for translation of the home visitation programme into daily practice (i.e., work patterns of PNs) [41]. However, PNs struggled a lot with the follow-up process and thus, the extent of arranging follow-up actions and monitoring older people over time might have been limited, as also found in another recent study [27], threatening fidelity of implementation. Besides time constraints, other causes may be inadequate guidelines or decision-aids for PNs to arrange the monitoring process, some older people did not want to undertake follow-up actions, and a lack of adequate ICT-support to facilitate registration of the follow-up process.

With respect to redesigning care delivery for older people, shifting of care from the GP to the PN was evaluated positively and appeared to be conducive to the delivery of proactive care, as PNs in general are more familiar with a preventive approach. Nevertheless, some GPs were still more inclined towards offering reactive care. This implies that over time, GPs may relapse into their usual way of delivering care upon request (because of time constraints, lack of benefits in terms of detected problems, etc.), stimulated by the disproportionate cost-benefit ratio of the home visitation programme as mentioned earlier and the predominantly reactive healthcare system in the Netherlands .

All older people were satisfied about the home visit, regardless of whether problems had been detected, mostly because it offered them the ability to express their daily concerns. This 'attention' aspect of the home visit has been recognised before and is considered insufficient for eliciting substantial effects on patient outcomes [42].

The development of a prospective process evaluation plan, underpinned by a theoretical framework, and using a mixed-method approach to data collection allowed for a high-quality and more thoroughly conducted process evaluation. Trustworthiness or credibility of the findings was enhanced using, among others, member checks, method triangulation (i.e., using multiple methods to collect data on a process evaluation question), and two independent coders during qualitative data-analysis. Nevertheless, the subjective experiences of PNs, GPs, and older people may have been subject to social-desirability bias or recall bias. Opinions of GPs might have been biased due to negotiations between insurers and care groups for a bundled payment system [43] for complex care for older people. Honest responding by PNs may have been promoted by the independent role of the researcher and relationship of trust created due to repeated contacts during the intervention period. Further, despite using a varied sample of older people, we could not entirely circumvent that older people tend to provide less detailed descriptions of their experiences [44]. Another limitation is that the structured registration forms were not always completely and accurately filled-out by PNs. This made them a less reliable source to assess for example implementation fidelity or dose delivered, and thereby also restricting method triangulation for certain process evaluation questions.

Conclusions

The current process evaluation offers useful insights for interpreting the results of the parallel quasi-experimental trial and for sustainability of the home visitation programme in general practices [45]. The largest threats to positive outcomes at the patient level are the low dose delivered and inadequate reach. According to PNs, beneficial effects of the home visitation programme were 'little' or 'not at all' present in the majority of visited older people (70.1%). Despite this, the home visitation programme was judged positively by both GPs and PNs and resulted in positive developments within the general practices. This suggests that the intervention does not have major shortcomings in itself, but the delivery offers room for improvement. Besides selecting the more frail community-dwelling older people with multiple and complex problems, alternative time-saving solutions for general practices may be sought in connecting general practices with initiatives in the neighbourhood or at the community level by developing welfare and care models. Regardless, the involvement of general practices is advocated [4,5] and GPs also believe the home visitation programme fits within their range of care services. Finally, PNs would benefit from on-going training to update their knowledge and skills, thereby enhancing implementation fidelity, and to allow for exchanging experiences with other PNs. An imbalance between the time investment and available financial reimbursement in proportion to the number of meaningful problems detected among older people requires attention to enable continuation of the home visitation programme over time. The development of future complex interventions in the primary care setting should take into account that a preplanned, theory-based process evaluation alongside the effect evaluation is inevitable to provide in-depth insight into the actual performance of the intervention in the intended context.

Abbreviations
CGA: Comprehensive Geriatric Assessment; [G]OLD: Getting OLD the healthy way; GP: General practitioner; PN: Practice nurse.

Competing interests
The authors declare that they have no competing interests.

Authors' contributions
IGPD as main applicant and MWJJ as project leader were involved in writing the grant proposal for the evaluation study, including the process evaluation. MMNS developed the process evaluation plan, with helpful comments of the co-authors. MMNS carried out the data collection on behalf of the process evaluation. MMNS drafted the manuscript with input from the other authors. All authors read, commented on and approved the final manuscript.

Acknowledgements
The process evaluation is part of a quasi-experimental study funded by the Netherlands Organisation for Health Research and Development (ZonMw 311070303) as part of The National Care for the Elderly Programme. Open access of this publication was financed by the Netherlands Organisation for Scientific Research ('NWO'). We are grateful to Marion de Mooij for her assistance in collecting and analysing the data. We thank all participating GPs, PNs, and older people for their participation in this study.

Author details
[1]Department of Family Medicine, School for Public Health and Primary Care (CAPHRI), Faculty of Health, Medicine and Life Sciences, Maastricht University, P.O. Box 616, 6200 MD Maastricht, The Netherlands. [2]Public Health Service South-Limburg, P.O. Box 2022, 6160 HA Geleen, The Netherlands. [3]Department of Health Services Research, School for Public Health and Primary Care (CAPHRI), Faculty of Health, Medicine and Life Sciences, Maastricht University, P.O. Box 616, 6200 MD Maastricht, The Netherlands. [4]Department of Patient and Care, Maastricht University Medical Centre, P.O. Box 5800, 6202 MD Maastricht, The Netherlands. [5]Tilburg School of Social and Behavioral Sciences, Scientific Centre for Care and Welfare (TRANZO), Tilburg University, P.O. Box 90153, 5000 LE Tilburg, The Netherlands. [6]Saw Swee Hock School of Public Health, National University of Singapore, MD3, 16 Medical Drive, Singapore 117597, Republic of Singapore.

References
1. Beswick AD, Rees K, Dieppe P, Ayis S, Gooberman-Hill R, Horwood J, Ebrahim S: Complex interventions to improve physical function and maintain independent living in elderly people: a systematic review and meta-analysis. Lancet 2008, 371:725–735.
2. Huss A, Stuck AE, Rubenstein LZ, Egger M, Clough-Gorr KM: Multidimensional preventive home visit programs for community-dwelling older adults: a systematic review and meta-analysis of randomized controlled trials. J Gerontol A Biol Sci Med Sci 2008, 63A:298–307.
3. MacAdam M: Frameworks of Integrated Care for the Elderly: A Systematic Review. Ontario: Canadian Policy Research Networks Inc; 2008.
4. Boeckxstaens P, De Graaf P: Primary care and care for older persons: position paper of the European forum for primary care. Qual Prim Care 2011, 19:369–389.
5. Lacas A, Rockwood K: Frailty in primary care: a review of its conceptualization and implications for practice. BMC Med 2012, 10:4.
6. Fletcher AE, Price GM, Ng ESW, Stirling SL, Bulpitt CJ, Breeze E, Nunes M, Jones DA, Latif A, Fasey NM, Vickers MR, Tulloch AJ: Population-based multidimensional assessment of older people in UK general practice: a cluster-randomised factorial trial. Lancet 2004, 364:1667–1677.
7. Metzelthin SF, Van Rossum E, De Witte LP, Ambergen AW, Hobma SO, Siper W, Kempen GIJM: Effectiveness of interdisciplinary primary care approach to reduce disability in community dwelling frail older people: cluster randomised controlled trial. Br Med J 2013, 347:f5264.
8. Vass M, Avlund K, Hendriksen C, Philipson L, Riis P: Preventive home visits to older people in Denmark. Why, how, by whom, and when? Z Gerontol Geriatr 2007, 40:209–216.
9. Adams WL, McIlvain HE, Lacy NL, Magsi H, Crabtree BF, Yenny SK, Sitorius MA: Primary care for elderly people. Why do doctors find it so hard? Gerontologist 2002, 42:835–842.
10. Van Hout HPJ, Jansen APD, Van Marwijk HWJ, Nijpel G: Prevention of adverse health trajectories in a vulnerable elderly population through nurse home visits: randomized controlled trial [ISRCTN05358495]. J Gerontol A Biol Sci Med Sci 2010, 65:734–742.
11. Stijnen MMN, Duimel-Peeters IGP, Jansen MWJ, Vrijhoef HJM: Early detection of health problems in potentially frail community-dwelling older people by general practices - project [G]OLD: design of a longitudinal, quasi-experimental study. BMC Geriatr 2013, 13:7.
12. Bodenheimer T, Wagner EH, Grumbach K: Improving primary care for patients with chronic illness. J Am Med Assoc 2002, 288:1775–1779.
13. Bodenheimer T, Wagner EH, Grumbach K: Improving primary care for patients with chronic illness. The chronic care model, part 2. J Am Med Assoc 2002, 288:1909–1914.
14. Boult C, Karm L, Groves C: Improving chronic care: the "guided care" model. Perm J 2008, 12:50–54.
15. Craig P, Dieppe P, Macintyre S, Michie S, Nazareth I, Petticrew M: Developing and evaluating complex interventions: the new medical research council guidance. Br Med J 2008, 337:a1655.
16. Oakley A, Strange V, Bonell C, Allen E, Stephenson J, RIPPLE Study Team: Process evaluation in randomised controlled trials of complex interventions. Br Med J 2006, 332:413–416.
17. Bradley F, Wiles R, Kinmonth A-L, Mant D, Gantley M: Development and evaluation of complex interventions in health services research: case study of the Southampton heart integrated care project (SHIP). Br Med J 1999, 318:711–715.
18. Stijnen MMN, Duimel-Peeters IGP, Vrijhoef HJM, Jansen MWJ: Process evaluation plan of a patient-centered home visitation program for potentially frail community-dwelling older people in general practice. Eur J Pers Cent Healthc 2013, 2:179–189.
19. Harachi TW, Abbott RD, Catalano RF, Haggerty KP, Fleming CB: Opening the black box: using process evaluation measures to assess implementation and theory building. Am J Community Psychol 1999, 27:711–731.
20. Reelick MF, Faes MC, Esselink RAJ, Kessels RPC, Olde Rikkert MGM: How to perform a preplanned process evaluation for complex interventions in

geriatric medicine: exemplified with the process evaluation of a complex falls-prevention program for community-dwelling frail older fallers. *J Am Med Dir Assoc* 2011, **12**:331–336.

21. Saunders RP, Evans MH, Joshi P: Developing a process-evaluation plan for assessing health promotion program implementation: a how-to guide. *Health Promot Pract* 2005, **6**:134–147.

22. Baranowski T, Stables G: Process evaluations of the 5-a-day projects. *Health Educ Behav* 2000, **27**:157–166.

23. Linnan L, Steckler A: Process evaluation for public health interventions and research. An overview. In *Process Evaluation for Public Health Interventions and Research*. Edited by Steckler A, Linnan L. San Francisco: Jossey-Bass; 2002:1–24.

24. May CR: A rational model for assessing and evaluating complex interventions in health care. *BMC Health Serv Res* 2006, **6**:86.

25. Bleijenberg N, Ten Dam VH, Drubbel I, Numans ME, De Wit NJ, Schuurmans MJ: Development of a proactive care program (U-CARE) to preserve physical functioning of frail older people in primary care. *J Nurs Scholarsh* 2013, **45**:230–237.

26. Melis RJF, Van Eijken MIJ, Boon ME, Olde Rikkert MGM, Van Achterberg T: Process evaluation of a trial evaluating a multidisciplinary nurse-led home visiting programme for vulnerable older people. *Disabil Rehabil* 2010, **32**:937–946.

27. Metzelthin SF, Daniëls R, Van Rossum E, Cox K, Habets H, De Witte LP, Kempen GIJM: A nurse-led interdisciplinary primary care approach to prevent disability among community-dwelling frail older people: a large-scale process evaluation. *Int J Nurs Stud* 2013, **50**:1184–1196.

28. Stijnen MMN, Jansen MWJ, Vrijhoef HJM, Duimel-Peeters IGP: Development of a home visitation programme for the early detection of health problems in potentially frail community-dwelling older people by general practices. *Eur J Ageing* 2013, **10**:49–60.

29. Edmonds WA, Kennedy TD: *An Applied Reference Guide to Research Designs. Quantitative, Qualitative and Mixed Methods*. Thousand Oaks, CA: Sage; 2013.

30. Creswell JW, Fetters MD, Ivankova NV: Designing a mixed methods study in primary care. *Ann Fam Med* 2004, **2**:7–12.

31. Clark JP: How to peer review a qualitative manuscript. In *Peer Review in Health Sciences*. Secondth edition. Edited by Godlee F, Jefferson T. London: BMJ Books; 2003:219–235.

32. Dutch College of General Practitioners: *NHG-Praktijkwijzer Ouderenzorg. Dutch College of General Practioners-Manual Care for Older People in General Practice*. Utrecht: NHG; 2010.

33. Thomas DR: A general inductive approach for analyzing qualitative evaluation data. *Am J Eval* 2006, **27**:237–246.

34. Hsieh H, Shannon SE: Three approaches to qualitative content analysis. *Qual Health Res* 2005, **15**:1277–1288.

35. Bouman A, Van Rossum E, Habets H, Kempen GIJM, Knipschild P: Home visiting program for older people with health problems: process evaluation. *J Adv Nurs* 2007, **58**:425–435.

36. Bleijenberg N, Hester-Ten Dam V, Steunenberg B, Drubbel I, Numans ME, De Wit NJ, Schuurmans MJ: Exploring the expectations, needs and experiences of general practitioners and nurses towards a proactive and structured care programme for frail older patients: a mixed-methods study. *J Adv Nurs* 2013, **69**:2262–2273.

37. Evans C, Drennan V, Roberts J: Practice nurses and older people: a case management approach to care. *J Adv Nurs* 2005, **51**:343–352.

38. De Lepeleire J, Iliffe S, Mann E, Degryse J: Frailty: an emerging concept for general practice. *Br J Gen Pract* 2009, **59**:e177–e182.

39. Iliffe S, Orrell M: Identifying unmet health needs in older people: comprehensive screening is not the answer. *Br J Gen Pract* 2006, **56**:404–406.

40. Hasson H, Blomberg S, Dunér A: Fidelity and moderating factors in complex interventions: a case study of a continuum of care program for frail elderly people in health and social care. *Implement Sci* 2012, **7**:23.

41. Glasgow RE, Emmons KM: How can we increase translation of research into practice? Types of evidence needed. *Annu Rev Public Health* 2007, **28**:413–433.

42. Van Haastregt JCM, Van Rossum E, Diederiks JPM, De Witte LP, Voorhoeve PM, Crebolder HFJM: Process-evaluation of a home visit programme to prevent falls and mobility impairments among elderly people at risk. *Patient Educ Couns* 2002, **47**:301–309.

43. Struijs JN, Baan CA: Integrating care through bundled payments — lessons from the Netherlands. *N Engl J Med* 2011, **364**:990–991.

44. Kirkevold M, Bergland A: The quality of qualitative data: issues to consider when interviewing participants who have difficulties providing detailed accounts of their experiences. *Int J Qual Stud Health Well-being* 2007, **2**:68–75.

45. Sibthorpe BM, Glasgow NJ, Wells RW: Emergent themes in the sustainability of primary health care innovation. *Med J Aust* 2005, **183**:S77–S80.

9

Telephone counselling by nurses in Norwegian primary care out-of-hours services

Vivian Midtbø[1]* ⓘ, Guttorm Raknes[1,2,3] and Steinar Hunskaar[1,4]

Abstract

Background: The primary care out-of-hours (OOH) services in Norway are characterized by high contact rates by telephone. The telephone contacts are handled by local emergency medical communication centres (LEMCs), mainly staffed by registered nurses. When assessment by a medical doctor is not required, the nurse often handles the contact solely by nurse telephone counselling. Little is known about this group of contacts. Thus, the aim of this study was to investigate characteristics of encounters with the OOH services that are handled solely by nurse telephone counselling.

Methods: Nurses recorded ICPC-2 reason for encounter (RFE) codes and patient characteristics of all patients who contacted six primary care OOH services in Norway during 2014. Descriptive statistics and frequency analyses were applied.

Results: Of all telephone contacts ($n = 61,441$), 23% were handled solely by nurse counselling. Fever was the RFE most frequently handled (7.3% of all nurse advice), followed by abdominal pain, cough, ear pain and general symptoms. Among the youngest patients, 32% of the total telephone contacts were resolved by nurse advice compared with 17% in the oldest age group. At night, 31% of the total telephone contacts were resolved solely by nurse advice compared with 21% during the day shift and 23% in the evening. The share of nurse advice was higher on weekdays compared to weekends (mean share 25% versus 20% respectively).

Conclusion: This study shows that nurses make a significant contribution to patient management in the Norwegian OOH services. The findings indicate which conditions nurses should be able to handle by telephone, which has implications for training and routines in the LEMCs. There is the potential for more nurse involvement in several of the RFEs with a currently low share of nurse counselling.

Keywords: Telephone counselling, Primary health care, After-hours care, Nurse, Reason for encounter, International classification of primary care, Norway

Background

The primary care out-of-hours (OOH) services in Norway are characterized by high contact rates by telephone [1, 2]. Telephone contacts are handled by local emergency medical communication centres (LEMCs). The LEMCs are most commonly staffed by registered nurses, who triage the contacts and refer the patients to the appropriate level of care. If the patient's condition does not require assessment by an on-call medical doctor, the nurse often handles the contact solely by telephone counselling. In most of the 200 or so Norwegian primary care OOH districts, the only way to contact the OOH services is by first calling the LEMC. In several of the largest cities patients can contact OOH casualty clinics at all times (24/7), and may turn up directly without calling the LEMC in advance. Direct attendance is, however, not encouraged. The OOH system is organized within the primary health care sector, owned by the municipalities, and serves as a gatekeeper to the hospitals and other secondary health care, which are owned by

* Correspondence: vivian.midtbo@uni.no
[1]National Centre for Emergency Primary Health Care, Uni Research Health, Box 7810, NO 5020 Bergen, Norway
Full list of author information is available at the end of the article

the state. Medical responsibility for the services is mainly assumed by general practitioners (GPs) who take shifts in their own OOH district, and by interns serving their compulsory general practice period.

Because of the challenging geography in parts of Norway, with poor roads, islands without road connection to the mainland, and scarcely-populated rural areas, the size of the OOH organisations varies considerably. The smallest organisation serves a population of less than a thousand people, while the largest casualty clinic in the capital, Oslo, serves more than 600,000.

The nurses' contribution to the LEMCs constitutes an important part of the primary care OOH services. It is estimated that there were approximately 1.8 million contacts with the OOH services in Norway in 2013 (contact rate 0.36 per inhabitant per year) and about 75% of these contacts were telephone contacts to an LEMC (0.27 contacts per inhabitant per year) [2]. Based on estimates, less than a third of these contacts were handled solely by nurse telephone counselling, with a wide variation between the LEMCs [2]. Nevertheless, this is an important and large volume activity that educates and counsels patients and caregivers, and reduces casualty clinic workload.

Previous literature on nurses' triage and telephone counselling in the OOH services has focused on the quality of communication and decisions [3–7], the safety of telephone triage [8–10], the use of protocols and decision support tools [11–16], the process of giving advice over the telephone versus meeting the patient face-to-face [17], patients' satisfaction with the advice, and their understanding and adherence to the advice [18–21]. Overall, previous research has found nurse telephone triage to be safe [8, 21]. Nonetheless, the nature of telephone triage makes it a vulnerable part of the service because the patient is not seen face-to-face. The level of nurse telephone advice differs between countries, ranging from about 23% in Norway [2, 22] to 40–50% in the Netherlands and UK [18, 23]. Studies have found that the quality of the nurses' advice is satisfactory [7], and that the patients understand and follow the advice given by the nurses [19–21, 24].

Because the organisation of primary care services varies, it can be difficult to directly compare nurse telephone triage between countries. Many of the European countries have a strong primary care health service, where triage nurses cover the whole range of contact types. In countries where the primary care service is less built out, such as in the United States, additional nurse triage services are often run from the specialized health care services, aimed at specific patient groups, such as paediatrics [24–26]. However, some findings are similar across continents. Studies from Europe, the United States, New Zealand and Australia all show that children

constitute a large group of the OOH contacts across the different continents [2, 24, 27–29]. Frequent RFEs in this group include fever, vomiting, colds and cough [24, 27, 28].

There is a lack of epidemiological studies documenting which medical problems and reason for encounter (RFE) are resolved and handled by nurses' telephone advice in the OOH services. Some European studies include information on the RFE using the ICPC-2 classification system [29–32]. In a Dutch study, researchers explored nurse telephone triage using the determinants of independent advice and return consultation [33]. Other than this, we have not found studies that investigate the characteristics of telephone contacts that were resolved by nurse telephone counselling.

Therefore, the present study aimed to identify which RFEs are most frequently handled by nurse telephone counselling in the OOH services. More specifically, we wanted to investigate which diagnostic chapters and single codes within the ICPC-2 are most frequently resolved by nurse telephone advice and, in addition, to examine a number of patient characteristics and the time of the encounter.

Methods

A cross-sectional design was applied to this study. Patient data for one year (2014) were collected from six OOH districts to estimate the incidence of nurse counselling at different RFEs.

Setting

The data were collected within a sentinel network called "The Watchtowers", which was established in 2006 by the National Centre for Emergency Primary Health Care [34]. The network includes the LEMCs in a representative sample of seven Norwegian OOH districts, consisting of 18 municipalities. Information on all contact, both by telephone and direct attendance, to the participating centres is recorded in an online database (Zoho Creator®) by the nurses on duty at that time. For the purposes of this study we included six of the seven Watchtowers. One was excluded due to major organisational changes during the time of data collection. Approximately 150 nurses worked in the LEMCs of the six Watchtowers during the period of data collection. Most nurses working in the LEMCs were registered nurses, and had prior clinical work experience before starting work in the LEMC. All nurses in the study were involved in both telephone nurse counselling and clinical patient management in the OOH services where they worked. This means that, in addition to operating the telephone in the LEMC, they also had duties in regard to taking care of patients in the casualty clinic, such as triage, performing clinical observations, assisting the GP and laboratory work (such as blood samples and measuring

C-reactive protein). The nurses rotated between operating the telephone and undertaking clinical work in the casualty clinic.

Participants and study size

Study size was determined by the number of dispensed patient contacts handled by nurses in the Watchtower project in 2014. Because the study focusses on contacts handled solely by nurse telephone advice, only telephone contacts were included in the study. Contacts of direct attendance at the OOH service, or with unknown mode of contact, were excluded from the study.

Variables

RFE was registered using the ICPC-2 (International Classification of Primary Care, 2nd edition). The ICPC-2 allows for classification of the patient's RFE, problems, diagnoses and interventions. The ICPC system was developed by WONCA [35]. It was published in 1987 and has been used in Norway from 1992. In the Watchtower project, RFE is recorded based on the patient's complaint or stated reason for contacting the OOH service. In order to minimize systematic variation, nurses at all participating casualty clinics have received standardized instructions on how to register ICPC-2 RFE codes in accordance with the official manual (http://www.kith.no/sokeverktoy/icpc-2/bok/kontaktarsak.html).

"Action taken" was classified in one of the following categories: (A) Telephone consultation/advice with a nurse or other health personnel, not a doctor, (B) Telephone consultation with a doctor, (C) Medical examination by a doctor, (D) Consultation with other than a doctor, (E) Call-out with a doctor and ambulance, and (F) Home visit by GP. The main focus of this study is on the contacts registered in the category: "Telephone consultation/advice with a nurse or other health personnel, not a doctor". For the purposes of analysis, we refer to this as "contacts handled solely by nurse telephone counselling/advice".

Mode of contact was classified in one of the following categories: (A) Telephone contact, (B) Direct attendance at the casualty clinic, (C) Contact with health professionals, (D) Contact with national emergency medical communication centres, or (E) Other.

Time of day was registered by three time categories: Daytime 08.00–15.29, afternoon 15.30–22.59, and night 23.00–07.59. We also recorded day of the week (Monday-Sunday), and the patient's gender and age (under one year of age was recorded as "0"). The urgency level was assessed by the nurse in accordance with the Norwegian Index for Medical Emergency Assistance (Index) [36] into one of three urgency levels defined by colour: Red (acute), yellow (urgent) and green (non-urgent). Because of the low numbers of yellow (n = 892) and red

(n = 19) urgency level cases handled by nurse telephone counselling we combined all levels of urgency in the analysis.

Because many of the ICPC-2 codes involve similar symptoms, we grouped some related ICPC-2 codes (see Additional file 1).

Data analysis

All patient contact data from 2014 were downloaded from the online database (Zoho Creator®) in January 2015. Excel was used to organize the data before importing the files into IBM SPSS statistics 22. Descriptive statistics and frequency analyses were used. In addition, logistic regression analysis was used to explore the relationship between nurse telephone counselling and time of day, and age of the patients. Nurse telephone counselling (yes/no) was the dependent variable; time of day and age group were independent, categorical variables. Data are presented as frequencies, rate per 100,000 inhabitants/year and proportion of total telephone contacts.

Ethics

The Watchtower project has been approved by the Regional Committee for Medical and Health Research Ethics, the Norwegian Social Science Data Services, and by the privacy ombudsman for research for Uni Research. The Watchtower database is owned and managed by our institution, the National Centre for Emergency Primary Health Care. No patient identifiable data were recorded at any time. The database was only accessible to the researchers in the project.

Results
Participants and contact characteristics

The six OOH districts included in the study had a combined population of 218,205 inhabitants as of 1 January 2014. During the study period, there were a total of 77,863 medical encounters, equivalent to 357 contacts per 1000 inhabitants per year. Of these, 16,394 attended the casualty clinic directly without contacting the LEMC beforehand, and 28 records had unknown mode of contact. Because the scope of this study is telephone contacts, direct attendance and unknown mode of contact were not included in the analysis. This gave a total of 61,441 encounters, equivalent to 282 telephone contacts per 1000 inhabitants per year, to be included in the analysis. These accounted for 79% of the total medical contacts.

14,155 (23%) of the telephone contacts were handled solely by nurse telephone counselling (65 contacts per 1000 inhabitants per year). The remaining telephone contacts were handled as follows: 10.2% had a telephone consultation with a doctor (29 contacts per 1000 inhabitants per year), 58.3% had a medical examination by a doctor (164 contacts per 1000 inhabitants per year), 1.2% had a consultation with other than a doctor (3 contacts per 1000 inhabitants per year), 2.6% had a call-out with a doctor and an ambulance (7 contacts per 1000 inhabitants per year), 1.4% had a home visit by GP (4 contacts per 1000 inhabitants per year), and 3% were other actions.

The age of the patients in the group that received nurse advice ranged from 0 to 103 years (median age of 25 years, mean age of 30.7 years), and women constituted 57.7% of the records. 1702 cases (12%) had no registered ICPC-2 code, and in 601 (4.2%) cases age was not registered.

Telephone contacts handled by nurse counselling in the different ICPC-2 chapters

Table 1 presents the distribution of telephone contacts handled by nurse telephone counselling in each ICPC-2 chapter. Encounters related to chapter A (General and unspecified problems) were most frequently resolved by nurse telephone advice, followed by L (Musculoskeletal), D (Digestive), S (Skin) and R (Respiratory problems).

In chapters H (Ear) and X (Female genital), more than 30% of the total telephone contacts were resolved by nurse advice. In contrast, in chapters U (Urological) and K (Cardiovascular) less than 15% of the total telephone contacts were resolved by nurse advice.

The distribution of the ICPC-2 chapters most frequently handled by nurse telephone counselling was quite similar for day and evening shifts, with some small differences for the night shifts. Chapter A (General and unspecified) was the chapter most frequently resolved by nurse telephone advice during all three shifts. Chapters D (Digestive) and P (Psychological) constituted more of the contacts resolved by nurse telephone advice during night shifts compared to day and evening shifts.

RFE ICPC-2 codes most frequently handled by nurse telephone counselling

For telephone contacts handled solely by nurse telephone counselling, 447 different ICPC-2 codes were recorded.

Table 2 presents the 15 RFE ICPC-2 codes most often handled solely by nurse telephone counselling. A03 (Fever) was most prevalent, accounting for 7% of all nurse advice in this study, and constituted 39% of all nurse advice given in chapter A. This was followed by D01 (Abdominal pain), R05 (Cough), H01 (Ear pain) and A29 (General symptoms). In eight of the RFE codes in Table 2 more than 30% of the total telephone contacts were resolved by nurse telephone advice. S18 (Laceration/cut) had the lowest total share in this group, with 11% of the total telephone contacts resolved solely by a nurse.

Table 3 presents the 30 RFE groups and non-grouped RFE codes most frequently handled by nurse telephone

Table 1 Telephone contacts handled by nurse counselling within each ICPC-2 chapter

ICPC-2 chapter		Nurse telephone advice (n = 14,155)			Proportion	
		Frequency	(%)	Incidence	%	(95% CIs)
A	General and unspecified	2683	(19.9)	1230	27	(26–28)
L	Musculoskeletal	1788	(12.6)	819	21	(20–21)
D	Digestive	1681	(11.9)	770	27	(26–28)
S	Skin	1444	(10.2)	662	25	(24–26)
R	Respiratory	1392	(9.8)	638	18	(17–19)
P	Psychological	710	(5.0)	325	28	(26–30)
H	Ear	568	(4.0)	260	35	(32–37)
N	Neurological	543	(3.8)	249	21	(19–22)
U	Urological	448	(3.2)	205	13	(12–14)
F	Eye	437	(3.1)	200	19	(17–20)
W	Pregnancy and family planning	185	(1.3)	85	28	(24–31)
X	Female genital	168	(1.2)	77	31	(27–35)
K	Cardiovascular	160	(1.1)	73	10	(8–11)
T	Endocrine/metabolic/nutrition	77	(0.5)	35	22	(17–26)
Y	Male genital	63	(0.4)	29	19	(15–23)
Z	Social problems	59	(0.4)	27	23	(18–28)
B	Blood	47	(0.3)	22	27	(20–34)

The numbers are presented as frequency, incidence per 100,000 inhabitants/year and the proportion of total telephone contacts handled by nurse counselling per chapter

Table 2 The 15 RFE ICPC-2 codes most frequently handled by nurse telephone counselling

ICPC-2 code		Nurse telephone advice (n = 14,155)			Proportion
		Frequency	(%)	Incidence	%
A03	Fever	1039	(7.3)	476	32
D01	Abdominal pain	471	(3.3)	216	18
R05	Cough	431	(3.0)	198	22
H01	Ear pain	311	(2.2)	143	37
A29	General symptom	295	(2.1)	135	31
R21	Throat symptom	266	(1.9)	122	17
L17	Foot/toe symptom	240	(1.7)	110	23
D10	Vomiting	235	(1.7)	108	45
L02	Back symptom	228	(1.6)	104	23
N01	Headache	222	(1.6)	102	23
A13	Concern/fear of medical treatment	217	(1.5)	99	33
A97	Administrative contact	204	(1.4)	93	35
S18	Laceration/cut	197	(1.4)	90	11
D11	Diarrhoea	193	(1.4)	88	46
S06	Rash localized	187	(1.3)	86	37
	Other	7717	(54.5)	3536	21
	ICPC-2 unknown	1702	(12.0)	780	28
	All nurse telephone advice	14,155	(100)	6487	23

The numbers are presented as frequency, incidence per 100,000 inhabitants/year and the proportion of total telephone contacts handled by nurse counselling per code

counselling. The RFEs in Table 3, General symptoms, were most frequently resolved by nurse advice, followed by the non-grouped RFE code A03 (Fever) and the groups Lower limbs symptom/injury/condition, Respiratory symptom/condition, Abdominal pain and Fears/concerns and worries. Table 3 includes 80% of all nurse advice given with a known ICPC-2 code (71% of all advice given when contacts with unknown ICPC-2 code are included). Furthermore, it includes 168 (38%) of the 447 ICPC-2 codes in the category of telephone contacts handled by nurse telephone counselling.

The ten RFE ICPC-2 codes most frequently handled by nurse telephone counselling within different age groups are presented in Table 4. A03 (Fever) and D01 (Abdominal pain) were among the top ten RFEs most often handled by nurse telephone advice in all six age groups. However, fever was significantly more prevalent in the youngest age group (0–5 years old), both in relation to other symptoms within this age group, and in relation to the prevalence of fever in the other age groups. It accounted for 21.6% of all advice given in the youngest age group, compared to 2.0–7.4% in the other age groups. H01 (Ear pain) was also a frequent symptom in the two youngest age groups, but was not among the symptoms most frequently handled by nurse telephone counselling in any of the other age groups. L17 (Foot/toe symptom) and N01 (Headache) were present in the

three age groups from 6 to 59 years, while L02 (Back symptoms) was prevalent in all the age groups from 16 years and upwards. R02 (Shortness of breath/dyspnoea) was found among the most frequent RFEs only in the two oldest age groups.

The five ICPC-2 codes most frequently handled by nurse telephone counselling in the age group 0–5 years old constituted about 40% of the total advice given in this group. Equivalent figures were 25% in the age group 6–15 years, and about 15% in the other age groups.

Factors potentially influencing the decision to handle contacts solely by nurse telephone counselling

Of the contacts handled by nurse counselling, 34% were during daytime, 48% in the evening and 18% at night. Patients in the age groups 0–5 years and 30–59 years received 24 and 25% of all nurse advice respectively.

Table 5 presents the share of telephone contacts handled by nurse telephone counselling, stratified by age groups, genders and time of day. The results of the logistic regression analysis are displayed in Table 6. There were significant differences in the likelihood of handling telephone contacts by nurse counselling between the different times of the day, and between the different age groups ($P < 0.001$ for all variables).

A larger share of the total telephone contacts was handled solely by nurses in the night shifts, compared with

Table 3 RFE groups and non-grouped ICPC-2 codes most frequently handled by nurse telephone counselling

RFE group/non-grouped ICPC-2 RFE code	Nurse telephone advice (n = 14,155)			Proportion
	Frequency	(%)	Incidence	%
General symptom	1053	(7.4)	483	23
Fever	1039	(7.3)	476	32
Lower limbs symptom/injury/condition	656	(4.6)	301	20
Respiratory symptom/condition	621	(4.4)	285	16
Abdominal pain	579	(4.1)	265	17
Fears, concerns and worries	567	(4.0)	260	33
Diarrhoea/Vomiting	499	(3.5)	229	44
Upper limb symptom/injury/condition	472	(3.3)	216	18
Ear symptom/condition	413	(2.9)	189	37
Neck/back symptom/condition	394	(2.8)	181	24
Skin itching/rash	389	(2.7)	178	35
Urinary tract symptom/condition	299	(2.1)	137	13
Skin injury	298	(2.1)	137	14
Throat symptom/condition	279	(2.0)	128	17
Eye symptom/condition	262	(1.9)	120	17
Head/face symptom/condition	243	(1.7)	111	22
Anxiety	231	(1.6)	106	33
Administrative contact	204	(1.4)	93	35
Mouth/teeth symptom/condition	177	(1.3)	81	41
Animal/human bite	168	(1.2)	77	37
Depression	150	(1.1)	69	25
Limited function/disability	143	(1.0)	66	34
Insect bite/sting	132	(0.9)	60	37
Respiratory infections	116	(0.8)	53	19
Constipation	116	(0.8)	53	49
Nose/sinus symptom/condition	106	(0.7)	49	24
Vertigo/dizziness	106	(0.7)	49	22
Alcohol/substance abuse/addiction	104	(0.7)	48	23
Chest symptom/condition	102	(0.7)	47	8
Allergy/allergic reactions	79	(0.6)	36	19
Other	2456	(17.4)	1126	21
ICPC-2 unknown	1702	(12.0)	780	28
All	14,155	(100)	6487	23

The 30 RFE groups and non-grouped ICPC-2 RFE codes most frequently handled by nurse telephone counselling, presented as frequency, incidence per 100,000 inhabitants/year and the proportion of total telephone contacts handled by nurse counselling per code/group

the evening and day shifts. Furthermore, the share of nurse telephone advice decreased as the patients' age increased. In the age group 0–5 years, the total share of

nurse telephone counselling was 32%, compared with 17% in the two oldest age groups. In the youngest age group, the share of total telephone contacts handled by nurse counselling increased from 27% in daytime, to 47% at night. In the two oldest age groups, equivalent numbers were 16% during the day and 21 and 22% during the night.

In the age group 80 years and above, 41% of the contacts were made by health personnel on behalf of the patient (the most frequent RFEs being A13 (Concern medical treatment), A28 (Limited function) and A96 (Death)), while this was the case in only 0.2% of the contacts in the youngest age group. There were no significant differences in the share of telephone contacts resolved by nurse advice between the weekdays Monday to Friday. However, there was a significant difference in the share of nurse advice during the week (mean nurse advice share: 25% (95% CIs 24–25)) compared to the weekend (mean nurse advice share: 20% (95% CIs 19–20)). In regard to the patients' gender, only small variations were found; during the night 32% of all female contacts were resolved by nurse telephone advice compared with 29% of the male contacts.

Discussion

The findings reveal that a large number of telephone contacts to the LEMCs were handled solely by nurse telephone counselling. The RFEs most frequently resolved by nurse telephone advice were fever, abdominal pain, cough, ear pain and general symptoms. Telephone contacts were more often resolved by nurse advice at night compared to day and evening, and more often during the week (Monday to Friday) compared to the weekends. A higher share of contacts with the youngest patients were handled by nurse telephone counselling compared with the oldest age group.

Of the total telephone contacts in our data material, 23% were handled solely by nurse counselling, which is equivalent to 65 nurse advice per 1000 inhabitants/year. This correlates with findings from previous years in the Watchtower project [2, 22]. It is also comparable with a study from the Netherlands where a nurse alone handled 27.5% of the telephone contacts [33]. Other studies from the Netherlands and UK have found that nurses handle as much as 40–50% of the contacts by nurse telephone advice [18, 23]. However, the literature seems somewhat divided on the effectiveness of nurse telephone triage. In one of the Dutch studies, it was indicated that high proportions of nurse telephone consultations were associated with increased probability of follow-up contacts, which in turn could lead to increased workload [18]. In contrast, studies from the UK found that nurse telephone consultation could reduce GP workload without an increase in adverse events [23]. Previous studies on

Table 4 RFEs most frequently handled by nurse telephone counselling within different age groups

Age group	ICPC-2 code		Nurse telephone advice		
			Frequency	(%)	Incidence
0–5 years (n = 3364)	A03	Fever	727	(21.6)	333
	R05	Cough	176	(5.2)	81
	H01	Ear pain	156	(4.6)	71
	D10	Vomiting	117	(3.5)	54
	S06	Rash localized	85	(2.5)	39
	S07	Rash generalized	74	(2.2)	34
	D11	Diarrhoea	62	(1.8)	28
	D01	Abdominal pain	50	(1.5)	23
	R21	Throat symptom	50	(1.5)	23
	S12	Insect bite/sting	49	(1.5)	22
	ICPC-2 unknown		356		
6–15 years (n = 1435)	A03	Fever	106	(7.4)	49
	H01	Ear pain	68	(4.7)	31
	D01	Abdominal pain	63	(4.4)	29
	L17	Foot/toe symptom	47	(3.3)	22
	S13	Animal/human bite	43	(3.0)	20
	R21	Throat symptom	42	(2.9)	19
	R05	Cough	39	(2.7)	18
	S18	Laceration/cut	33	(2.3)	15
	N01	Headache	32	(2.2)	15
	S06	Rash localized	32	(2.2)	15
	ICPC-2 unknown		131		
16–29 years (n = 2904)	D01	Abdominal pain	150	(5.2)	69
	R21	Throat symptom	101	(3.5)	46
	A03	Fever	69	(2.4)	32
	A29	General symptom	68	(2.3)	31
	L02	Back symptom	63	(2.2)	29
	R05	Cough	62	(2.1)	28
	L17	Foot/toe symptom	53	(1.8)	24
	N01	Headache	51	(1.8)	23
	A97	Administrative contact	45	(1.5)	21
	S18	Laceration/cut	45	(1.5)	21
	ICPC-2 unknown		314		
30–59 years (n = 3528)	D01	Abdominal pain	130	(3.7)	60
	L02	Back symptom	99	(2.8)	45
	R05	Cough	92	(2.6)	42
	A29	General symptom	88	(2.5)	40
	L17	Foot/toe symptom	82	(2.3)	38
	A03	Fever	74	(2.1)	34
	A97	Administrative contact	72	(2.0)	33
	A13	Concern/fear medical treatment	67	(1.9)	31
	N01	Headache	65	(1.8)	30
	P02	Acute stress reaction	52	(1.5)	24
	ICPC-2 unknown		414		

Table 4 RFEs most frequently handled by nurse telephone counselling within different age groups *(Continued)*

60–79 years (n = 1255)	A13	Concern/fear medical treatment	40	(2.8)	18
	A29	General symptom	40	(2.8)	18
	R05	Cough	40	(2.8)	18
	D01	Abdominal pain	39	(2.8)	18
	L02	Back symptom	32	(2.3)	15
	R02	Shortness of breath/dyspnoea	31	(2.2)	14
	A97	Administrative contact	30	(2.1)	14
	A03	Fever	28	(2.0)	13
	P01	Feeling anxious/nervous/tense	26	(1.8)	12
	N17	Vertigo/dizziness	25	(1.8)	11
	ICPC-2 unknown		153		
80 + years (n = 915)	A13	Concern/fear medical treatment	41	(4.5)	19
	A28	Limited function/disability	36	(3.9)	16
	A96	Death	31	(3.4)	14
	R02	Shortness of breath/dyspnoea	31	(3.4)	14
	A97	Administrative contact	27	(3.0)	12
	A29	General symptom	26	(2.8)	12
	A03	Fever	20	(2.2)	9
	D01	Abdominal pain	20	(2.2)	9
	L02	Back symptom	18	(2.0)	8
	L14	Leg/thigh symptom	16	(1.7)	7
	ICPC-2 unknown		104		

The numbers are presented as frequency and incidence per 100,000 inhabitants/year

the Norwegian OOH services conclude that two-thirds of the callers receiving nurse advice did not re-contact the OOH services, own GP or other sections of the healthcare services in the following week [19]. In the Norwegian OOH services, however, advising the patient to contact his or her own GP in practice hours is also an appropriate way of handling contacts that can wait. It is important to add that differences in the organization of the healthcare systems can make it difficult to directly compare study results between countries. In some European countries (e.g. UK and the Netherlands), and in the United States, self-referral to a hospital emergency department is possible. In Norway, a referral via the primary care sector is needed. Furthermore, in the Danish OOH service, it is mostly doctors who handle the phone calls, which is different from the other countries mentioned above, where nurses, physician assistants or secretaries handle the calls.

In our study, one fifth of all contacts handled by nurse telephone counselling were contacts regarding ICPC-2 chapter A (General and unspecified). The high frequency in this chapter can to some extent be explained by the code A03 (Fever). Fever was the symptom most often handled by nurse telephone counselling, and constituted 39% of all nurse advice given in chapter A. To the best of our knowledge, not many studies examine which

RFEs telephone nurses resolve by advice. Findings from the United States also show that, among parents contacting a children's careline regarding a child with fever, a majority followed nurse advice for home care, in spite of initially preferring to have their child seen by a medical doctor [25]. Furthermore, a Dutch study exploring determinants associated with nurse telephone advice alone presents similar findings to those found in our study [33]. A large share of contacts regarding earache, vomiting and fever were handled by nurse telephone consultations, consistent with our findings. Contacts regarding chest pain had the lowest share of nurse telephone advice, which is also similar to our study in which cardiovascular problems have the lowest share of contacts handled by nurse consultation. Furthermore, the Dutch study found that a greater share of telephone contacts was handled by nurse counselling at night, compared to day and evening. Contacts by the youngest age groups were more often handled by nurse advice compared to the older age groups. These findings are also in line with ours.

Several factors probably contribute to the large share of contacts handled in our study by nurse telephone counselling during the night, compared to day and evenings (Table 5); less resources at night-time, a desire not to wake the doctor on call, or the nurses may be stricter on what they would assign to be seen by a doctor during

Table 5 Proportion of nurse telephone counselling in different age groups and between the genders

Proportion of total telephone contacts handled by nurse telephone counselling

					Distribution % (95% CIs)				
		Total % (95% CIs)		Daytime		Evening		Night	
All nurse telephone advice (n = 14,155)		23	(23–23)	21	(20–21)	23	(22–23)	31	(30–32)
Age group									
0–5	(n = 3364)	32	(31–33)	27	(26–28)	32	(31–32)	47	(46–49)
6–15	(n = 1435)	25	(24–26)	21	(20–22)	24	(23–25)	43	(40–45)
16–29	(n = 2904)	23	(22–24)	21	(20–22)	22	(22–23)	29	(28–30)
30–59	(n = 3528)	20	(19–21)	18	(18–19)	19	(19–19)	28	(27–29)
60–79	(n = 1408)	17	(16–18)	16	(15–16)	16	(16–17)	21	(20–22)
80≤	(n = 915)	17	(16–18)	16	(15–17)	17	(16–18)	22	(21–24)
Age unknown	(n = 601)	56	(56–58)	55	(53–57)	61	(59–64)	45	(41–50)
Sum	(n = 14,155)								
Gender									
Women	(n = 8163)	24	(24–24)	21	(21–21)	24	(23–24)	32	(32–33)
Men	(n = 5975)	22	(22–22)	20	(20–20)	22	(21–22)	29	(28–29)
Gender unknown	(n = 17)	16	(12–19)	20	(14–25)	11	(6–16)	16	(7–24)
Sum	(n = 14,155)								

The table presents the proportion of total telephone contacts handled by nurse counselling in different age groups and between the genders. Presented as total and for the different times of the day

the night. Furthermore, our findings reveal that the major increase in nurse telephone advice during the night was due to changes in the two youngest age groups (Table 5). The lower share of nurse counselling during the weekend compared to the weekdays could be explained by the fact that it was not possible to advise the patients to contact their own GP the same day - or the day after, if a Saturday.

One reassuring finding is that the rate of nurse telephone advice declined as the patients' age increased, indicating

Table 6 Likelihood (odds ratio) of nurse telephone counselling by time of day and age of patient

Variables	OR	95% CI	P-value
Time of day			
Daytime shift	Ref.		
Evening shift	1.11	1.10–1.16	<0.001
Night shift	1.81	1.71–1.92	<0.001
Age group			
0–5	Ref.		
6–15	0.71	0.66–0.77	<0.001
16–29	0.63	0.59–0.67	<0.001
30–59	0.53	0.50–0.56	<0.001
60–79	0.43	0.40–0.46	<0.001
80≤	0.45	0.41–0.49	<0.001

Logistic regression analyses using daytime shift and age group 0–5 years as reference

that nurses at the LEMCs make safe decisions. The oldest age group is a complex group, often presenting with several and more severe symptoms and comorbidities compared with younger patients. However, on our data form it is only possible to register one symptom per patient. Consequently, we do not know if the older patients in our group presented with a mix of symptoms. Another factor might be that contacts from the oldest age group were made much more frequently by health personnel on behalf of the patient. This means that the patient's condition had often already been evaluated before contacting the OOH service. Furthermore, the youngest age group appeared to be more predictable regarding which RFEs the nurse resolved by nurse telephone advice. The five most commonly reported RFEs handled by nurse counselling in the youngest age group (fever, cough, ear pain, vomiting and localized rash), constituted around 40% of all advice given in this group. The type of contacts handled by nurse telephone counselling in the other age groups varied more.

Findings from Europe, the United States, New Zealand and Australia all show that children constitute a large group of the OOH contacts [2, 24, 27–29]. Studies from Denmark, Scotland and the Netherlands also report that the youngest age group receives telephone advice more frequently than the older age groups [29, 33, 37], and involves symptoms similar to those found in our study [33]. In a study from England reporting on young people's (aged 0–15) use of the telephone service NHS Direct, it was found that 44 to 49% of all calls were resolved solely by nurse advice [28]. The high share of nurse telephone counselling in this group of patients might emphasize the parents' need for advice and reassurance when their children are ill. Measures to meet this need could include public health centres to provide information and guidance to parents on the most usual symptoms and conditions that affect infants and young children.

Strengths and limitations

This study adds important knowledge on the telephone nurses' work in the Norwegian LEMCs. To our knowledge, this is the first study of its kind in Norway. One of the strengths of the study is the high numbers of observations. The data analysed were collected over a period of one year which minimises the influence of seasonal variations. Reports from previous years of the Watchtower project show that the quality of the data is good; in 2013 only 1% of the total records lacked at least one piece of information. Records lacking RFE ICPC-2 codes are not included in this number, as RFE is not marked as "compulsory" in the registering program.

In 2014, RFE ICPC-2 codes were missing in 11% of the total records, with a wide variation between individual OOH clinics, ranging from 2 to 21% [1]. These differences could reflect varying practices between the clinics in registration of the data. Of the contacts handled by nurse telephone counselling, 12% had no RFE ICPC-2 code registered. Even though the nurses have received standard training in how to register RFEs, there is still a potential for bias, for instance by recording a potential diagnosis instead of the symptom presented by the patient. However, symptoms are the dominating RFEs in our data material. The RFE mode of the ICPC system has also been found to be a reliable tool for registering RFEs in the primary care sector [38].

Although this study provides an important picture of the nurses' contributions to the LEMCs, and which contacts are handled solely by nurse telephone counselling, it would have been of great interest to analyse associations between characteristics of the individual nurses and nurse telephone counselling strategies. However, such data were not available.

Comparing the Watchtower data with the yearly statistics on reimbursement claims in the Norwegian OOH service, it is evident that there is under-reporting of cases in the Watchtower database. Results from 2014 show a 15% deviation in the numbers of doctor consultations [1]. Under-reporting of nurse telephone consultations in our data material is probably of the same size, if not greater. However, it is not possible to calculate accurate figures. Reasons for missing records could be related to different priorities during busy times in the LEMCs.

When the Watchtower project was initiated in 2006, it was designed to be a representative sample of the OOH services in Norway [34]. However, changes in population and community structures might cause the representativeness to be less accurate in 2014 compared with 2006. In our study, we also excluded one of the Watchtowers due to organisational changes at the time of data collection.

Nonetheless, because of the high numbers of observations, we believe that our data still provide a reliable picture of contacts handled by nurse telephone counselling in the Norwegian OOH services.

Conclusion

This study shows that nurses contribute significantly to patient management in the Norwegian OOH services. The findings can guide the process of developing training programmes for work in the LEMCs, especially in regard to the type of contacts the nurses have to manage and master. There is the potential for more nurse involvement in several of the RFEs which currently have a low share of nurse counselling. Finally, the study identifies areas that need further investigation. This includes the high share of nurse counselling provided during the night, compared to daytime, and the differences in the share of nurse advice between the youngest and the oldest age groups.

Abbreviations
GP: General practitioner; ICPC-2: International classification of primary care; LEMC: Local emergency medical communication centre; OOH: Out-of-hours; RFE: Reason for encounter

Acknowledgements
The authors would like to thank all the staff in the Watchtower project involved in registering the activity in the LEMCs.

Funding
This research was funded by the National Centre for Emergency Primary Health Care, Uni Research Health, Box 7810, NO 5020 Bergen, Norway.

Authors' contributions
VM contributed to the design of the study, analysis and interpretation of the data, and drafting and revising the article. GR contributed to the design of the study, acquisition and interpretation of the data, and revising the article critically for intellectual content. SH contributed to the design of the study, interpretation of the data and revising the article for intellectual content. All authors have approved the final version.

Ethics approval and consent to participate
The Watchtower project has been approved by the Norwegian Social Science Data Services and by the privacy ombudsman for research for Uni Research (statement no. 2007/17049).
The project was considered by the Regional Committee for Medical and Health Research Ethics (REC West, Bergen, statement no. 2012/1094) which concluded that there was no need for formal dispensation from professional secrecy requirements or consent to participate. This is according to national regulations, since the data were anonymised [39].

The database was only accessible to the researchers in the project. The Watchtower database is owned and managed by our institution, the National Centre for Emergency Primary Health Care. Researchers within the institution can use data from the Watchtower database for research projects. The leader of the Watchtower project gives the researchers access to the data needed for each specific project. The researchers do not need an ethical clearance to access these data, as this is already approved on behalf of the institution.

Consent for publication
Not applicable.

Competing interests
The authors declare that they have no competing interests.

Author details
[1]National Centre for Emergency Primary Health Care, Uni Research Health, Box 7810, NO 5020 Bergen, Norway. [2]Regional Medicines Information & Pharmacovigilance Centre (RELIS), University Hospital of North Norway, Box 79, NO 9038 Tromsø, Norway. [3]Raknes Research, Myrdalskogen 243, NO 5117 Ulset, Norway. [4]Department of Global Public Health and Primary Care, University of Bergen, Box 7804, NO 5018 Bergen, Norway.

References
1. Eikeland OJ, Raknes G, Hunskår S. Vakttårnprosjektet. Epidemiologiske data frå legevakt. Samlerapport for 2014. Rapport nr. 3–2015. [The Watchtower project. Epidemiological data from OOH services 2014]. Bergen: National Centre for Emergency Primary Health Care, Uni Research Health; 2015.
2. Eikeland OJ, Raknes G, Tønsaker S, Hunskår S. Vakttårnprosjektet. Epidemiologiske data frå legevakt. Samlerapport for 2013. Rapport nr. 3–2014. [The Watchtower project. Epidemiological data from OOH services 2013]. Bergen: National Centre for Emergency Primary Health Care, Uni Research Health; 2014.
3. Derkx HP, Rethans JJ, Muijtjens AM, Maiburg BH, Winkens R, van Rooij HG, et al. Quality of clinical aspects of call handling at Dutch out of hours centres: cross sectional national study. BMJ. 2008;337:a1264.
4. Derkx HP, Rethans JJ, Maiburg BH, Winkens RA, Muijtjens AM, van Rooij HG, et al. Quality of communication during telephone triage at Dutch out-of-hours centres. Patient Educ Couns. 2009;74:174–8.
5. Derkx HP, Rethans JJ, Knottnerus JA, Ram PM. Assessing communication skills of clinical call handlers working at an out-of-hours centre: development of the RICE rating scale. Br J Gen Pract. 2007;57:383–7.
6. Hansen EH, Hunskaar S. Telephone triage by nurses in primary care out-of-hours services in Norway: an evaluation study based on written case scenarios. BMJ Qual Saf. 2011;20:390–6.
7. Nyen B, Hansen EH, Bondevik GT. Kvaliteten på sykepleieres håndtering av telefonhenvendelser til legevakt. [The quality of nurses' handling of telephone contacts to the out-of-hours service]. Sykepleien Forskning. 2009; 3:220–6.
8. Huibers L, Smits M, Renaud V, Giesen P, Wensing M. Safety of telephone triage in out-of-hours care: a systematic review. Scand J Prim Health Care. 2011;29:198–209.
9. Giesen P, Ferwerda R, Tijssen R, Mokkink H, Drijver R, van den Bosch W, et al. Safety of telephone triage in general practitioner cooperatives: do triage nurses correctly estimate urgency? Qual Saf Health Care. 2007;16:181–4.
10. Lattimer V, George S, Thompson F, Thomas E, Mullee M, Turnbull J, et al. Safety and effectiveness of nurse telephone consultation in out of hours primary care: randomised controlled trial. The South Wiltshire Out of Hours Project (SWOOP) Group. BMJ. 1998;317:1054–9.
11. Mayo AM, Chang BL, Omery A. Use of protocols and guidelines by telephone nurses. Clin Nurs Res. 2002;11:204–19.
12. Holmström I. Decision aid software programs in telenursing: not used as intended? Experiences of Swedish telenurses. Nurs Health Sci. 2007;9:23–8.
13. O'Cathain A, Sampson FC, Munro JF, Thomas KJ, Nicholl JP. Nurses' views of using computerized decision support software in NHS Direct. J Adv Nurs. 2004;45:280–6.
14. Dowding D, Mitchell N, Randell R, Foster R, Lattimer V, Thompson C. Nurses' use of computerised clinical decision support systems: a case site analysis. J Clin Nurs. 2009;18:1159–67.
15. Kawamoto K, Houlihan CA, Balas EA, Lobach DF. Improving clinical practice using clinical decision support systems: a systematic review of trials to identify features critical to success. BMJ. 2005;330:765.
16. Ernesäter A, Holmström I, Engström M. Telenurses' experiences of working with computerized decision support: supporting, inhibiting and quality improving. J Adv Nurs. 2009;65:1074–83.
17. Purc-Stephenson RJ, Thrasher C. Nurses' experiences with telephone triage and advice: a meta-ethnography. J Adv Nurs. 2010;66:482–94.
18. Huibers L, Koetsenruijter J, Grol R, Giesen P, Wensing M. Follow-up after telephone consultations at out-of-hours primary care. J Am Board Fam Med. 2013;26:373–9.
19. Hansen EH, Hunskaar S. Understanding of and adherence to advice after telephone counselling by nurse: a survey among callers to a primary emergency out-of-hours service in Norway. Scand J Trauma Resusc Emerg Med. 2011;19:8.
20. Purc-Stephenson RJ, Thrasher C. Patient compliance with telephone triage recommendations: a meta-analytic review. Patient Educ Couns. 2012;87:135–42.
21. Blank L, Coster J, O'Cathain A, Knowles E, Tosh J, Turner J, et al. The appropriateness of, and compliance with, telephone triage decisions: a systematic review and narrative synthesis. J Adv Nurs. 2012;68:2610–21.
22. Hansen EH, Zakariassen E, Hunskaar S. Sentinel monitoring of activity of out-of-hours services in Norway in 2007: an observational study. BMC Health Serv Res. 2009;9:123.
23. Bunn F, Byrne G, Kendall S. The effects of telephone consultation and triage on healthcare use and patient satisfaction: a systematic review. Br J Gen Pract. 2005;55:956–61.
24. Light PA, Hupcey JE, Clark MB. Nursing telephone triage and its influence on parents' choice of care for febrile children. J Pediatr Nurs. 2005;20:424–9.
25. Bunik M, Glazner JE, Chandramouli V, Emsermann CB, Hegarty T, Kempe A. Pediatric telephone call centers: how do they affect health care use and costs? Pediatrics. 2007;119:305–13.
26. Keatinge D, Rawlings K. Outcomes of a nurse-led telephone triage service in Australia. Int J Nurs Pract. 2004;11:5–12.
27. St George I, Cullen M, Gardiner L, Karabatsos G. Universal telenursing triage in Australia and New Zealand. A new primary health service. Aust Fam Physician. 2008;3:476–9.
28. Cook EJ, Randhawa G, Large S, Guppy A, Chater AM, Pang D. Young people's use of NHS Direct: a national study of symptoms and outcome of calls for children aged 0–15. BMJ Open. 2013;3:e004106.
29. Leutgeb R, Laux G, Hermann K, Gutscher A, Szecsenyi J, Kuhlein T. Patient care in an out-of-hours care practice - A descriptive study of the CONTENT project. Gesundheitswesen. 2014;76:836–9.
30. Huibers LA, Moth G, Bondevik GT, Kersnik J, Huber CA, Christensen MB, et al. Diagnostic scope in out-of-hours primary care services in eight European countries: an observational study. BMC Fam Pract. 2011;12:30.
31. Moth G, Huibers L, Christensen MB, Vedsted P. Out-of-hours primary care: a population-based study of the diagnostic scope of telephone contacts. Fam Pract. 2016;33:504–9.
32. Raknes G, Hunskaar S. Reasons for encounter by different levels of urgency in out-of-hours emergency primary health care in Norway: a cross sectional study. BMC Emerg Med. 2017;17:19.
33. Moll van Charante EP, ter Riet G, Drost S, van der Linden L, Klazinga N, Bindels PJ. Nurse telephone triage in out-of-hours GP practice: determinants of independent advice and return consultation. BMC Fam Pract. 2006;7:74.
34. Hansen EH, Hunskaar S. Development, implementation, and pilot study of a sentinel network ("The Watchtowers") for monitoring emergency primary health care activity in Norway. BMC Health Serv Res. 2008;8:62.
35. Lamberts H, Wood M. The birth of the International Classification of Primary Care (ICPC) Serendipity at the border of Lac Léman. Fam Pract. 2002;19:433–5.
36. Norwegian Medical Association. Norsk indeks for medisinsk nødhjelp (Norwegian Index of Emergency Medical Assistance). 3rd ed. Stavanger: Laerdal Medical A/S- The Laerdal Foundation for Acute Medicine; 2009.

10

The effectiveness of a primary care nursing-led dietary intervention for prediabetes

Kirsten J. Coppell[1*] ⓘ, Sally L. Abel[2], Trish Freer[3], Andrew Gray[4], Kiri Sharp[1], Joanna K. Norton[1], Terrie Spedding[3], Lillian Ward[3] and Lisa C. Whitehead[5]

Abstract

Background: Primary care nurse-led prediabetes interventions are seldom reported. We examined the implementation and feasibility of a 6-month multilevel primary care nurse-led prediabetes lifestyle intervention compared with current practice in patients with prediabetes, with weight and glycated haemoglobin (HbA1c) as outcomes.

Methods: This study used a convergent mixed methods design involving a 6-month pragmatic non-randomised pilot study with a qualitative process evaluation, and was conducted in two neighbouring provincial cities in New Zealand, with indigenous Māori populations comprising 18.2% and 23.0%, respectively. Participants were non-pregnant adults aged ≤ 70 years with newly diagnosed prediabetes (HbA1c 41-49 mmol/mol), body mass index (BMI) ≥ 25 kg/m^2 and not prescribed Metformin. A structured dietary intervention tool delivered by primary care nurses with visits at baseline, 2–3 weeks, 3 months and 6 months was implemented in four intervention practices. Four control practices continued to provide usual care. Primary quantitative outcome measures were weight and HbA1c. Linear and quantile regression models were used to compare each outcome between the two groups at follow-up. Qualitative data included: observations of nurse training sessions and steering group meetings; document review; semi-structured interviews with a purposive sample of key informants ($n = 17$) and intervention patients ($n = 20$). Thematic analysis was used.

Results: One hundred fifty-seven patients with prediabetes enrolled (85 intervention, 72 control), 47.8% female and 31.2% Māori. Co-morbidities were common, particularly hypertension (49.7%), dyslipidaemia (40.1%) and gout (15.9%). Baseline and 6 month measures were available for 91% control and 79% intervention participants. After adjustment, the intervention group lost a mean 1.3 kg more than the control group ($p < 0.001$). Mean HbA1c, BMI and waist circumference decreased in the intervention group and increased in the control group, but differences were not statistically significant. Implementation fidelity was high, and it was feasible to implement the intervention in busy general practice settings. The intervention was highly acceptable to both patients and key stakeholders, especially primary care nurses.

Conclusions: Study findings confirm the feasibility and acceptability of primary care nurses providing structured dietary advice to patients with prediabetes in busy general practice settings. The small but potentially beneficial mean weight loss among the intervention group supports further investigation.

Keywords: Prediabetes, Dietary modification, Weight loss, Structured intervention implementation, General practice, Primary care nursing, Indigenous population, Pragmatic clinical trial, Outcome and process assessment, Qualitative evaluation

* Correspondence: kirsten.coppell@otago.ac.nz
[1]Edgar Diabetes and Obesity Research, Department of Medicine, Dunedin School of Medicine, University of Otago, PO Box 56, Dunedin 9054, New Zealand
Full list of author information is available at the end of the article

Background

Diabetes prevalence continues to increase worldwide [1, 2]. Effective prediabetes management strategies to reduce increasing diabetes-related costs, both societal and individual are urgently needed. Amongst New Zealand adults aged ≥15 years the prevalence of diabetes and prediabetes is 7.0% and 25.5%, respectively [3]. Of those with prediabetes, each year an estimated 5–10% develop type 2 diabetes mellitus (T2DM) [4, 5], with most eventually developing the condition, particularly those who are overweight or obese [6].

In New Zealand screening for diabetes and prediabetes is recommended as part of cardiovascular risk assessment for men aged ≥45 years and women aged ≥55 years, and at younger ages for high risk groups, including indigenous Māori, Pacific, Indo-Asian, obese, those with a family history of diabetes and women with previous gestational diabetes [7]. It is assumed that general practitioners (GPs) and primary care nurses will deliver effective nutrition advice for the management of prediabetes and prevention of diabetes. However, although good clinical trial evidence demonstrates lifestyle advice prevents progression from prediabetes to T2DM [8, 9], similar results have not been demonstrated in 'real-world' general practice settings [10], partly because few studies have examined the translation of diabetes prevention clinical trial evidence into the primary care setting [11].

Of the few primary care-based diabetes prevention lifestyle interventions, most have utilised GPs [12], dietitians [13] or multidisciplinary teams with nutritionists, exercise specialists and lifestyle coaches [14–17], which are costly. Yet approaches to cholesterol-lowering dietary advice in the general practice setting in the 1980s and 1990s and a recent general practice-based weight loss study suggest it is better if a nurse takes the lead for lifestyle advice with the GP in a supportive role [18, 19].

This paper reports on the results of the Prediabetes Intervention Package (PIP) in primary care pilot study which aimed to examine the implementation and feasibility of a multilevel primary care nurse-led prediabetes lifestyle intervention compared with current practice on weight and glycated haemoglobin in patients with prediabetes, at 6 months.

Methods

This primary care-based prediabetes intervention study used a convergent mixed methods design [20], combining a 6-month pragmatic non-randomised quantitative pilot study [ACTRN12615000806561] with a qualitative process evaluation to assess intervention implementation.

Setting

The study was conducted in general practices and community settings in two neighbouring provincial cities in

New Zealand with populations of 57,240 (18.2% Māori) and 73,245 (23.0% Māori) in 2013 [21]. Māori, the indigenous population of New Zealand, have high rates of prediabetes (30.4%) and diabetes (9.8%) [3].

In New Zealand primary medical care is delivered by GPs in mostly group, but some solo practices. Almost all practices have government capitation funding with varying levels of patient co-payment, depending on age and socioeconomic status of patients and the practice's business model. Most GP practices employ primary care nurses and belong to a Primary Health Organisation (PHO). PHOs are not-for-profit organisations that provide primary health services either directly or through their provider members. There was a single PHO in the study region.

For this study, member general practices employing primary care nurses were recruited. For operational reasons and to minimise potential contamination between the two arms of the trial, four intervention practices were located in one city and four control practices in the other. Practice patient characteristics were similar between arms, and included those with a high proportion of Māori and those with a high deprivation index score [22].

Participants and recruitment

Eligible participants were non-pregnant adults aged ≤70 years with newly diagnosed prediabetes (HbA1c 41-49 mmol/mol or fasting plasma glucose 6.1–6.9 mmol/L) [7], a body mass index (BMI) above 25 kg/m^2, not prescribed Metformin and able to communicate in English. Newly diagnosed prediabetes meant a diagnosis within the previous 6 months and no documented appointment to discuss prediabetes management following a positive test. Diagnosis followed either screening due to identified risk of prediabetes or cardiovascular risk assessment [7].

Practice patient management systems identified and generated a list of existing eligible patients. Eligible patients received a study invitation letter from their practice and a follow-up phone call from the primary care nurse. An appointment was arranged with those agreeing to participate. Patients subsequently diagnosed with prediabetes who fulfilled the eligibility criteria were invited to participate in the study at time of diagnosis. Patient recruitment occurred between August 2014 and April 2015.

Intervention

The intervention was informed by a literature review of lifestyle interventions and designed in collaboration with the PHO. The focus was to provide patients and their family/whānau[1] with an understanding of healthy eating principles and enhance empowerment around dietary choices. The multilevel package comprised six components:

1. Health professional training and support - evidence-based culturally appropriate training package for primary care and community nurses, with dietitian support.

The intervention primary care and community education nurses participated in a 6-h theoretical and practical training course, which included nutrition principles, dietary assessment, goal setting, the context within which nutrition advice is given and how to measure height, weight and waist circumference. Course dietary content was based on successful translation of diabetes treatment and prevention guidelines into a clinical trial setting in the Lifestyle Over and Above Drugs in Diabetes (LOADD) study [23]. Primary care dietary assessment, internal and external factors affecting food choices, cultural influences on diet, behaviour change and effective communication of dietary information were included in the course, which was delivered by study investigators (KC, KS and JN) with input from a local dietitian. A training manual provided reference material and research protocols.

A follow-up 2-h session was held to review study protocols, answer questions and make any necessary practical changes to the protocol. A further 2-h update course was run at 6 months, using case studies delivered by intervention primary care nurses to illustrate particular dietary consultation challenges.

A dietitian arranged monthly case review meetings with the primary care nurses. Similarly, a liaison nurse (TS) visited participating nurses at least monthly to assess intervention adherence and provide advice. Dietitian and nurse visits alternated, and both were available by email and phone to answer questions or discuss specific cases.

2. Individual patient education - dietary assessment, goal setting and dietary advice sessions

After providing written consent, patient participants were offered an initial 30 min dietary session with the primary care nurse and encouraged to bring family/whā-nau. Immediately prior to their nurse appointment, they completed a brief dietary assessment. We used Starting the Conversation (STC):Diet, a validated eight-item simplified food frequency instrument designed for use in primary care and health-promotion settings [24]. STC:Diet was minimally modified, with permission, for the New Zealand context. We changed the word 'sodas' to 'soft drinks', and added a traffic light system to indicate healthy, not-so-healthy and unhealthy dietary habits. The nurse reviewed the STC:Diet responses; asked additional dietary prompt questions (developed by KS and JN); sought additional contextual information, such as household membership

and budget, who purchased household foods and specific dietary requirements/ choices such as vegetarianism; and took anthropometric measures (height, weight and waist circumference). We called these additional questions the Detailed Dietary Assessment (DDA). A weight goal of a 5–10% loss over 6 months was calculated. Responses to the STC:Diet and DDA informed three dietary goals, negotiated with the participant, and individualised tailored dietary advice. Funded 15 min follow-up appointments were arranged 3 weeks later, then at 3 and 6 months.

3. Key messages and consistent opportunistic reminders

The three dietary goals were recorded in the practice patient management system for each participant. This facilitated opportunistic targeted advice and guidance by participants' GPs, thus reinforcing dietary information provided by the nurses. The goals were reviewed and updated accordingly, at follow-up nurse appointments.

4. Nutritionally supportive primary care environment

Prior to study beginning, each intervention practice was visited to discuss ways to enhance dietary messages provided by nurses. Specifically, the dietary information provided in pamphlets, magazines and posters in the waiting rooms were reviewed and updated, so dietary messages were appropriate and consistent. Provision of magazines that supported reputable dietary messages and active living, hobbies and sports, and posters promoting fruit and vegetables, such as those offered by Vegetables.co.nz (www.vegetables.co.nz), were encouraged.

5. Community-based group education for patients and their family/whānau

Community group nutrition education courses consisted of six weekly sessions of 1–1.5 h each. Courses were delivered by community nurses from the local Sports Trust at various times and locations and aimed to provide generic nutrition knowledge and advice. Content was developed by the research dietitian (KS), in conjuction with Sports Trust personnel. Topics included prevention of progression to diabetes, food groups, label reading, eating out, menu planning and food safety.

6. Written Patient Resources

Readily available patient resources were utilised. The key resource was the Diabetes New Zealand booklet, *Diabetes and healthy food choices* [25], used successfully in the LOADD study [23], where participants found the information clearly presented and easily understood.

Control practices (usual care)

Primary care nurses at control practices continued to provide dietary advice to patients with prediabetes in their usual way. Usual care is based on the Prediabetes Advice guidance circulated to all general practices by the New Zealand Ministry of Health in August 2013 [26]. Lifestyle advice is based on goal setting, a weight loss of 0.5-1 kg per week and a long term loss of at least 5% in those who are overweight or obese, healthy eating, aiming for 30 min of moderate intensity exercise most days, regular follow-up and a repeat HbA1c test following 3 months of 'lifestyle therapy', then 6–12 monthly. This typically consists of unstructured advice and sometimes a 'green prescription' [27], which is a nationwide initiative designed to increase physical activity (http://www.health.govt.nz/our-work/preventative-health-wellnes s/physical-activity/green-prescriptions).

Physical activity - intervention and control practices

All participating patients were given standard advice on physical activity, that is, 30 min of physical activity of moderate intensity on most, if not all, days of the week. Each participant was also given a 'Be Active Every Day' pamphlet [28].

Quantitative data

The primary outcome measures were weight and HbA1c. Other outcome measures included waist circumference, body mass index, blood pressure and lipids. The patient management system was modified to facilitate the recording of study data at baseline and 6 months. Most data were collected as part of routine primary care practice, and included demographic and medical details, lifestyle information (smoking, alcohol, diet and physical activity), blood pressure, anthropometric measures (height, weight and waist circumference) and laboratory measures (HbA1c, glucose, lipids, urate and liver enzymes). Additional non-routine intervention data included dietary assessment, dietary goals and weight goal.

Participating nurses were trained on standard practices for measuring anthropometry and blood pressure. General practice stadiometers, weighing scales and sphygmomanometers were calibrated. A Lufkin Executive thinline (2 m) tape measure was provided to each practice for measuring waist circumference. Shoes were removed before conducting anthropometric measurements. Weight was measured with patients wearing one layer of light clothing and waist circumference was measured with the tape measure against the skin. Nurses were asked to take duplicate measures.

Sample size calculations

A standard deviation of 18 kg for weight and a correlation between baseline and follow-up weights of 0.95 were obtained using data from the 2008/09 New Zealand Adult Nutrition Survey [29] and 2005 data from the Otago Diabetes Register [30], retrospectively. To detect a difference of 4 kg in weight (equivalent to a 5% relative difference in weight loss for a patient initially weighing 80 kg) at 6 months with 90% power using a two-sided test at the 5% level, required 42 people in each group with complete data. After incorporating design effects based on a mean cluster size of 21 (based on 4 practices in each arm) and an intraclass correlation (ICC) of 0.03, and allowing for a 20% loss to follow-up, required 84 people in each arm of the study at baseline.

Statistical analysis

Demographic and health characteristics were compared between the two groups using Chi-squared and Fisher's Exact tests at baseline and follow-up, without adjusting for practice cluster effects. Similarly retention at 6 months was compared within each group. Linear regression models were used to compare each outcome between the two groups at follow-up, except for GGT for which quantile regression was used due to extreme skew. Each outcome was adjusted for baseline values, sex, alcohol consumption, family history of T2DM, and ethnicity. The number of clusters was small, and Huber-White robust standard errors were used with Froot's extension for clustering at the practice level. Bias corrected confidence intervals were obtained from 1000 bootstrapped samples for each outcome (random number seeds were specified for each outcome in the statistical analysis plan prior to all analyses). Standard model diagnostics were used including assessing residual normality and homoscedasticity using histograms and scatterplots of residuals. Log-transformations were investigated and used where this improved residual diagnostics. Multinomial logistic regression was used to compare weight change categories ($\geq 5\%$ weight loss; $< 5\%$ weight loss; no weight change or weight gain) with clustered robust standard errors. As this was a pilot study no formal adjustments were made for multiple comparisons. Stata 14.2 was used for all analyses with two-sided $p < 0.05$ considered statistically significant.

Process evaluation

A summative process evaluation using qualitative research methods was undertaken to explore, whether the prediabetes intervention was implemented as intended (intervention fidelity), the feasibility of implementing the intervention package in busy primary care settings and what aspects of intervention implementation worked well and what was challenging from both stakeholder and patient perspectives. Data were collected through three pathways: Observation of nurse training sessions and monthly steering group meetings with comprehensive note taking, document review, and interviews with key informants (n

= 17) and intervention patients ($n = 20$). Data were collected by SA, an independent health researcher with 20 years qualitative research experience in multi-ethnic communities, and who was not involved in the intervention design and implementation.

All interviewees gave prior written consent and all agreed to audio-taping. Interviews were semi-structured with open-ended questions (Additional file 1).

Key informants were purposefully selected [31] as key players in intervention implementation, and included all intervention primary care nurses ($n = 11$). All those approached agreed to participate. Interviews were undertaken at the workplace or another chosen venue between 30 June and 21 August 2015. Primary care nurses who worked together were interviewed in pairs. They were asked about their intervention role and experiences, perceptions of successes and challenges, and recommendations for future development. Comprehensive notes were taken at the interview and after re-listening to audio-recordings. Preliminary findings from analysis of these interviews were presented to participants as a group and feedback encouraged. Written notes from this session were included in the final dataset.

Patients who had completed the six-month intervention were purposefully selected to ensure a range of demographic profiles and glycaemic outcomes (Table 1). They were first approached by their primary care nurse and, if willing to participate, contact details were given to SA. Four declined; two were too busy and two gave no reason. SA phoned those wishing to participate to explain the research and arrange an interview. All were interviewed individually between 7 August and 15 December 2015 at their chosen location; their own home ($n = 17$) or the researcher's workplace ($n = 3$). Although they had the option of including a support person, none did. Interviews explored patients' experiences of the intervention, both enjoyable and challenging. Close attention was paid to cultural etiquette when interviewing Māori and Pacific patients. Total interview time was 45–60 min. At interview conclusion, patients were given a $NZ20 gift voucher in appreciation of their time. All patient interview audio-recordings were transcribed by an external transcriber who had signed a confidentiality agreement. Transcripts were read thoroughly by SA to check for accuracy. The data were anonymised and password protected.

Qualitative data analysis
The data were analysed using thematic analysis [32]. SA, LW and KC undertook multiple close readings of the transcripts. Data coding and initial theme development were undertaken by SA, reviewed by LW and KC and discussed together over the course of several meetings. Themes were derived inductively. Key informant and patient interview data were initially coded and analysed

Table 1 Demographic characteristics and glycaemic outcomes for the 20 intervention participants who were interviewed

Patient participants	Normoglycaemia	Prediabetes	Diabetes	Total
Māori female		4		4
Māori male	1	3	1	5
NZ European female	2	2	1	5
NZ European male	1	3		4
Pacific female		1		1
Pacific male		1		1
Total	4	14	2	20

separately, then combined, synthesised and final key themes and sub-themes agreed by these three researchers.

Results
Characteristics of patient participants
Figure 1 shows the flow of the 157 participants enrolled in the study. Baseline characteristics and retention rates are shown in Table 2. At baseline there were slightly more men, and almost one-third were Māori. A family history of T2DM was common (39.5%), as were diabetes-associated co-morbidities - hypertension (49.7%), dyslipidaemia (40.1%), gout (15.9%), ischaemic heart disease (9.6%) and stroke (4.4%). Among women, 5.4% had previous gestational diabetes. Baseline and 6 month measures were available for 91% control participants and 79% intervention participants.

Clinical outcomes
Table 3 shows the clinical outcomes at baseline and 6 months. Overall, the control group gained weight (0.8 kg), whereas mean weight for the intervention group decreased (1.3 kg), a 2.2 kg difference. After adjustment for baseline measures the intervention group lost a mean 1.3 kg more than the control ($p < 0.001$). Among the intervention group, 65% lost some weight, and 18% achieved at least a 5% weight loss compared with 32% and 5%, respectively, of those in the control group (unadjusted multinomial regression Wald $p < 0.001$). Small decreases in both HbA1c and waist circumference were observed in the intervention group, compared with small increases in the control group. These differences were not statistically significant. At 6 months four intervention participants and eight control participants had progressed to T2DM.

Implementation fidelity
Implementation fidelity was high. All intervention primary care nurses attended the training and update sessions. They delivered the brief dietary assessment, goal setting and appropriate dietary advice, as per the study protocol. This was confirmed, during key informant interviews, by

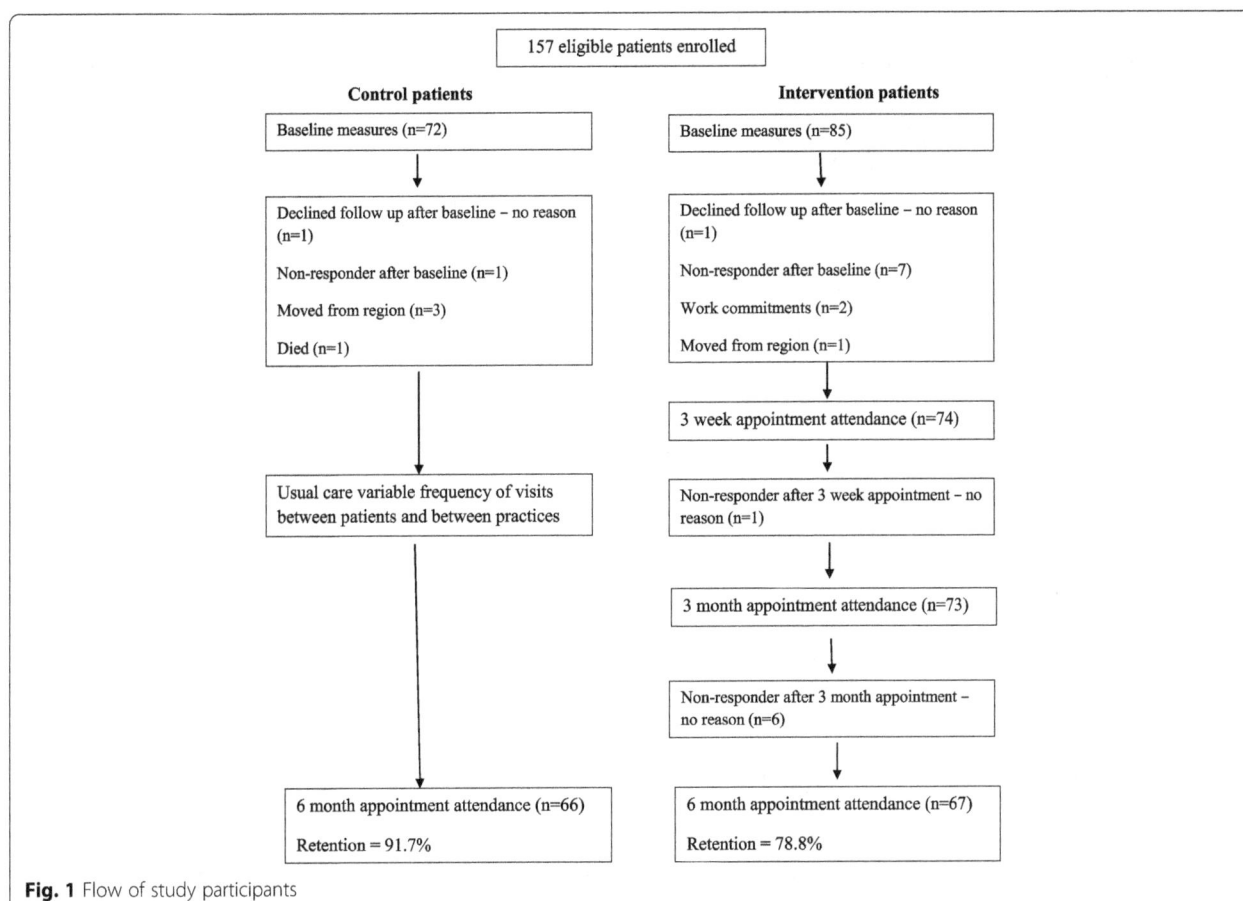

```
                          ┌─────────────────────────────┐
                          │  157 eligible patients enrolled  │
                          └─────────────────────────────┘

         Control patients                              Intervention patients

    ┌──────────────────────┐              ┌──────────────────────┐
    │ Baseline measures (n=72) │           │ Baseline measures (n=85) │
    └──────────────────────┘              └──────────────────────┘
```

Fig. 1 Flow of study participants

the support dietitian and liaison nurse, who independently checked in with each practice monthly to offer support to the nurses and ensure protocol compliance. The intervention practices reinforced healthy eating messages with appropriate seating, magazines in the waiting room and posters. Five separate group education courses were offered at a range of community settings and times to facilitate uptake and were delivered as planned, as confirmed by the group educators' manager. Eleven of the 20 patients interviewed visited their GP practice for other health issues during the intervention, eight of whom reported and greatly appreciated their GP providing additional encouragement.

Intervention feasibility

The process evaluation confirmed the feasibility of implementing the intervention in busy general practice settings. Primary care nurses reported that training ran smoothly, as did intervention implementation. They successfully recruited and mostly retained patients with prediabetes in the programme, and successfully incorporated the intervention into their busy workload, despite experiencing some time and study administrative pressures. The timing of the start of intervention implementation, when nurses needed sufficient time to familiarise themselves with this new additional role, was important to avoid clashes with increased seasonal-related workloads, such as flu vaccinations. Timely patient follow-up was affected when appointments fell in and around the festive season and patients were away or busy. GPs opportunistically encouraged their participating patients, utilising the information, including established dietary goals, recorded on the patient management system.

The community education component was also feasible, with group educators being very committed and adjusting usual service delivery processes to contribute to the study. Uptake was less than optimal, with 53% of intervention patients attending any sessions and one-third of these not completing the course. Modifications were recommended, including that six sessions be reduced to three or four.

Intervention acceptability

Key informants and patients alike found the intervention to be highly acceptable. It was described as *"well thought out and well planned as an initiative"* (KI-13, primary care nurse) and *"a very positive experience"* (KI-1, liaison nurse). One Māori woman recommended it *"roll out to*

Table 2 Demographic characteristics and diabetes-related co-morbidities of participants at baseline and 6-months. Data presented are number (%)

	Control				Intervention				Between groups p-values	
	At baseline (n = 72)	With follow-up data (n = 66)	No 6-month data (n = 6)	Retention p-value[a]	At baseline (n = 85)	With follow-up data (n = 67)	No 6-month data (n = 18)	Retention p-value[a]	At baseline[a]	At 6-months[a]
	n (%)	n (%)	n (%)		n (%)	n (%)	n (%)			
Age categories (years)										
≤ 49	11 (15)	11 (17)	0 (0)	0.719	13 (15)	8 (12)	5 (28)	0.226	0.724	0.582
50–64	40 (56)	36 (55)	4 (67)		42 (49)	35 (52)	7 (39)			
≥ 65	21 (29)	19 (29)	2 (33)		30 (35)	24 (36)	6 (33)			
Sex										
Female	28 (39)	25 (38)	3 (50)	0.672	46 (54)	38 (57)	8 (44)	0.429	0.077	0.370
Male	44 (61)	41 (62)	3 (50)		39 (46)	29 (43)	10 (56)			
Ethnicity										
Māori	22 (31)	19 (29)	3 (50)	0.471	27 (32)	19 (28)	8 (44)	0.001	0.456	0.942
NZ European & Other	48 (67)	45 (68)	3 (50)		52 (61)	47 (70)	5 (28)			
Pacific	2 (3)	2 (3)	0 (0)		6 (7)	1 (1)	5 (28)			
Family history of T2DM										
Yes	28 (40)	27 (42)	1 (17)	0.390	34 (40)	24 (36)	10 (56)	0.179	1.000	0.590
No	42 (60)	37 (58)	5 (83)		50 (60)	42 (64)	8 (44)			
Alcohol consumption										
Above guidelines	8 (13)	8 (14)	0 (0)		6 (8)	5 (9)	1 (6)	1.000	0.573	0.560
Within guidelines	54 (87)	50 (86)	4 (100)		65 (92)	49 (91)	16 (94)			
Smoking										
Current	12 (17)	9 (14)	3 (50)	0.147	18 (21)	12 (18)	6 (33)	0.340	0.193	0.336
Never	24 (33)	22 (33)	2 (33)		26 (31)	20 (30)	6 (33)			
Past – quit >12 months	31 (43)	30 (45)	1 (17)		27 (32)	24 (36)	3 (17)			
Past – quit <12 months	5 (7)	5 (8)	0 (0)		14 (16)	11 (16)	3 (17)			
Co-morbidities										
Hypertension										
Yes	39 (55)	36 (55)	3 (50)	1.000	38 (45)	30 (45)	8 (44)	1.000	0.260	0.296
No	32 (45)	29 (45)	3 (50)		47 (55)	37 (55)	10 (56)			
Ischaemic heart disease										
Yes	7 (11)	5 (8)	2 (40)	0.086	7 (8)	5 (7)	2 (11)	0.639	0.778	1.000
No	58 (89)	55 (92)	3 (60)		77 (92)	61 (91)	16 (89)			
Stroke										
Yes	2 (3)	1 (2)	1 (25)	0.122	5 (6)	4 (6)	1 (6)	1.000	0.699	0.367
No	62 (97)	59 (98)	3 (75)		78 (94)	61 (94)	17 (94)			
NAFLD										
Yes	4 (7)	4 (7)	0 (0)	1.000	1 (1)	1 (2)	0 (0)	1.000	0.166	0.192
No	57 (93)	53 (93)	4 (100)		79 (99)	61 (98)	18 (100)			

Table 2 Demographic characteristics and diabetes-related co-morbidities of participants at baseline and 6-months. Data presented are number (%) *(Continued)*

	Control				Intervention				Between groups p-values	
	At baseline (n = 72)	With follow-up data (n = 66)	No 6-month data (n = 6)	Retention p-value[a]	At baseline (n = 85)	With follow-up data (n = 67)	No 6-month data (n = 18)	Retention p-value[a]	At baseline[a]	At 6-months[a]
	n (%)	n (%)	n (%)		n (%)	n (%)	n (%)			
Gout										
Yes	13 (20)	13 (22)	0 (0)	0.574	12 (14)	8 (12)	4 (22)	0.271	0.378	0.158
No	51 (80)	47 (78)	4 (100)		73 (86)	59 (88)	14 (78)			

[a]Chi-squared test where at least 80% of cells have expected counts 5 or above, Fisher's Exact test otherwise

maraes[2] and a lot of the community groups" (Pt-15) alluding to the important need for improvements in dietary options at traditional meeting places and community events.

Five sub-themes relating to implementation acceptability and success were identified; strong relationships, primary care nurse empowerment, simplicity of approach, clear information and resources, and group support. Findings were consistent among primary care nurses working with differing communities and among patients with differing demographic and glycaemic outcome profiles.

1. Strong relationships

A major factor contributing to intervention acceptability and success was strong relationships between all parties.

The smooth implementation process was facilitated by good communication between the different stakeholder groups and a shared desire to address a significant health issue. Monthly steering group meetings involving stakeholder group representatives enabled issues to be discussed and addressed as they arose. The liaison nurse, a local specialist diabetes nurse, knew many primary care nurses and these pre-existing relationships appeared to facilitate her role.

Most patients expressed their strong appreciation of the opportunity to proactively address their recently diagnosed prediabetes and saw the care and attention provided by their primary care nurse and group educator and their enhanced relationship with them as a powerful enabler:

"It was the way she encouraged me, how she uplifted me. I am so grateful... So I think having the right

Table 3 Clinical and laboratory measures for participants at baseline and 6 months. Data presented are arithmetic means (SDs) number (%), unless otherwise stated

	Control (n = 66)		Intervention (n = 67)		Difference in mean changes in intervention group	
	Baseline Mean (SD)	6 months Mean (SD)	Baseline Mean (SD)	6 months Mean (SD)	Ratio (95% CI)	p-value
HbA1c (mmol/mol)	43.0 (2.2)	43.8 (6.2)	43.2 (2.2)	42.0 (3.6)	0.96 (0.92, 1.00)	0.096
Weight (kg)[a]	93.7 (15.1)	94.6 (15.5)	96.9 (21.5)	95.6 (23.8)	0.97 (0.95, 0.98)	< 0.001
BMI (kg/m^2)[b]	33.0 (6.0)	33.3 (6.1)	35.1 (7.4)	34.5 (8.1)	–	
Waist circumference (cm)	104.0 (17.9)	106.0 (12.2)	109.4 (15.2)	107.7 (16.3)	0.97 (0.94, 1.00)	0.101
Systolic blood pressure (mmHg)	132.7 (17.0)	135.0 (16.8)	133.0 (13.7)	131.2 (13.8)	0.97 (0.92, 1.05)	0.422
Diastolic blood pressure (mmHg)	81.2 (10.9)	80.3 (10.7)	79.6 (9.1)	79.2 (9.2)	1.00 (0.94, 1.04)	0.949
Total cholesterol (mmol/l)	5.3 (1.3)	5.2 (1.3)	5.3 (1.4)	5.2 (1.1)	1.00 (0.95 1.08)	0.933
HDL-cholesterol (mmol/l)	1.2 (0.3)	1.2 (0.4)	1.3 (0.5)	1.3 (0.5)	1.02 (0.96, 1.09)	0.595
Triglycerides (mmol/l)	2.4 (1.8)	2.4 (1.7)	2.1 (1.1)	2.2 (1.3)	0.95 (0.79, 1.24)	0.596
Alanine transaminase (IU/L)	33.7 (20.3)	33.4 (18.2)	28.5 (15.2)	26.0 (12.3)	0.91 (0.75, 1.03)	0.206
Aspartate aminotransferase (IU/L)	25.6 (10.3)	25.6 (11.3)	23.9 (7.5)	22.9 (9.7)	0.95 (0.73, 1.12)	0.649
Gamma glutamyl transpeptidase (IU/L)[c]	39.0 (31.5)	41.0 (33.0)	32.0 (61.0)	31.0 (53.0)	−4.00 (−8.19, 2.22)	0.369
Urate (mmol/l)	0.39 (0.11)	0.37 (0.09)	0.36 (0.07)	0.37 (0.08)	0.02 (−0.01, 0.25)	0.799

Statistical comparisons are from linear regression models, except for GGT where a quantile regression model was used to model medians, adjusting for baseline values, sex, alcohol consumption, family history of T2DM, and ethnicity and adjusting standard errors for clustering within practices
[a]6-month weight measurement was missing for one intervention participant. [b]Ratio not analysed as weight was the preferred body mass outcome. [c]Log-transformed

people at the forefront there just to open you up, you know, and acknowledging where I am at." (Pt-8, Pacific woman).

"Just by talking with them it makes you want to motivate yourself, you know. And you realise that they're not doing it for them, they're doing it for you. And to have that support that you don't know is out there, that's brilliant, that's absolutely brilliant" (Pt-9, Māori man).

2. Nurse empowerment

Primary care nurses felt the information, strategies and structured approach, along with nurse and dietitian expert advice and support, equipped them well to provide dietary advice to their patients with prediabetes. They felt newly empowered to work more effectively and intensively with these patients *"Spending time with them and giving them the education. I found that really rewarding"* (KI-15 primary care nurse).

3. Simple approach

Primary care nurses and patients both praised the intervention's simplicity. The nurses found focusing on small manageable goals both practical and realistic.

"I was quite happy to say to people 'what we're going to do, the changes, it's all simple.....and I think they went away not thinking it was a humongous ask on the food changes." (KI-12, primary care nurse).

Patients also appreciated focussing on simple, achievable, individually tailored dietary goals which they felt made making dietary improvement entirely manageable.

"It wasn't stop this, stop that. It was cut down on this, cut down, little steps... The favourite saying is 'little steps'. And that's probably one of the most helpful sayings I've ever heard." (Pt-9, Māori man).

"That (setting achievable goals) was explained and there was a fair bit of time put into that... You know, especially around Māori or Polynesian people, food can be a blessing and not a blessing. (Laughter). But it's certainly hard to change things that you've done all your life. And I think the nurses that I had anyway were very helpful and supportive...[they] had good ideas." (Pt-13, Māori man).

4. Clear information and resources

The clarity and consistency of information and resources also contributed to intervention acceptability.

This was significant for many patients as they grappled with the implications of their diagnosis. One reported finally gaining clarity after being confused by the plethora of dietary information received when supporting her husband who had had diabetes.

There's so much out there now that just totally throws you every which way and you don't know what's right and what's wrong. And it took away some of those falsehoods that were out there... It was easy to follow, it was easy to understand. The complication was taken out of it. (Pt-1, European woman).

They gave us all the resources to say you have options in how you want to change your lifestyle... That's what I took out of it, is that the information was readily available and the guidance was there, and the help. I have nothing but praise for all parties involved. (Pt-11, Pacific man)

5. Group support

Although six of the 20 interviewed patients reported being uncomfortable in groups and did not attend or did not complete a group education course, the rest enjoyed being with people who were *"in the same boat"*. They liked hearing other people's stories, sharing their own experiences with an interested audience, exchanging ideas and strategies, and being motivated by others. For some, this was another facet of support enabled by the intervention.

"The good thing was it brought you in contact with other people in your situation. That's a major, that's a good thing, you know" (Pt-2, Māori man).

Challenges
A number of challenges to implementing the intervention were identified. These were described primarily by key informants, as many patients spoke only positively about the implementation process, irrespective of their weight or glycaemic outcome. All patients, however, identified challenges they encountered when making dietary changes in answer to a separate question, which will be reported elsewhere. The main challenge identified by key informants was the need for greater information exchange between the primary care and community group educator teams. Neither group appeared to have a full understanding of what the other offered. While both groups had been present at the training sessions, at that time the group education courses had not been finalised. Key informants felt strengthening this linkage could enhance intervention cohesion and possibly group education attendance.

There was remarkable consistency between key informant and patient feedback on other implementation challenges. While primary care nurses did accommodate intervention sessions into their busy schedules, some nurses and patients felt more time was needed, particularly during the initial appointment when study procedures had to be complete. Both nurses and patients also suggested that the 3-month gap between the third and fourth appointments was too long, possibly leading to patients losing motivation. More sessions or monthly phone check-ins were recommended.

Developing goals that were realistic and manageable for patients with low food budgets was a significant challenge for primary care nurses. Some nurses called on the dietitian's expertise in these cases and developed effective pragmatic strategies but this was an ongoing challenge for patients with very low budgets. A few patients also identified this as a real challenge. One man, who had been made redundant and struggled financially, repeated several times that this was his biggest barrier and cautioned health professionals not to put unrealistic dietary expectations on people with limited financial resource:

"Look, the barrier to those goal settings is budget, you know... So when you see on TV people saying they're eating unhealthily, what they're doing, what we're doing is we're eating to a budget planned to survive for the week.... So don't go telling poor people, you're going to get diabetes if you eat this and this and this, so we want you to eat this food, but it's too expensive for you to buy, you know." (Pt-2, Māori man).

Discussion

Our structured prediabetes dietary intervention was able to be competently delivered by primary care nurses within the busy general practice setting following a 6-h training session, a 2-h case study nutrition update and monthly dietitian support for up to 9 months. We found this primary care nurse-delivered intervention led to twice as many intervention participants losing weight at 6 months compared with control participants. Overall the intervention group lost 1.3 kg while the control group gained 0.8 kg, a 2.2 kg difference between the groups, and 18% of intervention participants lost at least 5% of their baseline weight compared with 5% of control participants ($p < 0.001$). HbA1c decreased in the intervention group and increased in the control group. While there were clinically significant changes for some individuals, the difference between the two groups was small and not statistically significant. This study was not powered to examine progression to T2DM, but promisingly the number of intervention participants who progressed

to T2DM at 6 months ($n = 4$) was half that of control participants ($n = 8$).

The less than expected mean weight loss and insignificant change in HbA1c may reflect insufficient intensity of the intervention as both nurses and patients recommended additional sessions or monthly phone check-ins, particularly between months 3 and 6 of the intervention. This is a highly likely explanation considering that during the first 6 months of the DPP lifestyle intervention, case managers met with individual participants at least 16 times during the first 24 weeks of the study, [33] compared with only 4 appointments during our 6 month intervention. However, although mean weight loss was relatively small in our study, it is clinically meaningful, as in the DPP for each kilogram of weight loss, the risk of progressing to diabetes was reduced by 16% [34].

Effective evidence-based management of prediabetes in the primary care setting is potentially a key strategy to help stem the diabetes epidemic worldwide. This is an international challenge [35]. Primary care nurses are ideally suited to lead lifestyle changes, often building on an already established relationship, but for many nurses appropriate nutrition knowledge and skills, and resources are lacking [36]. The results from our feasibility study are encouraging when compared with the relatively few studies where primary care nurses have been upskilled and trained to deliver a prediabetes intervention programme. An evaluation of the Dutch Diabetes Federation 'Road map towards diabetes prevention' one-year nurse-led intervention found that while the level of reported physical activity increased in the intervention group compared with the control group, there was no difference in BMI at 2 years between the groups [37]. In contrast, among 105 participants in the Polish arm of DE-PLAN, a European-wide primary healthcare intervention based on the principles of the Diabetes Prevention Study [9], weight significantly decreased by 2.27 kg ($p < 0.001$) at 1 year [38] but increased by 1.14 kg at 3 years. While our 79% attendance at all four programme primary care nurse visits was less than ideal, it appears to be as good as [39] or better than other programmes [13, 37, 38]. Further, of six intervention participants who attended the 3-month but not 6-month visit, one achieved normoglycaemia at 3 months, and may have deemed it unnecessary to continue in the programme. For three others, HbA1c declined noticeably for two, and remained the same for another, suggesting they too had gained some benefit from two or three nurse-led intervention visits.

The qualitative process evaluation found that extending primary care nurses' dietary knowledge and practice base, and incorporating this into the everyday work of primary care, was not only feasible but also effective and rewarding. Further, the intervention was implemented as intended and highly acceptable to both nurses and patients. A central theme was the importance of strong cooperative relationships at all levels for effective, successful intervention implementation. A significant enabler was good communication and relationships between the funding PHO and primary care practices, between the primary care nurses and their liaison nurse and dietitian, and between the patients and their nurses and groups educators. The pre-existing and ongoing relationship between the nurse and patient was portrayed as one of trust and respect, and appeared to be an important underpinning success factor. The importance of effective communication when providing lifestyle advice and support has been increasingly recognised. Good relationships with primary care professionals were identified as an important component of dietary advice and support among those seeking treatment for obesity [40]. Conversely, Ball et al. [41] identified the lack of an established and ongoing relationship with a dietitian, and advice that was too directive and not individualised as key negative issues in a group of patients recently diagnosed with T2DM receiving nutrition advice from a dietitian. These findings are consistent with those of Ciechanowski et al. [42] who found that poor communication between healthcare providers and patients with diabetes may have a negative effect on treatment adherence. Indeed, in a small qualitative study, women with diabetes rated patient-provider communication as the most important factor influencing their adherence to diabetes treatment [43].

The significant influence of cultural and socioeconomic factors on diet is well documented [44–46]. Our intervention was not prescriptive, but facilitated a structured approach taking into account individuals' different socioeconomic and cultural environments, which enabled nurses to work with patients to first readily identify less than ideal dietary patterns, then develop individualised achievable goals and activities to improve their dietary practices. This approach appeared to work well for the Māori and Pacific participants interviewed. A recent study exploring perspectives on dietary diabetes education and healthy food choices among Pakistani people with T2DM [47] similarly concluded that dietary education that aims at establishing a connection to the everyday life of patients can facilitate successful and sustainable changes in dietary practices.

Recommendations from the process evaluation to further improve the intervention implementation process and its reach included increasing the patient's primary care nurse sessions from four to six; decreasing the group education sessions from six to four and ensuring good information flow between primary care nurses and community educators. These have been incorporated into the subsequent implementation of the intervention in further general practices in the study region.

Important considerations underpinned our study design. We used a convergent mixed methods design to assess the intervention [20] to take into account the pragmatic real-world setting and the principles of implementation science [48]. In real-world settings external factors that cannot be controlled may influence intervention implementation and effect, and this was a key reason for including a qualitative process evaluation. Qualitative evaluations of interventions are seldom reported but, as we found, can provide valuable insight into the intervention process, and the feasibility and acceptability of interventions [49–51].

Key strengths of this study were the ability of practices to fully embed the intervention within usual care, and the full engagement of primary care nurses at both intervention and control practices. This allowed the intervention to be adequately assessed, and facilitated improvements, a necessary step in the development and testing of general practice delivered lifestyle intervention for patients with diabetes [52, 53]. A high level of participation among Māori was also an important and critical strength, given the high prevalence of diabetes among this indigenous group [3]. A limitation was that primary care nurses, who first approached potential patient participants for the process evaluation, may have been more likely to choose those with whom they had good relationships. However, there were no other avenues for researchers to approach patients. Also, as we did not interview GPs, our assessment of their involvement was ascertained indirectly via participating nurses and patients. This study was a pragmatic non-randomised feasibility study, and the effectiveness of the intervention cannot yet be confirmed. While it is likely that weight loss among the intervention group was due to our primary care nurse-led dietary intervention, an alternative explanation is regression to the mean. Baseline weight measures differed between the two groups (93.7 kg and 96.9 kg), and at 6 months the mean weight for the intervention group (95.6 kg) was still greater than the control group at either time.

Conclusions

Study findings confirm the feasibility and acceptability of primary care nurses providing structured dietary advice to patients with prediabetes in busy primary care practices. Consideration of socioeconomic and cultural factors enabled realistic achievable nutrition goals to be established. Although this was a 6-month pragmatic pilot study, improvements in anthropometric measures and the positive trusting relationships between patients and primary care nurses suggest this programme is a worthwhile potentially long term primary care-based diabetes prevention intervention. Increased intensity of the intervention may be necessary to achieve greater weight loss, and definitive randomised controlled trials are required to assess intervention effectiveness.

Endnotes
[1]Māori language word for extended family
[2]a traditional Māori tribal meeting place

Abbreviations
BMI: Body Mass Index; DDA: Detailed Dietary Assessment; GP: General Practitioner; HbA1c: Glycated haemoglobin; ICC: Intraclass Correlation; LOADD: Lifestyle Over and Above Drugs in Diabetes study; PHO: Primary Health Organisation; PIP: Prediabetes Intervention Package in primary care; STC:Diet: Starting the Conversation:Diet; T2DM: Type 2 Diabetes Mellitus

Acknowledgements
We acknowledge the contributions of Rachael Engelbrecht, Primary Care Nurse, Greendale Family Health Centre, Diane Stride, Dietitian, Dahl Gurdit-Singh, Sport Hawke's Bay, and Janet Hill, Health Hawke's Bay who assisted with the implementation of the intervention and study.
We sincerely thank the commitment of practice study co-ordinators and nurses who provided useful comments when developing the intervention package – Robyn O'Keefe, Michele Doole, Sacha Turfrey-Halstead and Kris Banks (Greendale Family Health Centre), Robyn Brynildsen and Joyce Freer (Maraenui Medical Centre), Cath Matthews and Margaret Twydle (Tamatea Medical Centre), Kerriann Paling, Arlene Perry and Jane van Wyk (The Doctors, Napier), and Lisa Penhall, Amanda McInnes and Jane Denby (Sport Hawke's Bay Active Living Advisers). We also acknowledge Chris Petersen and Helen Morris, Health Hawke's Bay, who have made the necessary requirements to capture study data from the Patient Management System, and Roger Coleman, Sport Hawke's Bay. This study was supported in kind by the Hawke's Bay District Health Board.

Funding
This study was supported by health service funding from the New Zealand Ministry of Health, a Hawke's Bay Medical Research Foundation grant-in-aid and a New Zealand Society for the Study of Diabetes research award. No funding body had any role in the design of the study and collection, analysis, and interpretation of data and in writing the manuscript.

Authors' contributions
KC conceived the study. KC, TF, SA and LCW obtained funding to conduct the study. KC, TF, KS, JN, SA, AG and LCW contributed to the conception and design. LMW provided important cultural advice and guidance. KC, KS and JN were responsible for developing the dietary tool and compiling written dietary resources. TF and TS managed the implementation of the study. AG was responsible for the sample size calculations and statistical analysis plan. KC and SA drafted the manuscript which was critically revised for important intellectual content by all authors. All authors have read and approved the final version of the manuscript.

Authors' information
SA is an independent health researcher with 20 years qualitative research experience in multi-ethnic communities, and led the qualitative study, with input from LCW, a professor of nursing research. SA and LCW were not involved with the development and implementation of the intervention.

Consent of for publication
Not applicable.

Competing interests
The authors declare that they have no competing interests.

Author details
[1]Edgar Diabetes and Obesity Research, Department of Medicine, Dunedin School of Medicine, University of Otago, PO Box 56, Dunedin 9054, New Zealand. [2]Kaupapa Consulting Ltd, Napier 4110, New Zealand. [3]Health Hawke's Bay – Te Oranga Hawke's Bay, PO Box 11141, Hastings 4158, New Zealand. [4]Department of Preventive and Social Medicine, Dunedin School of Medicine, University of Otago, PO Box 56, Dunedin 9054, New Zealand. [5]School of Nursing and Midwifery, Edith Cowan University, 270 Joondalup Drive, Joondalup 6027, Australia.

References
1. Danaei G, Finucane M, Lu Y, Singh G, Cowan M, Paciorek C, for the Global Burden of Metabolic Risk Factors of Chronic Diseases Collaborating Group (Blood Glucose), et al. National, regional, and global trends in fasting plasma glucose and diabetes prevalence since 1980: systematic analysis of health examination surveys and epidemiological studies with 370 country-years and 2·7 million participants. Lancet. 2011;378:31–40.
2. Global Burden of Disease Study 2013 Collaborators. Global, regional, and national incidence, prevalence, and years lived with disability for 301 acute and chronic diseases and injuries in 188 countries, 1990-2013: a systematic analysis for the global burden of disease study 2013. Lancet. 2015;386:743–800.
3. Coppell KJ, Mann JI, Williams SM, Jo E, Drury PL, Miller JC, et al. Prevalence of diagnosed and undiagnosed diabetes and prediabetes in New Zealand: findings from the 2008/09 adult nutrition survey. N Z Med J. 2013;126:23–42.
4. Tabák AG, Herder C, Rathmann W, Brunner EJ, Kivimäki M. Prediabetes: a high-risk state for diabetes development. Lancet. 2012;379:2279–90.
5. Eades CE, Leese GP, Evans JM. Incidence of impaired glucose regulation and progression to type 2 diabetes mellitus in the Tayside region of Scotland. Diabetes Res Clin Pract. 2014;104:e16–9.
6. Nathan DM, Davidson MB, DeFronzo RA, Heine RJ, Henry RR, Pratley R, et al. Impaired fasting glucose and impaired glucose tolerance: implications for care. Diabetes Care. 2007;30:753–9.
7. Ministry of Health. New Zealand primary care handbook 2012 (updated 2013): cardiovascular disease risk assessment. Wellington: Ministry of Health; 2013.
8. Knowler W, Barrett-Connor E, Fowler S, Hamman R, Lachin J, Walker E, et al. For the diabetes prevention program research group. Reduction in the incidence of type 2 diabetes with lifestyle intervention or metformin. N Engl J Med. 2002;346:393–403.
9. Tuomilehto J, Lindstrom J, Eriksson JG, Valle TT, Hamalainen H, Ilanne-Parikka P, et al. Prevention of type 2 diabetes mellitus by changes in lifestyle among subjects with impaired glucose tolerance. N Engl J Med. 2001;344:1343–50.
10. Cefalu WT. Steps toward the meaningful translation of prevention strategies for type 2 diabetes. Diabetes Care. 2012;35:663–5.
11. Aziz Z, Absetz P, Oldroyd J, Pronk NP, Oldenburg B. A systematic review of real-world diabetes prevention programs: learnings from the last 15 years. Implement Sci. 2015;10:172. https://doi.org/10.1186/s13012-015-0354-6.
12. Sacerdote C, Fiorini L, Rosato R, Audenino M, Valpreda M, Vineis P. Randomized controlled trial: effect of nutritional counselling in general practice. Int J Epidemiol. 2006;35:409–15.
13. Weir DL, Johnson ST, Mundt C, Bray D, Taylor L, Eurich DT, et al. A primary care based healthy-eating and active living education session for weight reduction in the pre-diabetic population. Prim Care Diabetes. 2014;8:301–7.
14. Absetz P, Valve R, Oldenburg B, Heinonen H, Nissinen A, Fogelholm M, et al. Type 2 diabetes prevention in the "real world": one-year results of the GOAL implementation trial. Diabetes Care. 2007;30:2465–70.
15. Kilkkinen A, Heistaro S, Laatikainen T, Janus E, Chapman A, Absetz P, et al. Prevention of type 2 diabetes in a primary health care setting. Interim results from the Greater Green Triangle (GGT) diabetes prevention project. Diabetes Res Clin Pract. 2007;76:460–2.
16. Vadstrup E, Frolich A, Perrild H, Borg E, Roder M. Lifestyle intervention for type 2 diabetes patients - trial protocol of the Copenhagen type 2 diabetes rehabilitation project. BMC Public Health. 2009;9:166. https://doi.org/10.1186/1471-2458-9-166.

17. Vadstrup ES, Frølich A, Perrild H, Borg E, Røder M. Effect of a group-based rehabilitation programme on glycaemic control and cardiovascular risk factors in type 2 diabetes patients: the Copenhagen type 2 diabetes rehabilitation project. Patient Educ Couns. 2011;84:185–90.

18. Neil HAW, Roe L, Godlee RJP, Moore JW, Clark GMG, Brown J, et al. Randomised trial of lipid lowering dietary advice in general practice: the effects on serum lipids, lipoproteins, and antioxidants. BMJ. 1995;310:569–73.

19. Wadden TA, Volger S, Sarwer DB, Vetter ML, Tsai AG, Berkowitz RI, et al. A two-year randomized trial of obesity treatment in primary care practice. N Engl J Med. 2011;365:1969–79.

20. Pluye P, Hong QN. Combining the power of stories and the power of numbers: mixed methods research and mixed studies reviews. Annu Rev Public Health. 2014;35:29–45.

21. Statistics New Zealand, 2013 Census QuickStats about a place. http://archive.stats.govt.nz/Census/2013-census/profile-and-summary-reports/quickstats-about-a-place.aspx?url=/Census/2013-census/profile-and-summary-reports/quickstats-about-a-place.aspx&request_value=14074#14074. Accessed 4 Dec 2017.

22. Atkinson J, Salmond C, Crampton P. NZDep2013 index of deprivation. Wellington: Department of Public Health. Wellington: University of Otago; 2014.

23. Coppell K, Kataoka M, Williams S, Chisholm A, Vorgers S, Mann J. Nutritional intervention in patients with type 2 diabetes who are hyperglycaemic despite optimised drug treatment—lifestyle over and above drugs in diabetes (LOADD) study: randomised controlled trial. BMJ. 2010;341:c3337.

24. Paxton A, Strycker L, Toobert D, Ammerman A, Glasgow R. Starting the conversation performance of a brief dietary assessment and intervention tool for health professionals. Am J Prev Med. 2011;40:67–71.

25. Diabetes New Zealand. Diabetes and healthy food choices. Wellington: Diabetes New Zealand Inc. 2007. https://diabetes.org.nz/pamphlet-order-form/. Accessed 4 Dec 2017.

26. Ministry of Health. Prediabetes advice. Wellington: Ministry of Health; 2013.

27. Elley CR, Kerse N, Arroll B, Robinson E. Effectiveness of counselling patients on physical activity in general practice: cluster randomised controlled trial. BMJ. 2003;326:793.

28. Ministry of Health. Be Active Every Day. Wellington: Ministry of Health; 2010. https://www.healthed.govt.nz/resource/be-active-every-day-physical-activity-adults. Accessed 4 Dec 2017.

29. University of Otago and Ministry of Health. A focus on nutrition: key findings of the 2008/09 New Zealand adult nutrition survey. Wellington: Ministry of Health; 2011.

30. Coppell KJ, Anderson K, Williams S, Manning P, Mann J. Evaluation of diabetes care in the Otago region using a diabetes register, 1998-2003. Diabetes Res Clin Pract. 2006;71:345–52.

31. Patton MQ. Qualitative evaluation and research methods. 3rd ed. Newbury Park: Sage; 2002.

32. Braun V, Clarke V. Using thematic analysis in psychology. Qual Res Psychol. 2006;3(2):77–10.

33. Maruthur NM, Ma Y, Delahanty LM, Nelson JA, Aroda V, White NH, et al. Diabetes prevention program research group. Early response to preventive strategies in the Diabetes Prevention Program. J Gen Intern Med. 2013;28:1629–36.

34. Hamman RF, Wing RR, Edelstein SL, Lachin JM, Bray GA, Delahanty L, et al. Effect of weight loss with lifestyle intervention on risk of diabetes. Diabetes Care. 2006;29:2102–7.

35. Ard J. Obesity in the US: what is the best role for primary care? BMJ. 2015;350:g7846.

36. Kris-Etherton PM, Akabas SR, Bales CW, Bistrian B, Braun L, Edwards MS, et al. The need to advance nutrition education in the training of health care professionals and recommended research to evaluate implementation and effectiveness. Am J Clin Nutr. 2014;99(5 Suppl):1153S–66S. https://doi.org/10.3945/ajcn.113.073502.

37. Hesselink AE, Rutten GE, Slootmaker SM, de Weerdt I, Raaijmakers LG, Jonkers R, et al. Effects of a lifestyle program in subjects with impaired fasting glucose, a pragmatic cluster-randomized controlled trial. BMC Fam Pract. 2015;16:183. https://doi.org/10.1186/s12875-015-0394-7.

38. Gilis-Januszewska A, Lindström J, Tuomilehto J, Piwońska-Solska B, Topór-Mądry R, Szybiński Z, et al. Sustained diabetes risk reduction after real life and primary health care setting implementation of the diabetes in Europe prevention using lifestyle, physical activity and nutritional intervention (DE-PLAN) project. BMC Public Health. 2017;17:198. https://doi.org/10.1186/s12889-017-4104-3.

39. Costa B, Barrio F, Cabré JJ, Piñol JL, Cos X, Solé C, DE-PLAN-CAT Research Group, et al. Delaying progression to type 2 diabetes among high-risk Spanish individuals is feasible in real-life primary healthcare settings using intensive lifestyle intervention. Diabetologia. 2012;55:1319–28. https://doi.org/10.1007/s00125-012-2492-6.

40. Brown I, Thompson J, Tod A, Jones G. Primary care support for tackling obesity: a qualitative study of the perceptions of obese patients. Br J Gen Pract. 2006;56:666–72.

41. Ball L, Davmor R, Leveritt M, Desbrow B, Ehrlich C, Chaboyer W. The nutrition care needs of patients newly diagnosed with type 2 diabetes: informing dietetic practice. J Hum Nutr Diet. 2016;29:487–94.

42. Ciechanowski PS, Katon WJ, Russo JE, Walker EA. The patient-provider relationship: attachment theory and adherence to treatment in diabetes. Am J Psychiatry. 2001;158:29–35.

43. Matthews SM, Peden AR, Rowles GD. Patient-provider communication: understanding diabetes management among adult females. Patient Educ Couns. 2009;76:31–7.

44. Aitaoto N, Campo S, Snetselaar LG, Janz KF, Farris KB, Parker E, et al. Formative Research to Inform Nutrition Interventions in Chuuk and the US Pacific. J Acad Nutr Diet. 2015;115:947–53. https://doi.org/10.1016/j.jand.2014.11.018.

45. Belon AP, Nieuwendyk LM, Vallianatos H, Nykiforuk CI. Perceived community environmental influences on eating behaviors: A Photovoice analysis. Soc Sci Med. 2016;171:18–29. https://doi.org/10.1016/j.socscimed.2016.11.004.

46. Larson N, Story M. A review of environmental influences on food choices. Ann Behav Med. 2009;38(Suppl 1):S56–73. https://doi.org/10.1007/s12160-009-9120-9.

47. Hempler NF, Nicic S, Ewers B, Willaing I. Dietary education must fit into everyday life: a qualitative study of people with a Pakistani background and type 2 diabetes. Patient Prefer Adherence. 2015;9:347–54. https://doi.org/10.2147/PPA.S77380.

48. Fixsen DL, Naoom SF, Blase KA, Friedman RM, Wallace F. Implementation research: A synthesis of the literature. Tampa: University of South Florida, Louis de la parte Florida Mental Health Institute, The National Implementation Research. Network; 2005.

49. Rogers S, Humphrey C, Nazareth I, Lister S, Tomlin Z, Haines A. Designing trials of interventions to change professional practice in primary care: lessons from an exploratory study of two change strategies. BMJ. 2000;320:1580–3.

50. Victora CG, Habicht JP, Bryce J. Evidence-based public health: moving beyond randomized trials. Am J Public Health. 2004;94:400–5.

51. Whitehead LC, Crowe MT, Carter JD, Maskill VR, Carlyle D, Bugge C, Frampton CM. A nurse-led interdisciplinary approach to promote self-management of type 2 diabetes: A process evaluation of post-intervention experiences. J Eval Clin Pract. 2017;23:264–71. https://doi.org/10.1111/jep.12594.

52. Maindal HT, Bonde A, Aagaard-Hansen J. Action research led to a feasible lifestyle intervention in general practice for people with prediabetes. Prim Care Diabetes. 2014;8:23–9. https://doi.org/10.1016/j.pcd.2013.11.007.

53. Evans PH, Greaves C, Winder R, Fearn-Smith J, Campbell JL. Development of an educational 'toolkit' for health professionals and their patients with prediabetes: the WAKEUP study (ways of addressing knowledge education and understanding in pre-diabetes). Diabet Med. 2007;24:770–7.

11

Assessing treatment fidelity and contamination in a cluster randomised controlled trial of motivational interviewing and cognitive behavioural therapy skills in type 2 diabetes

Nicholas Magill[1*†] ⓘ, Helen Graves[2†], Nicole de Zoysa[2], Kirsty Winkley[2], Stephanie Amiel[3], Emma Shuttlewood[3], Sabine Landau[1] and Khalida Ismail[2,4]

Abstract

Background: Competencies in psychological techniques delivered by primary care nurses to support diabetes self-management were compared between the intervention and control arms of a cluster randomised controlled trial as part of a process evaluation. The trial was pragmatic and designed to assess effectiveness. This article addresses the question of whether the care that was delivered in the intervention and control trial arms represented high fidelity treatment and attention control, respectively.

Methods: Twenty-three primary care nurses were either trained in motivational interviewing (MI) and cognitive behavioural therapy (CBT) skills or delivered attention control. Nurses' skills in these treatments were evaluated soon after training (treatment arm) and treatment fidelity was assessed after treatment delivery for sessions midway through regimen (both arms) using the Motivational Interviewing Treatment Integrity (MITI) domains and Behaviour Change Counselling Index (BECCI) based on consultations with 151 participants (45% of those who entered the study). The MITI Global Spirit subscale measured demonstration of MI principles: evocation, collaboration, autonomy/support.

Results: After training, median MITI MI-Adherence was 86.2% (IQR 76.9–100%) and mean MITI Empathy was 4.09 (SD 1.04). During delivery of treatment, in the intervention arm mean MITI Spirit was 4.03 (SD 1.05), mean Empathy was 4.23 (SD 0.89), and median Percentage Complex Reflections was 53.8% (IQR 40.0–71.4%). In the attention control arm mean Empathy was 3.40 (SD 0.98) and median Percentage Complex Reflections was 55.6% (IQR 41.9–71.4%).

Conclusions: After MI and CBT skills training, detailed assessment showed that nurses had basic competencies in some psychological techniques. There appeared to be some delivery of elements of psychological treatment by nurses in the control arm. This model of training and delivery of MI and CBT skills integrated into routine nursing care to support diabetes self-management in primary care was not associated with high competency levels in all skills.

(Continued on next page)

* Correspondence: nicholas.magill@kcl.ac.uk
[†]Equal contributors
[1]Department of Biostatistics and Health Informatics, Institute of Psychiatry, Psychology and Neuroscience, King's College London, 16 De Crespigny Park, London SE5 8AF, UK
Full list of author information is available at the end of the article

(Continued from previous page)

Keywords: Treatment contamination, Randomised controlled trial, Diabetes, Self-management

Background

Psychological treatments are complex interventions, which are generally defined as treatments that comprise several interacting components or active ingredients [1]. In randomised controlled trials (RCTs) of such interventions, the standard intention-to-treat analysis can estimate the causal effect of treatment offer on outcome but does not shed any light on whether the two competing treatment offers were delivered to participants as intended. Process evaluations are a set of methodologies for assessing the implementation, mechanisms, and context of an intervention [2]. Process evaluation of an RCT has become increasingly important because it may help to explain why an intervention was or was not effective [3]. In trials of psychological treatments the most commonly studied process is fidelity. This is defined as the consistency of what was implemented with what was intended [4]. Related to this concept is that of clinician competency, which is a clinician's ability to implement a technique [5]. Its assessment is particularly important in trials where treatment is delivered by a non-specialist.

Randomised controlled trials of psychological treatments are increasingly assessing clinician competency, using methods such as audio recordings, clinical notes, and random observations of delivered therapy. These are frequently done in the active intervention arm but rarely in the control condition. The implication of this is that such process evaluation in trials may be missing the problem of treatment contamination, where participants in the control group receive elements of the active intervention [6]. An evaluation of what treatment participants in the control group receive is important in trials and especially when the comparator is an attention control that can contain some active ingredients.

The context of the assessment of treatment fidelity described in this article is a trial of a psychological treatment for people who suffer from type 2 diabetes (T2D) with suboptimal glycaemic control [7]. Suboptimal control is common amongst people with T2D despite medical and educational interventions [8–10]. Reasons are multifactorial and include psychological barriers such as denial, depression, stigma, and fears around insulin [11, 12]. The need for psychological care to help motivate patients towards lifestyle adjustment has been emphasised in national guidelines [13], and psychological interventions have demonstrated promise in improving outcomes in T2D [14]. The rationale for the Diabetes 6

(D6) trial was based on the need to find cost-effective ways of competently delivering diabetes-informed psychological treatments. Emerging evidence suggests that allied healthcare professionals can be trained to provide basic psychological interventions and that this is associated with an improvement in glycaemic control in type 1 diabetes. For example, hospital diabetes nurses have been trained to deliver diabetes-specific psychological therapy competently and primary care nurses have successfully been trained to use motivational techniques to improve oral medication adherence in people with T2D [15, 16]. In addition, a study of nurse-delivered motivational interviewing (MI) in primary care showed that nurses had some basic competency but this did not develop over time [17].

The D6 study was a cluster RCT evaluating the effectiveness of an intervention combining motivational interviewing (MI) and cognitive behavioural therapy (CBT) skills compared to an attention control which did not include any psychological components. One reason for using cluster randomisation at the level of the primary care nurse was to avoid treatment contamination that was anticipated if a given nurse were asked to provide both control and active treatments. The psychological interventions were both evidence-based approaches aimed at producing behavioural change, with evidence suggesting that integrating MI and CBT may be beneficial [18]. The treatment in the control arm consisted of standard diabetes care, with primary care nurses scheduled to meet participants for the same number of times and same duration as those in the active intervention arm. Participants were offered six face-to-face sessions followed by six sessions in a format agreed with the nurse. The primary aim of the trial was to investigate the effect of psychological treatment offer on glycated haemoglobin. Recruitment criteria included evidence of suboptimal control prior to entry into the study and current receipt of standard care.

The D6 trial provided an opportunity to assess treatment fidelity, using audio recordings of treatment sessions. This enabled an examination of whether nurses could be trained to deliver psychological therapy competently to participants within the active intervention arm. It also allowed an assessment of whether participants allocated to the attention control arm received psychological therapy – that is, whether contamination occurred. This article describes the fidelity assessment of the treatments delivered to participants in the two trial arms and represents a secondary analysis.

The aims of this study were to: i) assess whether D6 nurses achieved competencies in psychological therapy delivery at the end of the training period, ii) describe differences between end of training and delivery of intervention, iii) compare the levels of receipt of psychological treatment (MI and CBT skills) between the active intervention and control arms, and iv) determine to what extent the intervention and control treatments represented high fidelity MI and CBT or standard diabetes care, respectively.

Methods
Setting and trial design
The trial was set within 23 primary care surgeries in south London. Large surgeries (≥6000 patients) were invited to participate if they had a nurse providing diabetes care. Interventions were allocated at the surgery level (clusters). Ethical approval was granted by the King's College Hospital Research Ethics Committee (reference 09/H0808/97) and by the respective Primary Care Trusts (reference RDLSLBex 534 and 2010/403/W). Informed written consent was obtained from all individual participants included in the study. The trial was registered with ISRCTN (ISRCTN75776892) on 19 May 2010.

The training programme
The training programme for nurses in the intervention arm of the RCT was developed and delivered by an experienced clinical psychologist using both didactic and practicum strategies. Nurses were trained in six MI/CBT skills: active listening, managing resistance, directing change, supporting self-efficacy, addressing health beliefs, and shaping behaviours. The initial interactive training workshops were conducted over 12 3-hourly sessions and the nurses were given a handbook for ongoing reference. The focus was on increasing patients' motivation to improve their diabetes control and then collaboratively addressing key self-care behaviours such as medication adherence, blood sugar testing, physical activity, and dietary changes.

Techniques taught in MI and CBT
MI is a collaborative, person-centred approach to working with people in order to elicit and strengthen their motivation and commitment to change [19]. It has been found to be more effective than traditional advice-giving in the treatment of a range of behavioural problems and diseases, including diabetes [20]. CBT has been found to be effective at improving adjustment to diagnosis and self-management of diabetes [21]. It aims to achieve this by helping people to identify and restructure unhelpful

cognitions, teaching behavioural strategies, and supporting people to develop helpful coping strategies.

Clinical supervision
Nurses in the intervention group attended monthly supervision with the trial psychologist either in person at monthly group sessions or over the telephone if they were not able to attend throughout the delivery of the intervention. E-mail support was also offered for individual cases.

Assessment of treatment fidelity and competency
All nurses who participated in the D6 study were required by protocol to record their treatment consultations with participants digitally. A sample of recordings from nurses in the intervention arm from shortly after the end of training was used to assess competency. Another sample of recordings from both trial arms that was representative of participants' treatment receipt was selected in order to assess fidelity.

The definition, assessment, and difficulties of addressing treatment fidelity in research studies have been extensively discussed elsewhere in the literature [22–24]. A definition that is consistently used, and will be used for the purpose of this study, is that fidelity comprises both adherence and competence [24]. Adherence refers to whether the appropriate procedures were followed for that clinical intervention whereas competence refers to whether these procedures were implemented to an adequate level.

The Motivational Interviewing Treatment Integrity (MITI) Scale, version 3.1.1 [25, 26], was utilised to measure competence and skills used in both groups of nurses. A Global Spirit score is intended to capture the overall demonstration of MI principles, and a Global Empathy score is intended to capture the extent to which the clinician understands, or attempts to understand, the patient's perspective. Further measures of clinician behaviours include the use of simple reflections, complex reflections, open questions, and closed-ended questions. Scores are also calculated for MI adherent and non-adherent counselling behaviours. The possible ranges and threshold levels for subscales (as specified by the scale's authors) are given in Table 1.

The Behaviour Change Counselling Index (BECCI) [27] was designed to assist trainers in assessing a clinician's competence in using behaviour change counselling in consultations. It was included here in order to assess nurses' competence in eliciting patients' thoughts and cognitions, therefore addressing the CBT element of the intervention. BECCI comprises 11 items which are scored from zero to four (0 = *action carried out not at all*; 1 = *minimally*; 2 = *to some extent*; 3 = *a good deal*; 4

Table 1 Minimums, maximums, and proficiency and competency thresholds for the MITI and BECCI scales [26, 27]

MITI summary scores	Minimum (lowest score)	Maximum (highest score)	"Beginning proficiency" thresholds	"Competency" thresholds
Global Spirit and Global Empathy	1	5	Average of 3.5	Average of 4
Reflection-to-Question Ratio	0	–	1	2
Percent Open Questions	0	100	50%	70%
Percent Complex Reflections	0	100	40%	50%
Percent MI-Adherent	0	100	90%	100%
BECCI summary score				
Practitioner Score	0	4	–	–

= *a great deal*). The mean of these is used as the overall Practitioner Score.

This article describes the evaluation of nurses' competency in delivering the D6 intervention, which was done soon after the end of training, and the assessment of treatment fidelity during the delivery of treatment to participants. The nurse competency sample included one tape recording for each intervention nurse (11 nurses). For the assessment of treatment fidelity two samples were made. The first sample (69 recordings from 21 nurses) was used for quantifying the reliability of the ratings made by the clinical psychologists working on this study. The second sample was larger (266 recordings from 151 patients and 17 nurses) and was used for the fidelity assessment, which was the main focus of this article.

Nurse competency assessment

The nurse trainer, who was MITI trained, assessed post-training adherence and competency of all nurses in the intervention group using the MITI and BECCI rating scales. One tape recording of a treatment consultation was submitted by each nurse soon after the end of training and then rated on each of the two scales. Nurses were rated as not MI adherent if MITI MI-Adherence was lower than 90% (the "Beginning proficiency" threshold, see Table 1) and MITI Empathy was lower than 3 (which is defined as representing modest success of clinician trying to understand the patient's perspective [26]). These subscales were chosen because MI-Adherence and Empathy have been shown to be predictive of treatment success [28, 29]. The "Beginning proficiency" and "Competency" thresholds in the MITI manual (Table 1) were considered too high in the context of this study, where consultations included clinical communications that would not be part of a standard MI consultation (for example a physical examination, prescribing, and checking adherence). Any nurses rated as not MI adherent were given extra training and then reassessed. Nurses who were judged to be adherent but who did not meet the higher MITI threshold levels were expected to continue to improve with extra supervision.

Sampling for inter-rater reliability assessment

A researcher assessed every tape recording and removed duplicates and recordings where session number could not be identified. Of the tape recordings that were from treatment sessions two to four, and where there was a recording of a treatment session that lasted 20 min or more, stratified probability sampling was used to select three recordings from each nurse. Within each nurse stratum, the first tape recording was chosen at random and the second recording was then chosen at random after removing recordings from the previously-selected individual and session from the sample set. The same technique was used to sample the third recording.

The sample comprised 69 tape recordings (representing 3.4% of the total number of all treatment sessions, and 4.0% of sessions where a recording had been made). A 20-min window in the middle of the recording was rated using the MITI (by raters A and B). Of this sample, 32 recordings were rated using the BECCI by raters B and C. Recordings in this sub-sample featured in both the reliability assessment and fidelity assessment (described in next section). Rater C listened to and coded a 20-min window in the middle of the recording whilst rater B assessed the entire recording (raters B and C's assessments were originally intended for different purposes). Raters received suitable training for whichever scale they used and were blind to treatment allocation. This sample was used in order to check the inter-rater reliability of raters who assessed recordings in the fidelity study.

Sampling for fidelity assessment

The sampling procedure for the fidelity assessment selected tape recordings from participants who had at least one recording from sessions two, three, and four, and where treatment centre was identifiable (there was no minimum duration of session length). This set included 353 recordings from 154 participants (31 participants with one recording; 47 with two; and 76 with three). Random sampling stratified by participant was used to select two recordings from each of the participants with all three recordings. If only one or two recordings were available for a given participant then these were chosen for subsequent fidelity assessment.

The sample included 266 usable tape recordings (127 recordings in intervention arm) from 17 nurses' consultations with 151 participants and 11 recordings where the conversation could not be heard. The usable recordings represented 13.1% of all treatment sessions and 15.4% of sessions where a recording was made. The whole duration of each recording was rated using the MITI (rater A) and BECCI (rater B). Raters were blind to treatment allocation.

Data analysis
Statistical analyses were conducted using Stata version 14. In order to assess inter-rater reliability for the MITI global scores and BECCI Practitioner Scores, intra-class correlation coefficients (ICCs) were estimated using a mixed model. The model included a fixed effect for rater, a random effect for tape recording, and a random effect for primary care nurse in order to account for clustering. It assessed consistency between individual ratings by estimating ICCs at the participant-within-nurse level. The MITI global scores and BECCI Practitioner Score were summarized within the intervention arm shortly after the end of training and during delivery of intervention. Mixed effects regression models with random effects for primary care nurse and participant or Somers' D tests with sampling from the highest level of the cluster structure (i.e. primary care nurse) were used to compare the fidelity of the psychological therapy delivery between participants in the two trial arms.

Results
Nurse and participant sample characteristics
Twenty-three primary care nurses participated in the trial, with 11 randomised to the intervention arm, and 12 to control. They were all female, with a mean age of 48 (SD 8.5) years. Fourteen (61%) of the nurses were white, six (26%) black, and 3 (13%) Asian or other ethnicity.

In terms of previous training in psychological therapies, nine had no previous experience (4 intervention, 5 control), two had completed a module as part of a degree course (1 intervention, 1 control), two had completed some training in MI as part of a smoking cessation course (1 intervention, 1 control), two had undertaken one day or less of MI training (1 intervention, 1 control), one had completed some MI training as part of the Co-Creating Health Programme (intervention), and one had some experience as part of a nursing qualification (intervention). Data on previous training were not available for six nurses.

The participant sample from which the tape recordings were drawn (treatment fidelity assessment sample)

included 151 adults with T2D (45% of the total number of participants who entered into the trial), of whom 74 (49%) were in the psychological treatment trial arm. Mean age was 59.4 (SD 11.1) years and 77 (51%) were female. Sixty-eight (45%) were white, 60 (40%) black, 13 (9%) Asian, and 10 (7%) of another ethnicity. Median duration of diabetes was 9 (IQR 6–13) years and mean pre-intervention glycated haemoglobin was 80.1 mmol/mol (SD 18.9) or 9.5% (SD 1.7).

Nurse competency
The nurse trainer assessed post-training treatment adherence and competency using the MITI and BECCI rating scales. One nurse was not considered MI adherent post training (using MITI MI-Adherence and Empathy subscales) and therefore was given extra training by the clinical psychologist. Upon reassessment she was deemed MI adherent in the therapy. Mean MITI and BECCI competency scores post-training are presented in Table 2.

Inter-rater reliability
Estimates of intraclass correlation coefficients for the global MITI scores and BECCI Practitioner Score are reported in Table 3. These estimates suggested that inter-rater reliability was good (between 0.60 and 0.74) or excellent (> 0.75) for both scales, according to previously defined thresholds [30]. Reliability was greater for MITI, where all ratings were for the 20-min section in the middle of each recording, compared to BECCI, where one coder rated 20-min windows and another rated the full duration of recordings.

Fidelity assessment
MITI domain scores summarised by trial arm along with the results of the mixed model or Somers' D tests comparing trial arms are given in Table 4. Estimated standardised mean differences for the MITI global scores were 1.11 (Spirit) and 0.83 (Empathy). There was strong evidence of group differences in favour of the intervention for the global scores of Spirit and Empathy, the percentage of questions that were open, and of percentage of

Table 2 Competency scores assessed post-training

Domain	Post-training
MITI Global Spirit (mean; SD)	3.42 (0.67)
MITI Global Empathy (mean; SD)	4.09 (1.04)
Reflection-to-Question Ratio (median; IQR)	0.67 (0.45–0.82)
Percent Open Questions (median; IQR)	45.5 (25.0–72.2)
Percent Complex Reflections (median; IQR)	9.1 (0–28.6)
Percent MI-Adherent (median; IQR)	86.2 (76.9–100)
BECCI Practitioner Score (mean; SD)	2.78 (0.50)

Table 3 Intraclass correlation coefficients for MITI global scores and BECCI Practitioner Score

Domain	ICC	95% confidence interval
MITI Global Spirit	0.89	0.83–0.93
MITI Global Empathy	0.91	0.86–0.94
BECCI Practitioner Score	0.71	0.52–0.85

sessions that were MI adherent. There was no evidence of a group difference in percentage of reflections that were complex or the reflection-to-question ratio.

Numbers and proportions of sessions in the intervention arm that were rated as above MITI's "Beginning proficiency" and "Competency" thresholds for each domain are summarised in Table 5 [26]. This table summarises how many treatment sessions were assessed as meeting these thresholds within each of the trial arms.

Mean BECCI Practitioner Score in the control arm was 1.07 (SD 0.48) and in the intervention arm was 1.42 (SD 0.51). A z-test from a mixed effects model showed a significant difference in the BECCI Practitioner Scores between the treatment arms ($z = 3.22$, $p < .01$, 95% CI 0.15–0.62). The estimated standardised mean difference was 0.75.

Discussion

This article describes the assessment of the delivery of a nurse-led psychological therapy in the context of a cluster RCT aimed at improving persistent suboptimal glycaemic control in people with T2D. Treatment fidelity and contamination were evaluated by comparing the levels of MI and CBT skills in the two trial arms. At the end of training, nurses in the intervention group were considered competent in D6 skills at a basic level (according to "Beginning proficiency" thresholds) and it appears that there was improvement in some MI skills during delivery of the intervention. For example, MITI Global Spirit and the proportion of reflections that were complex improved. The active intervention delivered to trial participants was statistically superior in Spirit and Empathy, open questions, MI-Adherence, and behaviour

change scores compared to attention control. There were no group differences in the proportion of complex reflections or the reflection-to-question ratio. In clinical terms the differences between the trial arms were smaller than expected. The levels of treatment fidelity suggested that some participants in the psychotherapy arm did not receive high fidelity treatment, whilst some in the attention control arm received aspects of the psychological intervention.

In the active intervention arm, findings were partly consistent with the practice of MI, where the clinician collaborates with, supports, and allows the patient to take control of the need for change by listening empathically and using open-ended questions. This was demonstrated by high levels of Spirit and Empathy and a clear majority of treatment sessions being MI-Adherent. The superiority of MI-Adherence and Empathy when comparing the trial arms was particularly important as these have been shown to be predictive of treatment success [28, 29]. However, there were some challenges in providing high fidelity psychotherapy. Specifically, approximately only half of reflections were complex, a similar proportion of questions were open, the ratio of reflections to questions was slightly lower in the intervention group compared to control, and the level of achieved behaviour change fidelity (from the BECCI) was rated between "minimal" and "to some extent".

There were a number of possible reasons why nurses may not have exceeded MITI's "Beginning proficiency" levels. The most apparent of these is that the nurses did not self-select to take part in D6. All primary care surgeries meeting the eligibility criteria in the five boroughs were invited to participate. Of those that agreed, the surgery allocated a nurse to take part in the study. Some nurses were more enthusiastic about their participation than others. It is also possible that the skills that showed the lower fidelity levels reflected particular aspects of MI or CBT that are difficult to teach to clinicians who are not specialists in psychological treatment. An interview study with the nurses suggested that not all may be suited to the acquisition of psychological skills [31]. For

Table 4 MITI summary scores during treatment delivery by treatment allocation group

MITI Domain	Attention control group (mean; SD)	Intervention group (mean; SD)	z-test (from mixed model)	95% confidence interval for mean difference
Global Spirit	2.63 (1.12)	4.03 (1.05)	$z = 4.50$, $p < .001$	0.81, 2.06
Global Empathy	3.40 (0.98)	4.23 (0.89)	$z = 4.55$; $p < .001$	0.49, 1.23
	Attention control group (median; IQR)	Intervention group (median; IQR)	z-test (from Somers' D)	
Reflection-to-Question Ratio	0.50 (0.33–0.71)	0.44 (0.32–0.61)	$z = -0.55$; $p = .58$	
Percent Open Questions	23.1 (13.3–37.5)	46.5 (33.3–57.1)	$z = 4.17$, $p < .001$	
Percent Complex Reflections	55.6 (41.9–71.4)	53.8 (40.0–71.4)	$z = 0.12$, $p = .90$	
Percent MI-Adherent	21.4 (10.0–35.0)	63.4 (33.3–83.3)	$z = 3.68$; $p < .001$	

Assessing treatment fidelity and contamination in a cluster randomised controlled trial of motivational...

123

Table 5 Numbers and proportions of sessions rated as above MITI's "Beginning proficiency" and "Competency" thresholds for domains by treatment allocation group

MITI Domain	"Beginning proficiency"		"Competency"	
	Attention control group (n; %)	Intervention group (n; %)	Attention control group (n; %)	Intervention group (n; %)
Global Spirit	34 (24.5)	92 (72.4)	30 (21.6)	88 (69.3)
Global Empathy	71 (51.1)	103 (81.1)	71 (51.1)	103 (81.1)
Reflection-to-Question Ratio	17 (12.2)	9 (7.1)	4 (2.9)	0 (0)
Percent Open Questions	13 (9.4)	54 (42.5)	5 (3.6)	9 (7.1)
Percent Complex Reflections	106 (76.3)	98 (77.2)	87 (62.6)	78 (61.4)
Percent MI-Adherent	1 (0.7)	26 (20.5)	1 (0.7)	25 (19.7)

example, nurses expressed concern about over-stepping their professional roles, feeling that it was inappropriate for them to deliver specialist psychological intervention and described feeling under pressure to participate in the research. Some felt undersupported by their primary care surgery and others resented the extra workload as a result of participating in the trial. Although the surgeries were remunerated for participation, the trial did not provide direct individual financial compensation. One solution to this problem may be to assess inherent competencies prior to training, enabling a process of selection whereby the most suitable nurses are recruited. This is a similar idea to that put forward in an assessment of treatment fidelity of nurse-led MI in pain rehabilitation, where the authors suggested that more rigour was necessary in the selection of MI counsellors [32]. It is not currently possible to distinguish whether D6 nurses possessed existing psychological skills, which were not especially built upon, or whether they learned skills to a basic level but then failed to improve materially upon them.

In the attention control arm, the moderate levels of Spirit and Empathy of MI, the ratio of reflections to questions, which was slightly higher than in the psychological treatment arm, and the fact that just over half of reflections were complex suggested that there was some delivery of MI. On the other hand, the behavioural change index summary score was low in this trial arm. The evidence of delivery of active intervention in the control arm was surprising given the design of the trial. Specifically, cluster randomisation was used in part to avoid a given clinician being trained in the delivery of psychological treatment and then introducing elements of this to participants in the attention control arm. The contamination that took place despite this design may have been due to a number of reasons. For instance, some primary care nurses already possessed skills that were consistent with psychological treatment. Two control nurses are known to have had experience of MI before the trial: one had received brief training in it and one had applied it to smoking cessation. Other reasons

include the impact of giving extra time to deliver standard care as part of the attention control design; finally, participation in the trial may itself have induced nurses to provide a slightly different type of standard care.

The primary analysis of D6 included a fidelity assessment of a small sample of therapy session recordings (n = 69) in both treatment groups, using both the MITI and the BECCI [7]. The researchers sampled three tape recordings from each nurse and rated only a 20-min window in the middle of each recording. Those findings showed a similar trend to those reported here, but the trial arm differences were estimated to be smaller and had larger standard errors. We consider that, despite the labour-intensive nature of the fuller assessment and the increased costs of employing trained raters (usually psychologists), it is worth rating treatment fidelity for participants (ideally a large sample or all of them) rather than clinicians in order to generate more representative observations of treatment receipt in a trial. Costs may come down with developments in machine learning and automated fidelity evaluation.

In summary, the results indicate that the intervention did not represent the highest level of psychotherapy fidelity, whilst those allocated to receive attention control appeared to receive some components of the intervention. The findings suggest that a large estimate of effectiveness of the intervention, where comparison groups are defined by treatment offer, may be unlikely. There may be utility in an efficacy analysis which estimates treatment effect amongst a sub-population who would receive either high fidelity psychological treatment or pure attention control if offered.

Conclusions

There were many factors that may have contributed to limited development in skills, including individual nurse characteristics and organisational factors such as lack of support and appropriate surgery infrastructure [31]. Future studies should focus on selection strategies for nurses that maximise chances of success, enhance the training of nurses, consider comparing the comparator treatments of standard care and attention control, or consider the possibility that primary care nurse acquisition of high-level MI and CBT skills is not a viable approach to improved self-management among diabetic patients with persistent suboptimal control. Similar RCTs should assess treatment fidelity in a large sample of participants and should evaluate both treatment receipt in the intervention arm and the absence of intervention in the control arm. This enables an assessment of what treatments participants received and allows researchers to account for this in an efficacy analysis.

Primary care nurses struggled to acquire and deliver psychological skills such as MI and CBT to a high level, despite the use of an intensive, manualised training programme with ongoing supervision by an experienced clinical psychologist. Further studies may be needed to determine whether, for patients to benefit from such therapies, a different skill set may be needed in the healthcare professional or a re-organisation of nurse practitioner time to allow for greater engagement in training and delivery.

Abbreviations

BECCI: Behaviour Change Counselling Index; CBT: Cognitive behavioural therapy; D6: Diabetes 6; ICC: Intraclass correlation coefficient; MI: Motivational interviewing; MITI: Motivational Interviewing Treatment Integrity; RCT: Randomised controlled trial; T2D: Type 2 diabetes

Acknowledgments

The authors would like to thank all the nurses and patients who participated in the D6 Study. They would also like to thank Pamela Macdonald, Amy Harrison, and Clare Tucker who contributed to the treatment fidelity ratings.

Funding

This report is independent research arising from a Programme Grant for Applied Research (RP-PG-0606-1142) and a Doctoral Research Fellowship (DRF-2014-07-002) supported by the National Institute for Health Research (NIHR). Sabine Landau and Khalida Ismail received salary support from the NIHR Biomedical Research Center at South London and Maudsley NHS Foundation Trust and King's College London. The views expressed in this publication are those of the authors and not necessarily those of the NHS, the NIHR or the Department of Health, UK.

Authors' contributions

NM and HG performed analyses and prepared the final manuscript. KI and SL supervised the project. KI together with KW, NdZ, SA, and ES conceived the study design and oversaw the project. All authors read and approved the final manuscript.

Competing interests

KI has received honorarium from Eli Lilly, Sanofi, Janssen, and Sunovion for giving educational lectures at educational events. NdZ has received honorarium from Eli Lilly for giving an educational lecture.

Author details

[1]Department of Biostatistics and Health Informatics, Institute of Psychiatry, Psychology and Neuroscience, King's College London, 16 De Crespigny Park, London SE5 8AF, UK. [2]Department of Psychological Medicine, Institute of Psychiatry, Psychology and Neuroscience, King's College London, London, UK. [3]Diabetes and Nutritional Sciences Division, School of Medicine, King's College London, London, UK. [4]Institute of Diabetes, Endocrinology and Obesity, King's Health Partners, London, UK.

References

1. Craig P, Dieppe P, Macintyre S, Michie S, Nazareth I, Petticrew M. Developing and evaluating complex interventions: the new Medical Research Council guidance. Int J Nurs Stud. 2013;50:587–92. Davies MJ, Heller S, skinner TC, et al. effectiveness of the diabetes education and self management for ongoing and newly diagnosed (DESMOND) programme for people with newly diagnosed type 2 diabetes: cluster randomised controlled trial. Br Med J 2008;336:491–5
2. Moore G, Audrey S, Barker M, Bond L, Bonell C, Hardeman W, Moore L, O'Cathain A, Tinati T, Wight D, Baird J. Process evaluation of complex interventions: Medical Research Council guidance. Br Med J. 2015;350:h1258.
3. Dunn G, Emsley R, Liu HH, Landau S, Green J, White I, Pickles A. Evaluation and validation of social and psychological markers in randomised trials of complex interventions in mental health: a methodological research programme. Health Technol Assess. 2015;19(93)
4. Moore G, Audrey S, Barker M, Bond L, Bonell C, Hardeman W, et al. Process evaluation of complex interventions: a summary of Medical Research Council guidance. In: Richards DA, Hallberg IR, editors. Complex Interventions in Health: An overview of research methods. London: Routledge; 2015.
5. Kohrt B, Ramaiya M, Rai S, Bhardwaj A, Jordans MD. Development of a scoring system for non-specialist ratings of clinical competence in global mental health: a qualitative process evaluation of the enhancing assessment of common therapeutic factors (ENACT) scale. Glob Ment Health. 2015;2:e23.
6. Torgerson DJ. Contamination in trials: is cluster randomisation the answer? Br Med J. 2001;322:355–7.
7. Ismail K, Winkley K, de Zoysa N, Patel A, Heslin M, Graves H, Thomas S, et al. Cluster randomised controlled trial of a nurse-led psychological intervention for type 2 diabetes: Diabetes-6 study. Br J Gen Pract. In press.
8. King P, Peacock I, Donnelly R. The UK prospective diabetes study (UKPDS): clinical and therapeutic implications for type 2 diabetes. Br J Clin Pharmacol. 1999;48:643–8.
9. Gæde P, Lund-Andersen H, Parving H-H, Pedersen O. Effect of a multifactorial intervention on mortality in type 2 diabetes. N Engl J Med. 2008;358:580–91.
10. Davies MJ, Heller S, Skinner TC, Campbell MJ, Carey ME, Cradock S, et al. Effectiveness of the diabetes education and self management for ongoing and newly diagnosed (DESMOND) programme for people with newly diagnosed type 2 diabetes: cluster randomised controlled trial. Br Med J. 2008;336:491–5.
11. Ciechanowski PS, Katon WJ, Russo JE. Depression and diabetes: impact of depressive symptoms on adherence, function, and costs. Arch Intern Med. 2000;160:3278–85.
12. Peyrot M, Rubin RR, Lauritzen T, Snoek FJ, Matthews DR, Skovlund SE. Psychosocial problems and barriers to improved diabetes management: results of the cross-National Diabetes Attitudes, wishes and needs (DAWN) study. Diabetic Med. 2005;22:1379–85.
13. National Institute for Clinical Excellence. Type 2 diabetes in adults: management. NICE Guidelines 2015.
14. Alam R, Sturt J, Lall R, Winkley K. An updated meta-analysis to assess the effectiveness of psychological interventions delivered by psychological specialists and generalist clinicians on glycaemic control and on psychological status. Patient Educ Couns. 2009;75:25–36.
15. Ismail K, Thomas SM, Maissi E, Chalder T, Schmidt U, Bartlett J, Patel A, et al. Motivational enhancement therapy with and without cognitive behavior therapy to treat type 1 diabetes: a randomized trial. Ann Intern Med. 2008; 149:708–19.
16. Hardeman W, Lamming L, Kellar I, De Simoni A, Graffy J, Boase S, Sutton S, et al. Implementation of a nurse-led behaviour change intervention to support medication taking in type 2 diabetes: beyond hypothesised active ingredients (SAMS consultation study). Implement Sci. 2014;9:1–13.

17. Jansink R, Braspenning J, Laurant M, Keizer E, Elwyn G, van der Weijden T, Grol R. Minimal improvement of nurses' motivational interviewing skills in routine diabetes care one year after training: a cluster randomized trial. BMC Fam Pract. 2013;14:44.

18. Arkowitz HW, Westra HA. Integrating motivational interviewing and cognitive Behavioural therapy in the treatment of depression and anxiety. J Cogn Psychother. 2004;18:337–50.

19. Miller WR, Rollnick S. Motivational interviewing: preparing people for change. New York: Guilford Press; 2002.

20. Whittemore R, Melkus GD, Sullivan A, Grey M. A nurse-coaching intervention for women with type 2 diabetes. Diabetes Educ. 2004;30:795–804.

21. Ismail K, Winkley K, Rabe-Hesketh S. Systematic review and meta-analysis of randomised controlled trials of psychological interventions to improve glycaemic control in patients with type 2 diabetes. Lancet. 2004;363:1589–97.

22. Madson MB, Campbell TC. Measures of fidelity in motivational enhancement: a systematic review. J Subst Abus Treat. 2006;31:67–73.

23. Rakovshik SG, McManus F. Establishing evidence-based training in cognitive behavioral therapy: a review of current empirical findings and theoretical guidance. Clin Psychol Rev. 2010;30:496–516.

24. Fairburn CG, Cooper Z. Therapist competence, therapy quality, and therapist training. Behav Res and Ther. 2011;49:373–8.

25. Moyers TB, Martin T, Manuel JK, Hendrickson SML, Miller WR. Assessing competence in the use of motivational interviewing. J Subst Abuse Treat. 2005;28:19–26.

26. Moyers T, Martin T, Manuel J, Miller W, Ernst D. Revised global scales: motivational interviewing treatment integrity 3.1. 1 (MITI 3.1. 1). Unpublished manuscript, University of New Mexico, Albuquerque, NM. 2010. https://casaa.unm.edu/download/miti3_1.pdf.

27. Lane C, Huws-Thomas M, Hood K, Rollnick S, Edwards K, Robling M. Measuring adaptations of motivational interviewing: the development and validation of the behavior change counseling index (BECCI). Patient Educ Couns. 2005;56:166–73.

28. Apodaca TR, Longabaugh R. Mechanisms of change in motivational interviewing: a review and preliminary evaluation of the evidence. Addiction. 2009 May 1;104(5):705–15.

29. Moyers TB, Miller WR. Is low therapist empathy toxic? Psychol Addict Behav. 2013 Sep;27(3):878.

30. Cicchetti DV. Guidelines, criteria, and rules of thumb for evaluating normed and standardized assessment instruments in psychology. Psychol Assess. 1994;6:284–90.

31. Graves H, Garrett C, Amiel SA, Ismail K, Winkley K. Psychological skills training to support diabetes self-management: qualitative assessment of nurses' experiences. Prim Care Diabetes. 2016:376–82.

32. Mertens VC, Forsberg L, Verbunt JA, Smeets RE, Goossens ME. Treatment fidelity of a nurse-led motivational interviewing-based pre-treatment in pain rehabilitation. J Behav Health Serv Res. 2016;43(3):459–73.

12

Patients' and practice nurses' perceptions of depression in patients with type 2 diabetes and/or coronary heart disease screened for subthreshold depression

Alide D. Pols[1,2*] (iD), Karen Schipper[3], Debbie Overkamp[2], Harm W. J. van Marwijk[2,4], Maurits W. van Tulder[1] and Marcel C. Adriaanse[1]

Abstract

Background: Comorbid depression is common in patients with type 2 diabetes (DM2) and/or coronary heart disease (CHD) and is associated with poor quality of life and adverse health outcomes. However, little is known about patients' and practice nurses' (PNs) perceptions of depression. Tailoring care to these perceptions may affect depression detection and patient engagement with treatment and prevention programs. This study aimed to explore patients' and PNs' perceptions of depression in patients with DM2/CHD screened for subthreshold depression.

Methods: A qualitative study was conducted as part of a Dutch stepped-care prevention project. Using a purposive sampling strategy, data were collected through semi-structured interviews with 15 patients and 9 PNs. After consent, all interviews were recorded, transcribed verbatim and analyzed independently by two researchers with Atlas.ti.5.7.1 software. The patient and PN datasets were inspected for commonalities using a constant comparative method, from which a final thematic framework was generated.

Results: Main themes were: illness perception, need for care and causes of depression. Patients generally considered themselves at least mildly depressed, but perceived severity levels were not always congruent with Patient Health Questionnaire 9 scores at inclusion. Initially recognizing or naming their mental state as a (subthreshold) depression was difficult for some. Having trouble sleeping was frequently experienced as the most burdensome symptom. Most experienced a need for care; psycho-educational advice and talking therapy were preferred. Perceived symptom severity corresponded with perceived need for care, but did not necessarily match help-seeking behaviour. Main named barriers to help-seeking were experienced stigma and lack of awareness of depression and mental health care possibilities. PNs frequently perceived patients as not depressed and with minimal need for specific care except for attention. Participants pointed to a mix of causes of depression, most related to negative life events and circumstances and perceived indirect links with DM2/CHD.

Conclusion: Data of the interviewed patients and PNs suggest that they have different perceptions about (subthreshold) depressive illness and the need for care, although views on its causes seem to overlap more.

Keywords: Qualitative study, Depression, Type 2 diabetes mellitus, Coronary heart disease, Illness perceptions, Need for care

---

* Correspondence: a.pols@vumc.nl
[1]Department of Health Sciences, Amsterdam Public Health Research Institute,
Faculty of Science, Vrije Universiteit Amsterdam, Amsterdam, the Netherlands
[2]Amsterdam Public Health Research Institute, Department of General Practice
& Elderly Care Medicine, Amsterdam UMC, Vrije Universiteit Amsterdam,
Amsterdam, the Netherlands
Full list of author information is available at the end of the article

Background

Comorbid depression in patients with type 2 diabetes (DM2) and/ or coronary heart disease (CHD) is a major health issue. The risk of depression in these patients is approximately double compared to the general population [1, 2]. This comorbidity is associated with diminished self-care and medication adherence [3, 4], poorer quality of life [5], and increased mortality [6, 7]. Similar negative effects are seen with comorbid subthreshold depression [8], defined as clinically relevant depressive symptoms without fulfilling the criteria for major depressive disorder (MDD). Subthreshold depression is present in approximately one third of the patients with DM2 and/or CHD [9–11] and is the strongest predictor for the onset of MDD [12, 13].

Despite its negative impact, depression often remains under-recognized, under-discussed and undertreated in the general population [14]. The detection of comorbid depression in patients with long term physical conditions, like DM2 and CHD, is even more challenging as symptoms can overlap [15, 16]. Therefore, in clinical guidelines, various organizations have suggested screening for depression to improve detection rates [15, 17, 18]. However, at present, there is no substantial evidence that this approach is effective [19, 20]. Reducing the burden of depression by preventing the influx of new cases is a promising strategy, particularly through early recognition and treatment of patients at risk (indicated prevention), such as those with subthreshold depression. Meta-analyses have shown that preventative psychological interventions can overall reduce the incidence of MDD in comparison to control groups [12, 21].

Offering preventative psychological interventions in a stepped-care format could be an efficient approach, which also fits well with current task shifting and delegating trends. In primary care in the Netherlands, most GPs work with psychological practice nurses (those who provide low-intensity mental health care) and somatic practice nurses (those who largely focus on general physical care), who are generally located in the same building. This internationally unique integrated primary care team aims to provide local community-based continuity of care [22, 23]. In stepped-care, patients start with minimally intensive evidence-based treatments and progress is monitored systematically. Those who do not improve adequately, step up to a treatment of higher intensity [24]. Many guidelines endorse this stepped-care principle for depression treatment [15, 25, 26], but the evidence on the effectiveness of prevention is limited and conflicting. While effective in reducing the incidence of MDD in elderly or visually impaired populations [27–29], it was not superior to usual care in other elderly, diabetic or primary care populations [9, 30–32]. Recently, we conducted a randomized controlled trial in which we evaluated whether a pragmatic, nurse-led stepped-care program was effective in reducing the incidence of MDD at 12-months of follow-up in comparison with usual care among patients with DM2 and/or CHD and subthreshold depression (Step-Dep study) [33]. The stepped-care approach was not superior to usual care after one year [34]. Consecutively, qualitative research was conducted to gain a deeper understanding of these results. A process evaluation was conducted in which we explored both patients' and practice nurses' experiences with the Step-Dep program using the RE-AIM model which assesses five dimensions of an intervention: reach, efficacy, adoption, implementation, and maintenance [35]. We focused on barriers and facilitators of the implementation of the Step-Dep program [36] next to a more conceptual exploration of how DM2/CHD patients and practice nurses perceived comorbid depression.

More insight into patients' perceptions of depression in long-term conditions is of great value. Recent systematic reviews have suggested that the limited understanding we currently have contributes to many of the encountered difficulties in depression care [16, 37]. Differences between patients' and health care providers' perceptions further add to these difficulties [38]. As most patients with depression and DM2 and/or CHD are managed in primary care in the Netherlands, knowledge of these patients' and their health care providers' perceptions of this comorbidity is important, but only a few studies investigating this have been conducted [16, 39–44]. The most used theoretical framework in such studies on perceptions or illness representations is the Common Sense Self-Regulation Model of Health and Illness by Leventhal et al. [45]. This framework states that patients construct their own perceptions of the causes and consequences of the illness, its time-course, the feasibility of controlling or curing it, how it affects one's identity and emotions, and how well the illness is understood. This helps patients to make sense of their illnesses and serves as the basis for coping. Previous studies have mainly focused either on the patient perspective and their experienced relationship between these disorders (the 'cause' item of the model) [16, 39–42], or on health care providers' views of managing depression in these long-term conditions ('cure-control') [43, 44]. Studies exploring aspects like illness perceptions ('identity') and perceived need for care ('cure-control'), or comparing patients' and health care providers' perceptions are lacking. Yet, to improve patient engagement in future indicated prevention programs, knowledge on whether targeted patients perceive themselves as 'ill' and if they perceive a need for care, seems crucial. Moreover, better understanding of both caregivers' and patients' perspectives, as well as the differences between them, may enable prevention programs to be more tailored to these perceptions, potentially improving depression care [46]. Therefore, this study aimed to investigate patients' and practice nurses' perceptions of depression in patients with DM2 and/or CHD screened for subthreshold depression.

Methods
Step-dep study
This qualitative study was part of the Step-Dep study, which consisted of both a pragmatic cluster randomized controlled trial with economic evaluation, whose design [33], results [34] and process evaluation [36] have been described elsewhere. The qualitative process evaluation consisted of semi-structured face-to-face interviews with 24 participants of the intervention arm. As an extension to the 'reach' dimension of the RE-AIM model [35], which describes study participants' characteristics and compares them to the target population, patients' and practice nurses' perceptions of depression were thoroughly explored and reported in this article.

Participants and recruitment
We interviewed all the practice nurses involved in the implementation of the Step-Dep intervention. Amongst them were both psychological practice nurses and somatic practice nurses. Psychological practice nurses provide low-intensity mental health care for primary care patients. Somatic practice nurses provide chronic disease management in the GP practice of patients with physical long-term conditions like DM2, CHD, chronic obstructive pulmonary disease (COPD) and asthma. In the Netherlands, the educational programs for these two types of practice nurses are separate and generally take one year after an appropriate pre-registration education of four years at a University of Applied Sciences.

All Step-Dep study participants had a diagnosis of DM2 and/or CHD, hence the term 'patient' used in this paper. In addition, these patients screened positive on subthreshold or mild depression, which was defined as a Patient Health Questionnaire 9 (PHQ-9; range 0–27) score of six or more [47, 48] without evidence of a major depressive disorder according to the Mini International Neuropsychiatric Interview (MINI) [49, 50]. We used purposive sampling [51] to recruit a diverse sample of patients in order to elicit as many different views as possible on the pre-specified topics of the Common Sense Self-Regulation Model of Health and Illness model [45]. Based on a literature review of factors influencing depression incidence and outcome, we selected patients on: gender, age, presence of DM2 and/or CHD, self-reported history of depression, self-reported current depression, level of education, baseline depression severity (PHQ-9), baseline anxiety severity (HADS-a), baseline quality of life score (EQ5D), baseline social support

scores, locus of control scores. In addition, we selected patients from different urban and rural residential areas.

Both patients and practice nurses were asked by an investigator (AP or DO) to participate in the interviews by phone. All initially selected participants agreed to be interviewed, except for three patients, who were either suffering from a terminal illness or had a terminally ill partner. Three other patients were then asked and all agreed to participate.

Data collection
The interview topic guide (Appendix 1) was both based on the study aims of the process evaluation [36], and included the assessment of patients' and practice nurses' perceptions of (subthreshold) depression in DM2/CHD. For the latter, open-ended questions were formulated (Appendices 2 and 3) that drew upon the Common Sense Self-Regulation Model of Health and Illness [45]. We focused on illness perception ('identity'), need for care ('control-cure') and causes of depression and the interplay with their DM2/CHD ('cause'). These topics were considered to be most clinically relevant by the research-team, because of both patients' and practice nurses' interim feedback during the Step-Dep study, and the research questions that remained after its effectiveness analyses [34].

Two researchers (AP and DO) conducted all the interviews from September to November 2015. After consent, all interviews were anonymized, digitally recorded, transcribed verbatim and entered into Atlas.ti 5.7.1 for analysis and data management. Interviews took place at venues preferred by participants; at home (patients $n = 11$), at the GP practice (practice nurses $n = 8$) or at the VU University Medical Center in Amsterdam (patients $n = 4$, practice nurses $n = 1$) and lasted about 45 min each. AP kept at a reflective journal to be of aid in later analyses. A member check was performed and all participants but one (a patient who could not be reached despite multiple attempts) confirmed the content of the summary sent by mail to be representative of the interview [51]. Data saturation was reached after interviewing 11 patients. Four more patients were subsequently interviewed to confirm this [51]. All nine participating practice nurses in the intervention arm were interviewed, with data saturation reached after the eighth interview.

Data analysis
The process of data collection and analysis was iterative, as data analysis was concurrent with data collection to enable the incorporation and validation of relevant emerging themes into subsequent interviews. Elements from a responsive evaluation were used. This approach provides the opportunity to explore the multiple perspectives of involved stakeholders and to create a rich

and multi-layered understanding of a phenomenon [52]. An important notion in responsive evaluations is that stakeholders are involved in the study and that the perspective of patients is taken into account [52]. Along the research process, data were subject to a inductive thematic analysis [53, 54] .

First, codes were attached to citations related to specific (sub)topics (open coding), leading to a set of descriptive topics per transcript. Then, all codes of all transcripts were compared and redefined, and clustered into themes and subthemes (axial coding) and, overarching themes were formulated (selective coding). Next, similarities and differences between cases were identified (cross case analysis of constant comparison [55]). Patient and practice nurse transcripts were analyzed separately, but comparisons were made across data sets. Two researchers (AP and DO) analyzed the data individually, and relevant themes were agreed upon.

Results
Participants
Table 1 shows the patient and practice nurse characteristics as measured at baseline of the Step-Dep study. Of the 15 participating patients, eight were female. The average age was 62, ranging from 48 to 84 years. PHQ-9 scores at inclusion varied from seven to 16 and were 10.9 on average. 11 patients reported a history of depression and five patients a current depression. Of the nine practice nurses interviewed, six were psychological practice nurses, three were somatic practice nurses and one of the latter had been a psychological practice nurse before. The average number of treated Step-Dep patients per practice nurse was 11 and varied from 3 to 24. Additional data can be found in Table 1.

Main themes
The results of this study are presented by three main themes: 1) illness perception, 2) need for care and 3) causes of depressive symptoms. As the focus of this study was on perceptions of mental health, this is implied in both the concept of (mental) illness perception and need for (mental health) care. An overview of the main findings per theme and the corresponding interview questions can be found in Table 2. For each theme, the most illustrative quotes were selected. Per quote, the main interviewee characteristics are described; P is used for patients and N for practice nurses. Full (anonymized) interviewee details can be found in Appendix 4.

Illness perception
In general, patients and practice nurses perceived patients' depressive symptom severity prior to the start of Step-Dep as varying widely, ranging from 'not depressed' to 'severely depressed'. Patients' perceptions of their

Table 1 Patient (n = 15) and practice nurse (n = 9) characteristics at inclusion Step-Dep study

Patients		
Gender (n)	Female	8
	Male	7
Age	Range	48–84
	Mean	62
Chronic disease (n)	DM2	9
	CHD	10
	DM2 and CHD	4
Number of long-term conditions	Range	1–9
	Mean	3
Level of education (n)	Low	4
	Average	5
	High	6
History of depression (n)	Yes	11
	No	4
Self-reported depression (n)	Yes	5
	No	10
Depression severity PHQ-9 at inclusion	Range	7–16
	Mean	10,9
Anxiety HADS-A	Range	2–15
	Mean	8
Quality of life EQ5D	Range	0,39–0,92
	Mean	0,72
Social support	Range	34–55
	Mean	45
Locus of control	Range	5–21
	Mean	14
Practice nurses		
Gender (n)	female	7
Type (n)	Psychological practice nurse	6
	Somatic practice nurse	3
Number of patients treated during Step-Dep	Range	3–24
	Mean	11
Years of relevant professional experience as health-care provider	Range	3–30
	Mean	16,3

Abbreviations: CHD = Coronary Heart Disease, DM2 = Type 2 Diabetes Mellitus, PHQ-9 = Patients Health Questionnaire 9 score (range 0–27, higher scores indicating more severe depression), HADS-A = Hospital Anxiety and Depression Scale (range 0–21, with higher scores indicating more severe anxiety), EQ5D = EuroQol-5D (range 0–1, with higher scores indicating higher quality of life), social support (range 0–48, higher scores indicating more perceived social support), locus of control (range 0–20, higher scores indicating a more external locus of control)

Table 2 Overview of themes, questions and results

Themes	Questions	Results
Illness perception (identity)	Patient • How would you describe your mental state before starting Step-Dep? • If not depressed: please tell more about it? • If depressed: please tell more about it? Did it influence your life? PN • How did you view their mental state/ depressive symptoms? • Did patients recognize themselves in the depressed profile?	• Patients' and PNs' perceptions of depressive symptom severity varied from not to severely depressed and were not always congruent with PHQ-9 scores at inclusion • Almost all patients considered themselves at least mildly to moderately depressed • PNs frequently perceived their patients as 'not depressed' • Patients sometimes needed time to talk about and reflect on their mood • Work experience perhaps influenced PNs' perceptions of patients' depressive symptoms • Many patients did not initially realize that the mental state they were in was a level of depression • Patients preferred using their own words to describe their mental state, some terms were not connected to mood. • Sleeping was frequently pointed out as the most burdensome symptom
Need for care (cure/control)	Patient • Were you in need of care/ a preventive program to improve depressive symptoms? • How would it have been, if you had not received an invitation for Step-Dep? • What were your expectations/ hopes from the program? • What would your care of choice have been like? And to improve depressive symptoms? PN • Were the patients in need for care for depression? Other need for care? Why? Why not?	• Most interviewed patients experienced a need for care and preferred psycho-educational advice and talking therapy • PNs frequently said that patients had minimal need for specific care and mostly needed attention • In patients, perceived symptom severity corresponded with perceived need for care, but did not necessarily match help-seeking behaviour • Barriers to seek care: ○ Not realizing that mental state is a level of depression ○ Experienced stigma of depression ○ Unfamiliarity with mental health care ○ Experienced barriers discussing mental problems with GP
Depression causes (cause)	Patient • Is there a relationship with your chronic disease? How? • What do you think caused your depressive symptoms? • How is your mental state now? If improved: what are the reasons for that? PN • How do you view the relationship with the chronic disease? What coping strategies do patients have with a chronic disease? • What are causes of depressive symptoms? • If the depressive symptoms improved in your patients; what was the reason?	• Most patients and PNs appointed a mix of causes of depression • Most were related to negative life events and circumstances • Many PNs and patients perceived indirect links with long-term conditions via: ○ physical limitation ○ changed future perspectives ○ difficulties with acceptance of diagnosis of a long-term condition

symptom severity did not necessarily correspond with their individual PHQ-9 scores at inclusion. It was more common for the PHQ-9 scores to be higher than the perceived symptom severity than the other way around, but both occurred. When asked whether patients recognized themselves in the 'subthreshold depression' profile they were screened on, three patients responded at first that they had not felt depressed at all. One of them explained that she only screened 'positive' (with a relatively high score of 11) on the PHQ-9 by scoring on physical symptoms, unrelated to her mood, caused by her multiple chronic diseases. However, during the interviews, the other two patients eventually explained that they had been somewhat down or 'sombre'. In Dutch primary

care depression guidelines and patient information, 'sombre' is the most frequently used term to describe all severity levels of depression [56]. It seemed that these two patients needed time to feel comfortable enough to open up and reflect on their mood, which could be problematic in short consultations in primary care.

"It was not as if I was in a sombre mood when I decided to participate. [...] Well yes, that was when I was not feeling too happy..." (P2, female, CHD)

All the other interviewed patients did experience some level of depression and indicated that this had a significant impact on their daily lives. About half the patients thought their mood matched the subthreshold depressed profile well and confirmed that they had felt mildly to moderately depressed. Yet many others described themselves as fully depressed.

"I was feeling really miserable. Too often feeling sombre and too tired. A complete lack of energy, just a wreck. I had trouble sleeping and concentrating. I was just not happy. Not a fun person anymore, in my opinion. (laughs). There was no room for anything else. I think I was actually barely hanging on. Yes, I was certainly depressed." (P5, female, DM2)

Whereas almost all patients would have labelled themselves as at least mildly to moderately depressed, practice nurses frequently perceived their patients as 'not depressed'. Two very experienced psychological practice nurses, who treated more Step-Dep patients than other practice nurses, even reported that virtually none of their patients were depressed.

"But I did not consider them depressed. That is something you can sense, or taste almost. No." (N7, psychological PN)

One of these practice nurses questioned whether her perception of her patients' depressive symptoms was influenced by her working experience: *"As I am used to working with some more severe problems, I thought: 'Am I missing something here?'" (N2, psychological PN)*. In contrast, a few practice nurses called their patients chronically (mildly) depressed and one somatic practice nurse thought all her patients had severe depressive symptoms.

In terms of acknowledging, labelling and naming symptoms as part of 'depression', patients initially had difficulty realizing that their mental state was actually a level of depression. Filling out the PHQ-9 questionnaire as part of the screening process of Step-Dep and reflecting on that, seemed to help patients to identify their negative mental state as a (subthreshold) depression.

"Looking back, I wouldn't have thought that I was that... how should I phrase that...sombre. That actually shocked me at times. To realize that I seemed quite negative. And I actually was negative back then." (P9, male, DM2 & CHD)

The following extract illustrates how some practice nurses experienced this in their patients as well.

"Due to that questionnaire, they would say: 'My gosh, all this time, I have been depressed without knowing.'

The best example was this one patient who had a massive score and was like: 'My goodness, what is the matter with me?' Well, she had been feeling miserable, but had not connected the dots." (N3, psychological PN)

Many patients however, who did recognize their mental state as a mild to moderate depression, rejected the term 'sombre' to describe it. It felt like a stigma for some or just too exaggerated for others. The following quote illustrates this.

"Sombre would be exaggerating, but I sure wasn't cheerful. Not a happy lad and at the same time seeing a psychologist." (P11, male, DM2)

Almost all patients would spontaneously use other words to describe their low mood, even the patients that labelled themselves as 'fully depressed'.

"took a bad turn" (P10, male, DM2) "rough times" (P11, male, DM2) "continuous sorrow" (P13, male, CHD) "down and out" (P12, female, DM2 & CHD) "wrecked" (P12, female, DM2 & CHD)

Some of the terms they used, were not even necessarily connected to a depressed mood.

"loss of self-confidence" "stress" (P11, male, DM2) " burdensome worries" (P1, female, CHD) "burn-out" (P12, female, DM2 & CHD)

A striking number of patients reported troubled sleeping and described this as their most burdensome symptom. The following quotation illustrates a perceived link between trouble sleeping and depression.

"Trouble sleeping. You fall into a downwards spiral, you get so tired, chronically tired I would say. It makes it so easy to stay underneath the covers in the morning, drifting off to depression." (P15, female, CHD)

Need for care

Most interviewed patients indicated that they experienced a need for (mental health) care prior to the start of the Step-Dep study. In general, the perceived symptom severity matched the level of perceived need for care. Many practice nurses explained that the need for care varied considerably between patients, and usually corresponded with their perception of the patients' symptom severity. However, the general opinion amongst practice nurses was that the majority of patients had minimal need for specific care and mostly needed attention.

> "The majority did not have a need for care, no. And those who did, were so depressed that they needed clinical treatment." (N7, psychological PN)

The majority of patients cited practical advice and someone to talk to as their preferred modes of care. Practical advice entailed ways to improve their mood, for example through physical exercise and activity planning, and often concerned handling sleeping problems.

> "Just talking to someone, every other week, for half an hour or an hour. To get some practical advice of (name practice nurse) on how to cope with trouble sleeping for example. For her to say: 'Why don't you try this', that really works." (P15, female, CHD)

Many patients did not have a clear idea who the person 'to talk to' would be, but psychotherapists were most frequently mentioned.

> "I did not know much about it, except for the term 'psychotherapy'." (P7, male, DM2)

Whereas patients mainly emphasized their need for practical psycho-educational advice and talking therapy, practice nurses reported that patients predominantly needed attention.

> "I often reckoned that maybe they just needed some attention. Not to be negative or anything. Just to have somewhere and someone to talk to without sparing that someone, like they would have to with a partner or family member. The freedom to just talk. A need for attention." (N2, psychological PN)

Such mismatches in patients' and practice nurses' views on how much and which care is needed potentially jeopardizes patient engagement in offered care.

An interesting finding from the patients' interviews was that the perceived symptom severity and the corresponding perceived need for care did not necessarily match patients' own predictions of or actual help-seeking behaviour. While most patients experienced a need for care, many did not and would not have asked for it. Patients explained that they experienced barriers that withheld them from seeking care. These appointed barriers were often also perceived by practice nurses. Many of the barriers indicated dealt with the taboo and social stigma of depression. The following quotation illustrate a variety of these.

> "Being a true 'Twent' (Dutch word for someone from the eastern province of the Netherlands) I never reveal what I am truly feeling." (P10, male, DM2)

> "I never would have asked for that kind of help myself. Growing up, I was taught not to complain. Especially not about mental problems, because that is just all in your head and therefor something you should resolve on your own. [...] To overcome the idea of 'You used to be normal, yet now you have become a psychiatric patient' [...] The stigma already completely surrounds you." (P7, male, DM2)

> "So many of them were of a certain age, when society used to say 'Take it like a man, stop complaining.' And so many would lead their lives according to these social codes, bearing their problems in silence." (N1, psychological PN)

In addition, as patients would often not realize that they were depressed, they were unaware that they could ask for help.

> "I wonder if I would have looked for any help, since I was just so used to feeling like that. I just feel so much better now. It makes me think: 'Darn, things were definitely not alright back then.' But, it was normal for me." (P5, female, DM2)

> "But in the end, there were quite a few who did have a need for care. But apparently, they had not acted upon it yet. It had not reached their frontal lobe yet, so to say. Not up to the point where they would say: 'I need to do something about this, I should make an appointment.'"(N3, psychological PN)

Patients also mentioned barriers that practice nurses did not. Some patients explained that they were unfamiliar with mental health care and its possibilities for help. Other patients mentioned difficulties talking to their GPs about mental problems. Patients felt that GPs mainly focused on physical disease, or they experienced a lack of time and space, or a lack of continuity of care to discuss mental issues with their GP.

> "I guess because I was unfamiliar with that area of health care, I would not have looked for it." (P9, male, DM2 & CHD)

> "In my experience, GP's are always short on time. That makes it really difficult to discuss that kind of problems. Because GPs, like mine, are so busy already and work part-time too, that you always see a different one, which I find very disturbing." (P1, female, CHD)

Causes of depressive symptoms

Both patients and practice nurses indicated various causes of depressive symptoms, both related and unrelated to long-term conditions, and most said that a mix of these leads to depression. The most frequently mentioned causes were serious life-events like divorce, bereavement or childhood traumas, as well as negative circumstances like job loss or work pressure. Other, less frequently named causes were personal traits like personality, genes or character, aging and loneliness.

"Those life events obviously had an impact on their quality of life and appealed to their coping mechanisms." (N1, psychological PN)

"It was caused by job insecurity, financial problems or by thyroid medication that needed adjusting. They would appoint very specific problems and say: 'The way I felt, was a reaction to those problems.' Circumstances, yes." (N2, psychological PN)

Many patients and practice nurses experienced indirect links between long-term conditions and depression. Physical limitations caused by DM2, CHD or other chronic diseases, along with their impact on daily life, were seen as the most prominent indirect causes of depression. Interviewees did not necessarily presume a 'linear' relation between the severity of these limitations and depressive symptoms. Changed prospects of the future due to a chronic disease formed another important indirect cause. Further, both patients and practice nurses explained how 'mourning' the diagnosis of a chronic illness could lead to depression, in which acceptance problems played a dominant role.

"I used to walk 20 to 25 km with a friend every other week. That used to be so easy for me, but I can't anymore. The fact that we had to turn around, that I couldn't finish that specific walk and had to take a short-cut back... That had a considerable impact. It did not cheer me up at all, to the contrary." (P6, male, CHD)

"But even in those people with severe limitations, it would not necessarily have that much of an impact. I am remembering this lady who was severely limited, but was so incredibly active. (laughs) In her case, it did not influence her mood, per se." (N4, psychological PN)

"I don't really feel those glucose levels. I know the diabetes is there and I realize its

consequences, which is possibly the most frightening aspect for me. People say that it is a secret assassin, and that is true, actually." (P10, male, DM2)

"It is a kind of 'mourning' process that you have to go through, to reach a state of acceptance of your losses, like your energy levels, at work, things you used to be able to do. You have to learn to accept that you won't be able to do all of that anymore. Well, that was my biggest problem." (P7, male, DM2)

Very few patients and practice nurses directly linked DM2 and/ or CHD to depression.

"That (her and her husband's chronic diseases) absolutely has it effect on the things you want to do or the way you feel. I do believe that." (P12, female, DM2 & CHD)

"Well, I have seen how being chronically ill just leads to a depressed mood." (N8, somatic PN)

There were also some patients and practice nurses who believed that depression is not related to DM2 or CHD.

"Well, it didn't even cross my mind, that is how important it is to me. I have a hint of diabetes. (laughs) I just use one pill a day. For me, it is such a none-issue, that it hadn't even occurred to me." (P11, male, DM2)

Only one practice nurse reckoned that the diagnosis of a long-term condition itself could have an anti-depressant effect.

"I did not see that presumed relation, or hardly. It is very well possible that people adjust their lifestyle, and realize the impermanence of life...that it is a wake-up call and acts as an anti-depressant." (N7, psychological PN)

Discussion

This qualitative study explored patients' and practice nurses' perceptions of the construct of 'depression' in patients with DM2 and/or CHD screened for subthreshold depression. Our overall analysis is that better understanding of how chronically ill patients make sense of depressive symptoms or illnesses, in view of their need for care and in view of how they see the symptoms in the context of their lives (the 'causes') is crucial for the implementation of mental health care into chronic disease care. Perhaps practice nurses can also be better trained for this.

Illness perception

In general, the interviewed patients considered themselves at least mildly depressed, whereas practice nurses, interestingly, frequently perceived patients as not depressed. This discrepancy is perhaps partially caused by the fact that psychological practice nurses are used to working with patients with quite severe depression and a clear request for help. Step-Dep patients, on the other hand, were pro-actively selected on the presence of subthreshold depression on a self-report questionnaire. Furthermore, previous research suggests that somatic practice nurses sometimes experience a lack of competence to adequately recognize and handle mental problems in chronically ill patients [36]. However, this could also be part of a more widespread phenomenon, as it is has been described before that many caregivers have the tendency to 'normalize' depression in patients with long-term conditions [43, 44]. In addition, some patients initially did not recognize their mental state as a level of depression, which might prohibit them from disclosing their depressive symptoms to caregivers. This has been observed in other studies as well [37, 39]. These studies suggest that patients might 'refuse' to recognize and acknowledge their depression due to an inner conflict of their ideal self-identity and perceiving themselves as a person with depression (ego dystonia in Freudian terms). In this study, we have also observed the opposite as in some patients sombre feelings would be present for so long, that they accepted these as normal (egosyntonic) and therefore failed to recognize these as a level of depression.

Perceived depressive symptom severity was not always congruent with PHQ-9 scores at inclusion. Both over- and underestimation by the PHQ-9 of depression severity was perceived. Even though the PHQ-9 is a validated instrument to screen for mild depression in the chronically ill using a cut-off of 6 [47, 48], our findings could indicate that, in these specific long-term conditions, the discriminative properties of this method were not optimal. A recent study in a population of patients with DM2/CHD, found optimal cut-off scores for minor and major depression to be within a small range of 8 and 10 respectively [57]. This suggests that the PHQ-9 might not be specific enough to distinguish minor from major depression for scores in this range. A higher cut-off score of 8 might be necessary in order not to over-diagnose mild depression in patients with DM2/CHD, as

symptom of the somatic diseases and depression, like fatigue and altered appetite, can overlap. Also, there is an association between depressive symptoms and distress related to long-term conditions [58], such as diabetes distress [59, 60]. A complex finding of our study was that even though patients explained they felt mildly to moderately depressed, they independently labelled their mental state differently than 'depression'. It seems likely that patients actually do suffer from depressive symptoms, but prefer using different labels like 'stress' or 'sleeping disorders', as they perceive these as less stigmatizing than 'depression'. However, since the specificity of the PHQ-9 with a cut-off of 6 was found to be only 55% [57], our findings raise questions over whether it discriminates enough between mild depression and mild forms of other psychological problems, like anxiety, burn-out or sleeping disorders.

In this study, many patients expressed both the heavy burden of sleeping problems and the wish to alleviate it. Problems with sleeping are classic symptoms of depression, but the associations between disturbed sleep and depression [61] or long-term conditions [62], like CHD and DM2, have also been well established. While the underlying mechanisms of the relationships between these conditions and their implications for rational therapeutics should be further explored [63], addressing sleeping problems seems a promising starting point for the delivery of mental health care for most patients with depressive symptoms.

Need for care

Perceived need for care coincided with perceived symptom severity, but often did not match help-seeking behaviour. Although most patients experienced a need for care, preferring psycho-educational advice and talking therapy, many would not have sought such care if it had not been offered pro-actively. Patients blamed several experienced barriers. The perceived stigma of depression was the most important barrier, but the initial lack of awareness about depression and mental health care options, and perceived difficulties to discuss mental health issues with GPs, were also mentioned. In previous studies, experienced stigma and taboo of depression were found to form important barriers to both help-seeking and disclosure of depressive symptoms [16, 37, 39, 43]. Whereas the appointed barriers apparently withheld patients from actively seeking care, it did not seem to withhold them from accepting care by participating in the Step-Dep program. Pro-actively offering care therefore appears to be an appropriate approach to overcome such barriers. However, we cannot exclude the possibility that the motivation to contribute to research was actually pivotal in their decision to participate in the program. The process evaluation of Step-Dep revealed that all patients appointed the contribution to research as (one of the) primary motivators to participate. Only less than half named the need to improve their mood as a primary motivation [36]. Yet, given the importance and magnitude of perceived stigma of depression, it seems more likely that naming the contribution to research instead of experienced depression as the main motivator felt less stigmatizing for some and the pro-active offer of care facilitated the acceptance of care.

Causes of depression

The interviewees in this study cited a mix of causes leading to depression. The perceived importance of the contribution of negative life events and circumstances to the development of depression is in line with findings from the review by Anderson et al. [37]. A direct causal link between long-term conditions and depression was largely not supported in our study. This is in contrast with the views of the elderly interviewed by Bogner et al. [42], who perceived that their long-term condition directly caused depression and vice versa. Patients in this and several other studies reported that long-term conditions can lead to depression, not the other way around. In these patients' views, long-term conditions caused depression indirectly, via the burden of physical limitations [16, 41], diminished future perspectives [16] and difficulties accepting the long-term condition diagnosis. The latter was frequently explained in our study as part of the 'mourning' process. Both patients and caregivers frequently referred to terms like 'mourning' and 'acceptance' when describing the response to chronic illness [64], which are originally derived from the Kubler-Ross' grief model [65]. These outcomes, however, are not supported by multiple studies showing that the diagnosis of DM2 by screening does not have significant psychological impact [66, 67]. Still, tuning into patients' perceptions of the causes might facilitate the conversation on depression. In chronic disease care, starting points could therefore be the impact of the diagnosis, physical limitations, or the impairment of future perspectives. However, patients who do not perceive any link between their long-term condition and depression might not disclose depressive symptoms in integrated care settings, which may be a barrier for such care.

Implications

It seems to be of great importance to better inform caregivers in chronic care about the risk of normalising depression and the magnitude of stigma patients experience about depression. Pro-actively educating patients in chronic care on possible comorbid depression and how to handle such symptoms might further help to diminish experienced stigma and create more patient awareness of depression. This might further facilitate integrated somatic and mental health care, as patients would get more acquainted with the concept of chronic caregivers discussing mental health, which is something patients do not necessarily expect, potentially interfering with the success of care integration [23]. Additionally, exploring in practice which terms and settings individual patients relate most to seem very relevant to improve the acceptance of mental health care. Addressing sleeping problems, for example, might be an easily accepted starting point for patients with (subthreshold) depression. More research on how to best identify mild depressive disorders in patients with DM2/CHD and what prompts patients to accept and seek care could contribute to the success of future depression prevention programs.

Strengths and limitations

An important strength of this paper is that both patients and practice nurses were interviewed. Deeper understanding was gained of the caregivers' and patients' views, which led to valuable complementary and contrasting data. The utilisation of two analysts, the systematic development of codes and code definitions, the use of a qualitative computer program, and complete data saturation while still conducting interviews, enhanced the quality of the data.

As the organization of care, for example concerning the role of practice nurses in primary care, might be different outside the Netherlands, these findings might be less applicable in other settings. Furthermore, the results are based on the perceptions of patients who participated in the Step-Dep study. It would be of much added value to interview screened patients who did not consent to participate in Step-Dep, as they might have different perceptions of the investigated themes. Additionally, since our interviewees were mainly native Dutch, cultural differences that may influence depression perceptions were not explored.

Conclusion

Data of the interviewed patients and practice nurses suggest that they have different perceptions about (subthreshold) depressive illness and the need for care, although views on its causes seem to overlap more.

Appendix 1

Table 3 Topic list

RE-AIM	Topic
Reach	Appropriateness Step-Dep patients (target population)
	Depression: recognition, severity, causes, improving factors
	Need for care
	Motivation to participate
	Access mental health care
Efficacy	Perceived effectiveness
	Perceived usefulness
Adoption	Information practices, caregivers
Implementation	Barriers & facilitators
	Deviations from protocol
	Reasons for dropout
	Prerequisites for implementation
Maintenance	Satisfaction
	Feasibility for future

Appendix 2

Table 4 Patients interview

Topic	Question
General	How was your experience participating in Step-Dep/ the program in your general practitioner practice?
	What was the best part for you?
	What was the weakest part for you?
Motivation	Why did you decide to participate in Step-Dep?
Mental state	How would you describe your mental state before starting Step-Dep?
	If not depressed: please tell more about it?
	If depressed: please tell more about it? Did it influence your life? What do you think caused it? Is there a relationship with your chronic disease? How? How is your mental state now? If improved: what are the reasons for that improvement?
	Did you feel the PHQ-9 reflected your mental state correctly? Why? Why not?
Need for care	Were you in need of care/ a preventive program to improve depressive symptoms?
	How would it have been, if you had not received an invitation for Step-Dep?
	What were your expectations/ hopes from the program?
	Did the program match your needs?
	What would your care of choice have been like? And to improve depressive symptoms?
	How would it have been for you to be offered a program at the time of diagnosis of your chronic disease?
Perceived effectiveness	Was the offered program useful to improve your depressive symptoms? Why? Why not? What was most useful to you? How do you see that in the long-term?

Table 4 Patients interview *(Continued)*

Topic	Question
	How were/was the consultations with the practice nurse/ self-help/ problem solving treatment/ referral to general practitioner for you?
Suggestions for future care	Would you recommend this program to others? Why? Why not? To whom?
	What would your suggestions be to improve Step-Dep?
	Is there anything you would like to add to the interview?

Appendix 3

Table 5 Practice nurses interview

Topic	Question
General	How did you experience executing Step-Dep?
	What is your opinion on the Step-Dep program?
	What were the main facilitators?
	What were the main barriers?
Reach	Were the selected patients appropriate for this prevention program? Why? Why not?
	How did you view their mental state/ depressive symptoms? Did patients recognize themselves in the depressed profile? What are causes for depressive symptoms? How do you view the relationship with the chronic disease? What coping strategies do patients have with a chronic disease?
	Were the patients in need for care for depression? Other need for care? Why? Why not?
Efficacy	Did the program match their need for care?
	Was Step-Dep effective in your opinion on preventing depression/ improving depressive symptoms for these patients? Why? Why not? How?
	What is your view on the program elements: consultations, self-help, problem solving treatment, referral to general practitioner?
	If the depressive symptoms improved in your patients; what was the reason for this improvement? Did the program play a part?
Implementation	Why did you decide to participate in Step-Dep?
	How do you view your competences to execute the program?
	Was it necessary to deviate from the protocol? Why? Why not?
	How was using the PHQ-9 for you? And as a screening/ monitoring/ decision tool?
	How much time would you need for the consultations/ self-help/ problem solving treatment?
Maintenance	Is this program (or elements) useful in daily practice for this group? Why? Why not?
	Would you use this program (or elements) in the future? Why? Why not?
	What would be necessary to implement this in your practice?
	How would you ideally see depression prevention?
	What is your opinion on offering a program like that at the time of diagnosis of the chronic disease?

Appendix 4

Table 6 Patient and practice nurse characteristics

Patients

Interview nr	Age	Sex	DM2/CHD	Educational level	Self-reported depression at baseline*	Self-reported History of depression	PHQ-9 score at inclusion
P1	66	f	CHD	high	no	yes	7
P2	61	f	CHD	high	no	yes	7
P3	63	f	Both	intermediate	yes	yes	9
P4	84	f	CHD	low	yes	no	10
P5	53	f	DM2	high	no	yes	16
P6	72	m	CHD	intermediate	no	yes	10
P7	56	m	DM2	high	no	yes	10
P8	73	f	Both	low	no	no	11
P9	55	m	Both	intermediate	no	yes	14
P10	48	m	DM2	intermediate	yes	yes	12
P11	61	m	DM2	low	yes	yes	8
P12	56	f	Both	high	yes	yes	14
P13	66	m	CHD	high	no	yes	7
P14	57	m	DM2	intermediate	no	no	14
P15	55	f	CHD	low	no	no	15

Practice nurses

Interview nr	Practice nurse type	Number of Step-Dep patients treated
N1	psychological practice nurse	24
N2	psychological practice nurse	15
N3	psychological practice nurse	13
N4	psychological practice nurse	10
N5	somatic practice nurse	3
N6	somatic practice nurse	6
N7	psychological practice nurse	15
N8	currently somatic practice nurse, previously psychological practice nurse	3
N9	psychological practice nurse	7

Abbreviations: *F* female, *M* male, *CHD* Coronary Heart Disease, *DM2* Type 2 Diabetes Mellitus, *PHQ-9* Patients Health Questionnaire 9 score. *Scores do not equal inclusion PHQ-9 scores due to time between inclusion and baseline

Abbreviations
CHD: Coronary heart disease; DM2: Type 2 Diabetes Mellitus; GP: General practitioner; PHQ-9: Patients Health Questionnaire 9; PN: Practice nurse

Acknowledgements
The authors would like to thank Lotte Bakker for the transcriptions of the interviews. We also would like to thank all the participating general practices and the research networks of general practitioners (ANH, THOON and LEON) for their participation and collaboration in the implementation and execution of the Step-Dep study. Furthermore, this study has been possible thanks to all interviewed participants. We would like to extend our gratitude to all Step-Dep participants.

Funding
This study is funded by ZonMw, the Netherlands Organisation for Health Research and Development (project number 80–82310–97-12110). The sponsor had no role in the design and conduct of the present study or in the writing of the manuscript.

Author's contributions
AP constructed the design of the study and drafted the manuscript. AP and DO performed all interviews and analyses. KS collaborated in constructing the design, supervised the analyses and revised the manuscript. MA, MvT and HvM collaborated in constructing the design and revised the manuscript. The final manuscript was read and approved by all authors.

Consent for publication
Not applicable.

Competing interests
The authors declare that they have no competing interests.

Author details

[1]Department of Health Sciences, Amsterdam Public Health Research Institute, Faculty of Science, Vrije Universiteit Amsterdam, Amsterdam, the Netherlands. [2]Amsterdam Public Health Research Institute, Department of General Practice & Elderly Care Medicine, Amsterdam UMC, Vrije Universiteit Amsterdam, Amsterdam, the Netherlands. [3]Amsterdam Public Health Research Institute, Department of Medical Humanities, Amsterdam UMC, Vrije Universiteit Amsterdam, Amsterdam, the Netherlands. [4]Division of Primary Care and Public Health, Brighton and Sussex Medical School, Mayfield House, University of Brighton, Brighton, UK.

References

1. Roy T, Lloyd CE. Epidemiology of depression and diabetes: a systematic review. J Affect Disord. 2012;142:S8–21.
2. Rudisch B, Nemeroff CB. Epidemiology of comorbid coronary artery disease and depression. Biol Psychiatry. 2003;54:227–40.
3. Lin EHB, Katon W, Von Korff M, Rutter C, Simon GE, Oliver M, et al. Relationship of depression and diabetes self-care, medication adherence, and preventive care. Diabetes Care. 2004;27:2154–60.
4. Gehi A, Haas D, Sharon Pipkin MAW. Depression and medication adherence in outpatients with coronary heart disease. Arch Intern Med. 2005;165:2508–13.
5. Ali S. The association between depression and health-related quality of life in people with type 2 diabetes: a systematic literature review. Diabetes Metab Res Rev. 2010;26:75–89.
6. van Dooren FEP, Nefs G, Schram MT, Verhey FRJ, Denollet J, Pouwer F. Depression and risk of mortality in people with diabetes mellitus: a systematic review and meta-analysis. PLoS One. 2013;8(3):e57058.
7. Barth J, Schumacher M, Herrmann-Lingen C. Depression as a risk factor for mortality in patients with coronary heart disease: a meta-analysis. Psychosom Med. 2004;66:802–13.
8. Sullivan M, O'Connor P, Feeney P, Hire D, Simmons DL, Raisch D, et al. Depression predicts all-cause mortality. Diabetes Care. 2012;35:1708–15.
9. Bot M, Pouwer F, Ormel J, Slaets JPJ, de Jonge P. Predictors of incident major depression in diabetic outpatients with subthreshold depression. Diabet Med England. 2010;27:1295–301.
10. Thombs BD, Bass EB, Ford DE, Stewart KJ, Tsilidis KK, Patel U, et al. Prevalence of depression in survivors of acute myocardial infarction. J Gen Intern Med. 2005;21:30–8.
11. Hance M, Carney R, Freedland K, Skala J. Depression in patients with coronary heart disease: a 12-month follow-up. Gen Hosp Psychiatry. 1996;18:61–5.
12. Cuijpers P, van Straten A, Smit F, Mihalopoulos C, Beekman A. Preventing the onset of depressive disorders: a meta-analytic review of psychological interventions. Am J Psychiatry. 2008;165:1272–80.
13. Davidson SK, Harris MG, Dowrick CF, Wachtler CA, Pirkis J, Gunn JM. Mental health interventions and future major depression among primary care patients with subthreshold depression. J Affect Disord Elsevier. 2015;177:65–73.
14. Cepoiu M, McCusker J, Cole MG, Sewitch M, Belzile E, Ciampi A. Recognition of depression by non-psychiatric physicians - a systematic literature review and meta-analysis. J Gen Intern Med. 2008;23:25–36.
15. National Collaborating Centre for Mental Health. Depression in adults with a chronic physical health problem. In: The NICE guideline of Treatmen and management; 2010.
16. DeJean D, Giacomini M, Vanstone M, Brundisini F. Patient experiences of depression and anxiety with chronic disease: a systematic review and qualitative meta-synthesis. Ont Health Technol Assess Ser. 2013;13:1–33.
17. Canadian Task Force on Preventive Health Care, Joffres M, Jaramillo A, Dickinson J, Lewin G, Pottie K, Shaw E, TM CGS. Recommendations on screening for depression in adults. CMAJ. 2013;185:753–4.
18. U.S. Preventive Services Task force, Agency for Healthcare Research and Quality, Rockville, Maryland U. Screening for depression in adults: U.S. preventive services task force recommendation statement. Ann Intern Med. 2009;151(11):784–92.
19. Thombs BD, de Jonge P, Coyne JC, Whooley MA, Frasure-smith N, Mitchell AJ, et al. Depression screening and patient outcomes in cardiovascular care a systematic review. JAMA. 2008;300(18):2161–71.
20. Pouwer F, Tack CJ, Geelhoed-Duijvestijn PHLM, Bazelmans E, Beekman AT, Heine RJ, et al. Limited effect of screening for depression with written feedback in outpatients with diabetes mellitus: a randomised controlled trial. Diabetologia. 2011;54:741–8.
21. van Zoonen K, Buntrock C, Ebert DD, Smit F, Reynolds CF, Beekman ATF, et al. Preventing the onset of major depressive disorder: a meta-analytic review of psychological interventions. Int J Epidemiol. 2014;43:318–29.
22. Magnée T, De BDP, De BDH. Verlicht de POH-GGZ de werkdruk van de huisarts? Ned Tijdschr Geneeskd. 2017;160:D983.
23. van Dijk-de Vries A, van Bokhoven MA, de Jong S, Metsemakers JFM, Verhaak PFM, van der Weijden T, et al. Patients' readiness to receive psychosocial care during nurse-led routine diabetes consultations in primary care: a mixed methods study. Int J Nurs Stud. 2016;63:58–64.
24. Bower P, Gilbody S. Stepped care in psychological therapies: access, effectiveness and efficiency. Narrative literature review Br J Psychiatry. 2005;186:11–7.
25. Spijker. Herziening van de multidisciplinaire richtlijnen angst en depressie. Tijdschr Psychiatr. 2010;52(10):715–8.
26. Nice THE. On G, treatment THE, of M. In: D, edition U. the Nice guideline on the treatment and depression the treatment and management of depression; 2009.
27. van't Veer-Tazelaar PJ, van HWJ M, van Oppen P, van HPJ H, van der Horst HE, Cuijpers P, et al. Stepped-care prevention of anxiety and depression in late life: a randomized controlled trial. Arch Gen Psychiatry. 2009;66:297–304.
28. Dozeman E, van Marwijk HWJ, van Schaik DJF, Smit F, Stek ML, van der Horst HE, et al. Contradictory effects for prevention of depression and anxiety in residents in homes for the elderly: a pragmatic randomized controlled trial. Int Psychogeriatrics. 2012;24:1242–51.
29. van der Aa HPA, van Rens GHMB, Comijs HC, Margrain TH, Gallindo-Garre F, Twisk JWR, et al. Stepped care for depression and anxiety in visually impaired older adults: multicentre randomised controlled trial. BMJ. 2015;351:h6127.
30. Zhang DX, Lewis G, Araya R, Tang WK, Mak WWS, Cheung FMC, et al. Prevention of anxiety and depression in Chinese: a randomized clinical trial testing the effectiveness of a stepped care program in primary care. J Affect Disord Netherlands. 2014;169:212–20.
31. Van der Weele GM, De Waal MWM, Van den Hout WB, De Craen AJM, Spinhoven P, Stijnen T, et al. Effects of a stepped-care intervention programme among older subjects who screened positive for depressive symptoms in general practice: the PROMODE randomised controlled trial. Age Ageing. 2012;41:482–8.
32. van Beljouw IM, van Exel E, van de Ven PM, Joling KJ, Dhondt TD, Stek ML, et al. Does an outreaching stepped care program reduce depressive symptoms in community-dwelling older adults? A randomized implementation trial. Am J Geriatr Psychiatry Elsevier Inc. 2014;23:807–17.
33. van Dijk SEM, Pols AD, Adriaanse MC, Bosmans JE, Elders PJM, van Marwijk HWJ, et al. Cost-effectiveness of a stepped-care intervention to prevent major depression in patients with type 2 diabetes mellitus and/or coronary heart disease and subthreshold depression: design of a cluster-randomized controlled trial. BMC Psychiatry. 2013;13:128.
34. Pols, AD, Van Dijk, SEM, Bosmans, JE, Hoekstra, T, Van Marwijk HWJ, Van Tulder, MW, Adriaanse M. Effectiveness of a stepped-care intervention to prevent major depression in patients with type 2 diabetes mellitus and/or coronary heart disease and subthreshold depression: a pragmatic cluster randomized controlled trial. PLoS One. 2017;12(8):e0181023.
35. Glasgow RE, Vogt TM, Boles SM. Evaluating the public health impact of health promotion interventions: the RE-AIM framework. Am J Public Health. 1999;89:1322–7.
36. Pols A, Schipper K, Overkamp D, van Dijk S, Bosmans J, van Marwijk H, Adriaanse M, van Tulder M. Process evaluation of a stepped-care program to prevent depression in primary care: patients' and practice nurses' experiences. BMC Fam Pract. 2017;18:26.
37. Alderson SL, Foy R, Glidewell L, Mclintock K, House A. How patients understand depression associated with chronic physical disease – a systematic review. BMC Fam Pract. 2012;13:41.
38. Saito M, Kawabata H, Murakami MMM. Factors in the awareness of depression, focusing on perceptual dissimilarities between PCPs and patients: an exploratory and qualitative research. Hokkaido Igaky Zasshi. 86:79–83.
39. Alderson SL, Foy R, Glidewell L, House AO. Patients understanding of depression associated with chronic physical illness: a qualitative study. BMC Fam Pract. 2014;15:37.
40. Gask L, Macdonald W, Bower P. What is the relationship between diabetes and depression? A qualitative meta-synthesis of patient experience of co-morbidity. Chronic Illn. 2011;7:239–52.

41. Simmonds RL, Tylee A, Walters P, Rose D. Patients' perceptions of depression and coronary heart disease : a qualitative UPBEAT-UK study. BMC Fam Pract. 2013;14:38.

42. Bogner HR, Dahlberg B. Vries HF De, Cahill E, Barg FK. Older patients' views on the relationship between depression and heart disease. Fam Med. 2008; 40(9):652–7.

43. Coventry PA, Hays R, Dickens C, Bundy C, Garrett C, Cherrington A, et al. Talking about depression: a qualitative study of barriers to managing depression in people with long term conditions in primary care. BMC Fam Pract. 2011;12:10.

44. Barley EA, Walters P, Tylee A, Murray J. General practitioners' and practice nurses' views and experience of managing depression in coronary heart disease: a qualitative interview study. BMC Fam Pract. 2012;13:1–10.

45. Cameron LDLH. The self-regulation of health and illness behaviour. London: Routledge; 2003.

46. E a B, Murray J, Walters P, Tylee A. Managing depression in primary care: a meta-synthesis of qualitative and quantitative research from the UK to identify barriers and facilitators. BMC Fam Pract. 2011;12:47.

47. Kroenke KSR. The PHQ-9: a new depression diagnostic and severity measure. Psychiatr Ann. 2002;32:509–15.

48. Lamers F, Jonkers CCM, Bosma H, Penninx BWJH, Knottnerus JA, van Eijk JTM. Summed score of the patient health Questionnaire-9 was a reliable and valid method for depression screening in chronically ill elderly patients. J Clin Epidemiol. 2008;61:679–87.

49. Sheehan DV, Lecrubier YSK. The MINI-international neuropsychiatric interview (MINI): the development and validation of a structured diagnostic psychiatric interview for DSM-IV and ICD-10. J Clin Psychiatr. 1998;59:22–33.

50. Van Vliet IM, De Beurs E. Het MINI Internationaal Neuropsychiatrisch interview (MINI): Een kort gestructureerd diagnostisch psychiatrisch interview voor DSM-IV-en ICD-10-stoornissen. Tijdschr Psychiatr. 2007;49(6):393–7.

51. Meadows LMJ. Evidence within the qualitative project. Nat Qual Evidence Tijdschr Psychiatr. 2007;9(6):393-7.

52. Abma TA, Stake RE. Responsive evaluation. roots and evolution New Directions for Evaluation. 2001;92:7–22.

53. Braun V, Clarke V. Using thematic analysis in psychology. Qual Res Psychol. 2008;3:77–101.

54. Green J, Thorogood N. Qualitative methods for Health Research. London: SAGE; 2014.

55. Hallberg L. The 'core' category of grounded theory: making constant comparisons. Int J Qual Stud Health Well-B. 2006;1(3):141–8.

56. Depressie N. M44 NHG-Standaard Depressie. Huisarts&Wetenschap. 2012;55: 252–9.

57. van der Zwaan GL, van Dijk SEM, Adriaanse MC, van Marwijk HWJ, van Tulder MW, Pols AD, et al. Diagnostic accuracy of the patient health Questionnaire-9 for assessment of depression in type II diabetes mellitus and/or coronary heart disease in primary care. J Affect Disord. 2015;190:68–74.

58. Nakaya N, Kogure M, Saito-Nakaya K, Tomata Y, Sone T, Kakizaki M, et al. The association between self-reported history of physical diseases and psychological distress in a community-dwelling Japanese population: the Ohsaki cohort 2006 study. Eur J Pub Health. 2013;24:45–9.

59. Snoek FJ, Bremmer MA, Hermanns N. Constructs of depression and distress in diabetes: time for an appraisal. Lancet Diabetes Endocrinol Elsevier Ltd. 2015;3:450–60.

60. Fisher L, Gonzalez JS, Polonsky WH. The confusing tale of depression and distress in patients with diabetes: a call for greater clarity and precision. Diabet Med. 2014;31:764–72.

61. Bao Y-P, Han Y, Ma J, Wang R-J, Shi L, Wang T-Y, et al. Cooccurrence and bidirectional prediction of sleep disturbances and depression in older adults: meta-analysis and systematic review. Neurosci Biobehav Rev. 2017;75: 257–73.

62. Itani O, Jike M, Watanabe N, Kaneita Y. Short sleep duration and health outcomes: a systematic review, meta-analysis and meta-regression. Sleep Med. 2016;32:246–56.

63. Bass J, Takahashi JS. Circadian integration of metabolism and energetics. Science. 2010;330(6009):1349–54.

64. Telford K, Kralik D, Koch T. Acceptance and denial: implications for people adapting to chronic illness: literature review. J Adv Nurs. 2006;55:457–64.

65. Kubler-Ross E. On death and dying. New York: Springer; 1969.

66. Adriaanse MC, Snoek FJ. The psychological impact of screening for type 2 diabetes. Diabetes Metab Res Rev. 2006;22:20–5.

67. Eborall HC, Griffin SJ, Prevost AT, Kinmonth A-L, French DP, Sutton S. Psychological impact of screening for type 2 diabetes: controlled trial and comparative study embedded in the ADDITION (Cambridge) randomised controlled trial. BMJ. 2007;335:486.

13

Nurses' perceptions towards the delivery and feasibility of a behaviour change intervention to enhance physical activity in patients at risk for cardiovascular disease in primary care

Heleen Westland[1]* ⓘ, Yvonne Koop[2], Carin D. Schröder[3], Marieke J. Schuurmans[6], P. Slabbers[4], Jaap C. A. Trappenburg[1] and Sigrid C. J. M. Vervoort[5]

Abstract

Background: Self-management support is widely accepted for the management of chronic conditions. Self-management often requires behaviour change in patients, in which primary care nurses play a pivotal role. To support patients in changing their behaviour, the structured behaviour change Activate intervention was developed. This intervention aims to enhance physical activity in patients at risk for cardiovascular disease in primary care as well as to enhance nurses' role in supporting these patients. This study aimed to evaluate nurses' perceptions towards the delivery and feasibility of the Activate intervention.

Methods: A qualitative study nested within a cluster-randomised controlled trial using semistructured interviews was conducted and thematically analysed. Fourteen nurses who delivered the Activate intervention participated.

Results: Three key themes emerged concerning nurses' perceptions of delivering the intervention: nurses' engagement towards delivering the intervention; acquiring knowledge and skills; and dealing with adherence to the consultation structure. Three key themes were identified concerning the feasibility of the intervention: expectations towards the use of the intervention in routine practice; perceptions towards the feasibility of the training programme; and enabling personal development.

Conclusions: Delivering a behaviour change intervention is challenged by the complexity of changing nurses' consultation style, including acquiring corresponding knowledge and skills. The findings have increased the understanding of the effectiveness of the Activate trial and will guide the development and evaluation of future behaviour change interventions delivered by nurses in primary care.

* Correspondence: H.Westland@umcutrecht.nl
[1]Julius Center for Health Sciences and Primary Care, University Medical Center Utrecht, HP Str. 6.131, PO 85500, 3508, GA, Utrecht, The Netherlands
Full list of author information is available at the end of the article

Background

Self-management support is widely accepted as an approach to improve health-related outcomes, enhance patients' involvement and decrease healthcare costs [1–3]. Self-management support by health care providers, such as primary care nurses, aims to equip patients with the essential skills to manage symptoms, treatment, physical and psychosocial consequences of chronic diseases and to change patients' health behaviour [4, 5]. Over the past decade, in most Western countries, disease management of some of the most prevalent chronic conditions, including diabetes mellitus type 2 and (risk of) cardiovascular disease (CVD), has shifted away from hospitals and towards primary care. In primary care, chronic care is increasingly reallocated from general practitioners towards primary care nurses [6]. Primary care nurses play a pivotal role in the management of chronic conditions, promoting self-management and offering follow-up consultations [6]. Therefore, they in a key position to support these patients in changing their health behaviour [6]. Like other behavioural interventions, self-management interventions are considered complex, containing multiple interacting components [7]. Self-management support requires nurses to adapt their traditional consultation style, which is focused on giving advice, informing and educating patients about their condition, towards a more coaching-oriented consultation style aimed at supporting patients in changing their behaviour [8–10]. Adapting their consultation style adequately implies that nurses need to change their behaviour, which is challenging to accomplish [8, 11–14]. Furthermore, in order to change and incorporate their adapted consultation style into their routine practice, nurses need to be facilitated and supported by their superiors, for instance through being autonomous, having enough time to integrate self-management into their consultations and having training opportunities [11, 12]. The effectiveness of self-management interventions is often evaluated in randomised controlled trials that are mainly focused on pre-specified outcomes rather than on in-depth exploration of the delivery and implementation process [15]. Insight into the perceptions of providers towards the delivery and feasibility of such interventions, as part of a process evaluation, might enhance our understanding of the effectiveness of complex interventions and shed some light on how the intervention works [16–19].

This study evaluated the perceptions of the providers towards the delivery and feasibility of a self-management intervention alongside the cluster-randomised controlled Activate trial. The Activate intervention is a nurse-led behaviour change intervention targeted at increasing physical activity in a large heterogeneous subgroup of patients, namely, those at risk for CVD. The research questions of this study were:

1. What are primary care nurses' perceptions of delivering the Activate intervention to patients at risk for CVD?
2. What are primary care nurses' perceptions of the feasibility of the Activate intervention for routine practice?

Methods
Study design
A qualitative study of nurses' perceptions of delivering the Activate intervention, nested within a cluster-randomised trial in primary care, was conducted.

The Activate intervention
To enhance behaviour change in both patients and nurses, the Activate intervention was developed using the Behaviour Change Wheel (BCW) [20]. A behavioural analysis was conducted for the behaviour of patients and the behaviour of nurses using the COM-B (capability, opportunity, motivation-behaviour) model [20]. Subsequently, intervention functions were selected, by which patients' level of physical activity and nurses' skills to provide support could be enhanced. The intervention functions were linked to a selection of behaviour change techniques (BCTs) to support behaviour change [20, 21].

Behavioural analysis of the patients resulted in a selection of 17 BCTs, which were integrated into the Activate intervention. The intervention consisted of four standardised nurse-led consultations to enhance physical activity spread over a 12-week period: one consultation in the first week with subsequent consultations after 2, 6 and 12 weeks. Consultations occurred in the patients' own general practice, with a duration of 20–30 min.

The intervention structure was described in a handbook for nurses. Nurses were asked to individualise the content of the consultations to the patients' unique circumstances, needs and preferences. Patients received a workbook, which included tips and tricks, useful websites, activity logs and action plans and were equipped with an accelerometer (personal activity monitor; Pam AM300) [22] in order to self-monitor their physical activity daily.

Behavioural analysis of the nurses resulted in a selection of 21 BCTs, which were integrated into a standardised comprehensive training programme to equip nurses with the skills to deliver the Activate consultations to patients. The training consisted of several components: a one-day training, two individual coaching sessions, instructional videos on how to apply the BCTs in the consultations, a handbook with example sentences and checklists (what to do when). Preparatory to the one-day training, nurses received a workbook, including study procedures and materials and were asked to view two online presentations to reinforce the procedures and the relevance of physical activity for patients at risk for CVD. The one-day training was held in a small group led by a health psychologist, and it focused on learning how to deliver the BCTs in each of the consultations. This training included theoretical background about how to promote behaviour change and included practising skills in delivering the consultation using an outlined structure, which included BCTs, by use of instructional videos and role-playing. To optimise and rehearse the gained skills, nurses received two individual coaching sessions by the health psychologist. For each coaching session, nurses recorded one of their consultations on which they received feedback on their performance during the coaching session. To strengthen their gained skills, nurses were encouraged to use the instructional videos, handbook and checklists.

Further details on the development and content of the intervention are described elsewhere [23].

The Activate intervention is currently being tested for its effectiveness in terms of number of minutes of moderate to vigorous physical activity within a 6-month follow-up period in a two-armed cluster-randomised controlled trial in primary care settings in the Netherlands comparing the Activate intervention with care as usual, according to the Dutch guideline of cardiovascular risk management. The Activate trial entails participation by 31 general practices, 36 primary care nurses and 195 patients (Activate trial, ClinicalTrials.gov NCT02725203). A total of 16 general practices (20 primary care nurses) were randomly allocated to the intervention group and a total of 15 general practices (16 primary care nurses) were randomly allocated to the control group.

Sample and recruitment

The study sample consisted of 20 primary care nurses from 16 general practices situated throughout the Netherlands who participated in the Activate trial and were allocated to the intervention group. Nurses were eligible to participate if they had experience with delivering the intervention, which was operationalised as having completed the training and delivered the intervention to at least two patients. Therefore, two nurses were excluded from this study, as they had delivered the intervention to fewer than two patients due to difficulties recruiting patients. One nurse was excluded because she had changed jobs during the study. After completing the intervention, all eligible nurses ($n = 17$) were invited through email to participate in this qualitative study. In total, 14 nurses (82.4%) agreed to participate, and 3 nurses refused to participate due to busy clinical practice.

To increase the likelihood of reflecting different nurse perspectives and to increase the representativeness of the data, maximum variation sampling was used in the recruitment phase of the Activate trial to obtain diversity with regard to nurses' age and years of working experience with patients at risk for CVD in primary care. Furthermore, we strived for maximum variation in the sample with regard to nurses' educational background, as some nurses -other than working as a registered nurse- had formerly worked predominantly as receptionists and practitioner assistants in general practices prior to their specialisation in primary care nursing.

Data collection

Face-to-face individual interviews were conducted using a semi-structured interview guide. This consisted of open questions asking about perceptions towards the training, intervention delivery, effect on patients' behaviour, changes in consultation style and feasibility of the intervention in practice (Additional file 1). Based on nurses' narratives, topics that were mentioned were explored in depth. The interview guide was developed by four researchers and peer reviewed by the research team to ensure feasibility and completeness of the topics. All interviews started with the same opening question: "What was the reason you agreed to participate in the Activate study?"

The interviews were conducted by three researchers. An expert on qualitative research was involved in the process to ascertain the methodological quality of the study.

The interviewers were unknown to the nurses, enabling them to express their experiences and opinions without inhibitions. Nurses were interviewed once at the general practice or at the nurses' homes based on nurses' preferences. Interviews ranged in duration from 35 to 62 min (mean: 48 min). All interviews were audio-recorded.

During and after the interviews, memos were made to describe observations, reflect on methodological issues, capture initial ideas about emerging themes and inform refinements of the interview guide. Furthermore, the interview techniques of the interviewers were discussed and they were trained by the research team to ameliorate the equivocality of the interviews. Nurses' baseline characteristics were collected in the Activate trial.

Ethical approval to conduct the interviews was awarded within the overall approval for the Activate trial, which was approved by the Medical Ethics Research Committee of the University Medical Center Utrecht (NL54286 .041.15).

Data analysis

All interviews were transcribed verbatim. Data were thematically analysed [24]. Data analysis started after the first three interviews. The transcripts were read and re-read, initial ideas for coding and refinements of the interview guide were discussed. After every three interviews, the transcripts were double-coded and the codes were assessed for similarities and differences by the research team. Subsequently the initial codes were collated into potential themes, and all relevant data were structured to each potential theme. Potential themes and subthemes were reviewed on consistency with the codes and entire data to ensure they reflect the entire data. Inconsistencies were discussed during joint meetings with the research team and themes were further developed and depicted in a thematic map of the data. Furthermore, the essence of each theme was further considered by the research team, themes were defined and illustrative quotes were selected.

Data saturation was reached after the twelfth interview; however, the data were complemented with two interviews to affirm the potential themes and ensure a maximum variation in the sample.

Data analysis was supported by NVivo 11.0 software (QSR International Pty Ltd., Version 11.0, 2011).

Trustworthiness

Credibility of data collection and analysis was enhanced by researcher triangulation and peer review in all phases of the study [25]. An expert on qualitative research was involved in the process to ensure accuracy and enhance data dependability [26]. Biweekly meetings with four team members to discuss data collection and analysis decisions enhanced methodological quality. In addition, an audit trail ensured the study's confirmability [25]. Memo writing and expert opinion supported

the analysis and enhanced study reliability [26]. The use of a 15-point checklist by Braun and Clarke [24] ensured correct application of the phases of thematic analysis; see Additional file 2. The consolidated criteria for reporting qualitative studies (COREQ) were used to facilitate reporting of the results [27]; see Additional file 3.

Results

Between October 2016 and March 2017, 14 nurses were interviewed. All nurses were female. Maximum variation was achieved for age (range 24–63 years; mean 48.9), years of experience working with patients at risk for CVD in primary care (range 2–14 years; mean 7.2) and educational background ($n = 11$; 73.3% registered nurses). Nurses' characteristics are presented in Table 1.

A thematic map was created to depict the emerged themes; see Fig. 1. Three themes emerged in answer to research question 1: nurses' perceptions towards delivering the Activate intervention:

- Nurses' engagement towards delivering the Activate intervention
- Acquiring knowledge and skills
- Dealing with adherence to the consultation structure

Research question 2: nurses' perceptions towards the feasibility of the Activate intervention for routine practice, was captured in three themes:

- Expectations towards the use of the intervention in routine practice

Table 1 Characteristics of participating primary care nurses

ID	Age range	Working experience (years)[a]	Educational background	Additional training	Included patients in the study (n)
R1	51–55	12	Former practice assistant	None	2
R2	41–45	14	Former practice assistant	MI, SQ	10
R3	61–65	2	Former practice assistant	None	3
R4	51–55	5	Registered nurse	MI	3
R5	51–55	5	Registered nurse	MI	11
R6	46–50	9	Registered nurse	None	5
R7	36–40	9	Registered nurse	None	10
R8	36–40	2	Registered nurse	MI	2
R9	56–60	2	Former practice assistant	MI	5
R10	51–55	11	Registered nurse	MI	7
R11	56–60	6	Former practice assistant	MI	5
R12	46–50	13	Registered nurse	MI, SQ	2
R13	21–25	3	Registered nurse	MI	3
R14	51–55	8	Registered nurse	MI, SM	5

Abbreviations: CVD cardiovascular diseases, MI motivational interviewing, SM self-management, SQ Socratic Questioning
[a]Working experience as a nurse in primary care with patients at risk for CVD

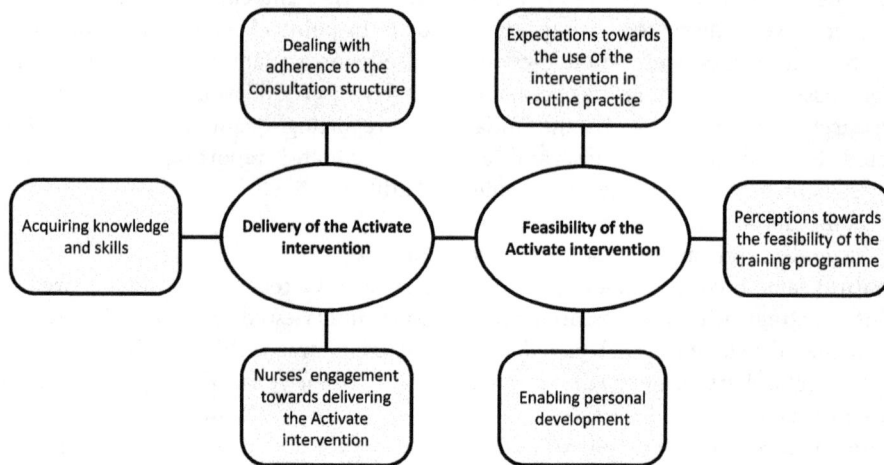

Fig. 1 Thematic map of nurses' perceptions of delivering and the feasibility of the Activate intervention

– Perceptions towards the feasibility of the training programme
– Enabling personal development

Nurses' engagement towards delivering the activate intervention

All nurses indicated that contributing to the improvement of patients' health outcomes was the core of their nursing role, which aligned with delivering an intervention to enhance patients' behaviour change. Reasons for participating in the Activate trial corresponded with their beliefs about the advantage of increased physical activity for lowering the risk of CVD and thus improving health outcomes. Based on their experience in supporting patients to change their health behaviour, all nurses expressed a need to increase their skills to enhance their support to patients in order to increase physical activity.

"The main reason was that it's difficult to motivate people to increase their physical activity. I could use some tools for how I could handle this the best way. Very often, questions about patients' motivation remain superficial, and I wanted to know how I am going to ask in-depth questions about their motivation?" (R10)

Directly after the training, all nurses felt engaged to deliver the intervention in their practice. Their engagement was supported by having been convinced that the intervention could be beneficial to patients.

"I felt that I could perform better in my job, that I could make a difference to people and that I have more to offer them." (R6)

Nurses expressed that, during the study period, their engagement towards delivering the intervention strongly depended on their experiences with delivering the intervention.

All nurses valued and felt rewarded by patients' success at increasing their level of physical activity and perceived this as an effect of their intervening activities. Patients' success had a positive impact on the nurses' job satisfaction and their engagement towards delivering the intervention.

"It is very nice to see that it just has an effect on people and that people feel fitter. That makes you excited and willing to continue. Ultimately, it is what you want to do: to help people further." (R13)

However, differences were seen in how nurses dealt with patients' lack of motivation to participate in the intervention or their lack of success at increasing their physical activity, and this negatively affected the engagement of some nurses. Patients' lack of motivation to participate often led to a postponed start for delivering the intervention or fewer practising opportunities. Some nurses felt rewarded by enhancement of their knowledge and skills to support patients, in particular with patients who they perceived as challenging to motivate. They perceived that actual delivery of the intervention increased their confidence and job satisfaction and helped them to positively continue with the study despite perceived difficulties with patient inclusion.

"Otherwise, you have nothing to discuss, right? If someone has 100% perseverance, then you are soon done. You have a lot more to discuss, that's nice. If someone says, 'I have already tried it ten times, but I

can't keep it up', well then you have something to look for."(R12)

Despite their high initial engagement, some nurses felt that their engagement towards delivering the intervention strongly depended on patients' motivation. Patients' unwillingness to participate as well as patients' lack of commitment to goal attainment resulted in some nurses questioning their efforts to support them, which affected their engagement negatively.

"For me, it's more fun to support a motivated patient who does his homework perfectly compared to a patient who brings a completely empty diary and says, 'Yes, I did not really keep up'. Then, you think this costs me forty-five minutes, and that patient actually does not do anything. It's a lot more fun when they say, 'I deliberately went cycling to reach my goal.' Yes, then you really feel like that's what I am doing it for." (R2)

While continuing their participation in the study, nurses had to deal with circumstances such as a high work load and absence due to sick leave or holiday, which often negatively influenced their engagement towards delivering the intervention.

Acquiring knowledge and skills

All nurses reported that the training, handbook, checklists, instructional videos and coaching sessions were essential to equip them with the necessary knowledge and skills to establish and deliver the intervention as intended, which strengthened their confidence and engagement in their support.

"After the training, I felt I had a lot of tools I could apply to patients. I was equipped with a lot of techniques for gaining effects in patients, and that feels good. Normally, I asked: 'are you physically active?' Now, I make it more specific and explore with the patient how to continue." (R6)

To strengthen their confidence, nurses reinforced their gained skills and knowledge by rehearsing the consultation structure using the instructional videos and the handbook.

Once their initial feelings of uncertainty towards their skills were overcome and their confidence improved, brief repetition of the handbook prior to a consultation was sufficient.

"I really regretted there was a long delay between the training and the first consultation. Then, things dwindled pretty fast since you are not practising it.

Only prior to my first and second patient I watched the instructional videos again. Then, I had the idea that I had a better grip on it." (R6)

Most nurses felt regular practice was the most beneficial factor for developing their skills; however, some nurses felt a need for additional training with the health psychologist to refine their skills.

Furthermore, focusing solely on physical activity without getting in conflict with other clinical demands, enabled them to develop their skills.

"This sure is special, whereas you normally don't do this, since there is a lot more in a consultation. But, yes, you notice that once you have more time, you can practise a lot." (R10)

Nurses' participation in the intervention, in particular the role-playing and coaching, exposed their habits with regard to their own consultation style and skills, such as solving patients' problems by giving advice and filling in for the patient. Once nurses became aware of their habits, they identified that changing their routines by applying the acquired knowledge and skills was challenging, as they easily fell back into their traditional style.

"Sometimes, I noticed I was the one searching for solutions. Of course, that was not how it was meant. That's very typical for nurses' way of doing things. Then I thought, well, I'm sitting here working, while the one in front of me should work."(R14)

"The feedback from the coach was a kind of eye-opener; I do things, but I did not ask in-depth questions...that made me think and I took that with me to the next consultation. I found that to be particularly useful." (R12)

Nurses valued that they could transfer their developed skills to other patients and to other behaviours, such as smoking cessation and dietary intake. This indirect benefit enhanced nurses' engagement to deliver the intervention.

"Now, it is very much focused on physical activity, but I think, in any case, helping people with behavioural change is something that you can see broader applications, like for other lifestyle topics." (R12)

Dealing with adherence to the consultation structure

To ensure fidelity of the intervention, nurses were aware that they had to adhere to the structure of the consultations as described in the handbook, even if they had personal doubts about specific elements. However, some nurses deliberately deviated from the consultation structure when they were not convinced of the effectiveness of a specific element or when they did not feel comfortable with an element. Furthermore, most nurses valued the use of the handbook in their consultations, as this allowed them to follow the structure and use example sentences more easily. Nurses often changed the wording of the sentences to something which they felt more comfortable with.

"There was a question about patients' confidence, which didn't make me very happy. But it is part of the intervention, I know. I have tried to ask it."(R12)

"But you don't talk like these sentences. I make my own sentences. But, yes, of course it helps. You don't literally say it like that though. Because then...the conversation is less fluent." (R1)

After the training, most nurses reported that adhering to the consultation structure was more difficult than expected, which reduced their confidence in their capabilities. Patients easily initiated other topics, as they were used to doing so in the routine consultations. That distracted the nurses from following the prescribed structure.

"I sometimes found it difficult to follow the script, prompting me to think, well, this is yet more difficult than I thought. So, then, my confidence decreased. I can certainly understand how it works on paper and that it works, but in practice it's different." (R8)

To enhance fidelity of the intervention, nurses were aware that they had to fill in the charts at the end of each consultation to check if they discussed all of the elements described in the handbook.

Expectations towards the use of the intervention in routine practice

Nurses' beliefs about the use of the intervention in their routine practice strongly depended on their beliefs about the effectiveness of the intervention to increase patients' level of physical activity and health outcomes. Nurses were convinced that the effectiveness of the intervention relied on patients' engagement to set goals and having a reasonable level of health literacy to understand the intervention materials.

"It works in patients who just need a helping hand to perform it. But the truly unmotivated patients who don't want to be active, those patients are not going to

be active using this method, no. They still have to do it themselves." (R2)

The nurses were convinced that the combination of the accelerometer, activity log and their subsequent and structural support incentivised patients' goal attainment in changing their physical activity, which strengthened their positive beliefs about the feasibility of the intervention in their routine practice.

"If you would send them home with an activity log but without consultations, then no one would fill it in. But now they have to come back. Then they must do it anyway, because of course they know it will be discussed then...I found the activity log was very good. Patients confirmed that. However, so were the consultations. So, basically, just the combination really made it work." (R2)

Nurses valued the consultation structure, including techniques such as goal setting, action planning, reviewing behavioural goals, feedback on behaviour, self-monitoring and problem solving, as being feasible to use in their routine practice. Most nurses found that goal setting and action planning enabled them to stimulate patients in formulating their goals and actions, which in turn facilitated patients' goal attainment. The use of the activity log to review patients' level of goal attainment facilitated them in giving feedback on their behaviour.

"You have to make it specific; otherwise, it won't work. If you make it very specific, patients also know: all right, that's my goal and here I go. And then you can say, 'I've done it or not' ... I was always aware of the fact that patients specified their planned actions. If patients said, 'I'm going to be active in five days', that's, of course, not very specific, so I tried to make it even more specific." (R13)

The use of self-monitoring tools such as the accelerometer and activity log were seen as additional motivators and incentives for patients, as they provided insight into patients' level of physical activity and challenged patients to goal attainment. The nurses believed that the use of such tools would help them to deliver the intervention in their routine practice.

"The accelerometer just provides insight, which makes your activity very specific. Actually, you normally don't really think about it that much."(R13)

Despite the log and accelerometer being highly valued by nurses, a few nurses questioned the usability of such tools in their routine practice as some patients did not completely understand the user instructions and faced practical and technical problems, such as losing the accelerometer or losing their activity data after the accelerometer automatically reset at midnight.

"I noticed that it was quite complicated for patients... the accelerometer was difficult to operate...And the fact that the accelerometer erased itself after midnight, then they couldn't read it out anymore." (R9)

Although all nurses believed that the intervention was feasible for routine practice, they thought that using the intervention in routine practice might conflict with other clinical demands during routine consultations. Initially, nurses needed more time to deliver the intervention, which may adversely influence the feasibility due to time constraints in their routine practice. However, nurses believed that mastering the necessary skills would enable them to gain more in-depth support, which eventually would save them time. To enhance the fit of the intervention in routine practice, nurses suggested shortening the number of in-depth questions.

"I think it takes too much time to do it in such an extensive way. You also need to check patients and discuss their medications, insulin and whatever." (R14)

"It may seem like it's very time consuming, but once you ask the right questions then I think you can get a lot of information in a short period of time, and it's a bit of an art to let the patients talk themselves." (R10)

Perceptions towards the feasibility of the training programme

All nurses felt appropriately trained and supported by the one-day training in combination with the instructional videos, handbook and checklists to deliver the Activate intervention. The nurses particularly valued the safe learning environment of the small-scale role playing, in which they directly received feedback.

"...first of all, the small-scale, practising with two... At least for me, it's an obstacle to practice a role-play in front of a group... and having someone to observe... who provided feedback. So, it was a very safe setting in which, without being judged or anything, you received objective feedback." (R11)

Although all nurses valued the coaching, some initially felt uncomfortable submitting a recorded consultation, and delayed doing so. However, afterwards, the nurses regretted postponing their submissions, because they felt that the feedback would have helped them in delivering other consultations. Some nurses could not overcome their uncomfortable feelings surrounding recording their consultations and did not submit any consultation.

"I just found it difficult to record it, and then it's indelible, and then you will send it, and people will listen to it. That's just a bit of an uncomfortable idea...Therefore, I was a little late with recording a consultation, which was a bit of a pity. So, I could not apply the feedback so much afterwards." (R7)

Enabling personal development

All nurses expressed that participating in the Activate trial enabled their personal development and enhanced their knowledge and skills to support patients in their behaviour change. The nurses tended to incorporate specific skills and elements of the intervention into their routine practice that they were convinced were effective for patients, such as setting specific and attainable goals and planning actions for goal attainment. Nurses became more critical towards patients' answers and used a more positive approach, focusing on solutions instead of traditionally addressing barriers for patients.

"I became more aware of the fact that it's important for someone to come up with their own solution, even though I am staggering with enthusiasm...if I take a step back, more can arise from oneself and that is very powerful in this work." (R8)

"Specifying patients' goal, that's really something I've learned. And giving feedback on that goal once they come again next time. Yes, I have learned that very well." (R6)

Discussion

This qualitative study explored the perceptions of primary care nurses towards delivering the Activate intervention and its feasibility in routine practice. Nurses were dedicated to deliver the intervention in order to improve health outcomes. Nurses felt engaged and rewarded by patients' success in increasing their physical activity. Patients' lack of motivation to participate in the intervention and lack of success negatively affected nurses' engagement. The training, training tools and delivery of the intervention facilitated nurses in acquiring the required knowledge and skills. Acquiring skills was challenging, as the nurses tended to relapse into their traditional habits. The nurses valued and tried to adhere to the intervention structure despite perceived difficulties, such as distraction by patients who initiated discussion of topics other than physical activity.

Nurses were positive towards the feasibility of the intervention in routine practice. Nurses thought that the consultations combined with the self-monitoring tools were effective to increase patients' physical activity and feasible to use in routine practice. However, the use of the intervention in routine practice might be hindered by complying with other clinical demands. Nurses felt appropriately trained and supported to deliver the intervention. Participation in the trial enabled their personal development and changed their routine practice, as they incorporated newly acquired skills, particularly those that they believed were efficacious, in their routine practice with other patients.

The challenges of changing nurses' behaviour in order to enhance the implementation of behaviour change interventions are widely reported [8, 11–14, 28]. Therefore, a training programme was developed using the BCW, targeting the COM-B components using BCTs [20]. Despite the provided comprehensive training to support their patients in their own context and facilitating them with extra consultation time, changing nurses' behaviour was complex. Delivering the intervention required nurses to shift from their traditional consultation style of being an expert, who gives advice and informs patients to a coaching consultation style that entails being supportive and facilitative to patients' needs and preferences [8, 29]. Nurses felt comfortable in their expert role and most nurses had previously received additional training in the motivational interviewing approach; however, they unanimously expressed their need to deepen their support and increase the effectiveness of their support. This suggests that the nurses were willing to acquire the necessary knowledge and skills and to participate in the Activate trial. Participation in the trial raised awareness of their traditional consultation style and facilitated a shift to a more patient-centred approach, allowing patients to take more responsibility rather than advising and telling patients what to do, which is in line with other studies [11, 13, 29]. Despite increased awareness, it appeared difficult to perpetuate these changes in consultation style, as all nurses thought they easily relapsed into their traditional consultation style and skills, as also seen in other studies [11].

The handbook with example sentences guided nurses in structuring their consultations and facilitated their adherence towards the intervention delivery, as also seen in other studies [13, 30]. Overall, nurses tended to adjust the content of the intervention if they had personal doubts about specific elements, and this finding aligned with other studies [12, 13]. This suggests that nurses'

beliefs are pivotal with regard to the extent to which they adopt the intervention into their practice. Nurses' tendency to tailor the intervention to their beliefs should be addressed during the training of nurses to maintain sufficient uniform delivery and underlines the need to assess nurses' fidelity of the delivery of the intervention [13, 31]. Nurses' engagement, confidence and job satisfaction were enhanced by patients' success at increasing their physical activity, nurses' personal development and transferability of knowledge and skills to other patients, as has previously been shown [11, 13, 32]. Nurses' job satisfaction is potentially linked to their intrinsic drive to help and assist patients. Nurses often thought that patients expect and prefer their traditional nursing role in behaviour change support. However, the patient-centred approach of the intervention requires reflection on their traditional role and adaption of their role towards facilitating and supporting patients in changing their behaviour. Changing a nurses' role is challenging as nurses are often wedded to what they do [11, 14]. This might complicate nurses' adoption of their gained knowledge and skills in routine practice [11].

The intervention structure and BCTs were relatively new to the nurses, as they were not specifically trained in applying and tailoring the BCTs prior to their participation in the Activate trial. Another study examining self-management support by primary care nurses in routine care found that nurses seldom focus on behaviour change and infrequently use effective techniques to support this change [33]. This strengthens the need for such training and support, because nurses are in a key position to deliver behaviour change interventions in primary care [11]. Previous studies have also found that appropriate training and support for nurses before and during delivery of the intervention is essential for the implementation of behaviour change interventions [11, 13, 32, 34]. This study showed that nurses particularly valued the small-scale role-playing in the training led by the health psychologist. The role-plays, including the feedback, allowed them to practise and directly reshape their consultation and BCT skills, and different scenarios that they perceived as difficult. This suggests that the training of nurses to deliver a behaviour change intervention should be comprehensive, interactive and delivered by a credible source, such as an expert trainer.

Despite that the nurses became more confident with their skills as they practised more often and that they were motivated to deliver the intervention as intended, they reported that recording the consultation felt uncomfortable, as they felt judged, which aligns with another study [35].

The Activate intervention included both self-monitoring tools and nurses' support, similar to other studies [36–39]. The nurses were convinced that combining the self-monitoring tools with offering subsequent consultations was effective in changing patients' physical activity and that the consultations were essential for enhancing patients' engagement to continue and adjust their goals. This is in line with a study by van der Weegen et al. [36], which found that a combination of a self-monitoring tool and nurse-led consultations was effective to increase physical activity in patients with diabetes mellitus type 2 and chronic obstructive pulmonary disease. That study also found that counselling by the nurses without use of the self-monitoring tool was not effective compared to routine care.

Strengths
This study was nested within a cluster-randomised controlled trial. Comprehensive process evaluations of complex interventions from the perspective of the providers of such interventions have been largely missing from the literature [7, 17, 18], but are increasingly being undertaken [12, 13, 34]. To prevent interpretation bias, such an evaluation should be conducted before the trial results are known. Furthermore, exploration of the perspectives of nurses may enhance implementation once the effectiveness has been established. To strengthen the trustworthiness of the study, the data were independently analysed by three researchers and supported by a qualitative research expert during the entire process. Furthermore, an audit trail, memo writing, expert opinion and the use of Braun & Clarke' checklist [24] and the COREQ [27] enhanced trustworthiness.

The interviewers were unknown to the nurses prior to the interviews, which might have positively affected data dependability, as it allowed the nurses to express their experiences and opinions without inhibitions.

Although the results of this study were based on fourteen nurses, maximum variation sampling of nurses' age, years of working experience with primary care patients at risk for CVD and nurses' educational background was used to increase the likelihood of diversity with regard to nurses' perspectives and contribute to the transferability of the results. Data saturation on all themes was achieved within these fourteen interviews, which also strengthened the transferability of the results.

Limitations
A few limitations need to be considered. Despite all efforts to include all seventeen eligible nurses, three nurses refused to participate. Furthermore, three nurses were not eligible, as they had either used the intervention on fewer than two patients or had changed jobs during the trial. These nurses might have expressed different perspectives, which could have affected the results. The interviews were conducted at a single point in time, namely, after the nurses completed the

intervention. The retrospective reflection of the nurses might not have revealed all of the individual processes with regard to delivery of the intervention and behaviour change. Furthermore, despite all efforts, for some interviews, there was a delay between the last trial consultation and the interview, potentially affecting nurses' memory to recall. However, the researchers provided the training tools and study materials and asked further questions during the interviews to help stimulate the nurses' memory.

Implications
This study identified areas of concern regarding the intervention delivery and feasibility of behaviour change interventions in routine practice. First, to improve implementation, nurses need to be convinced that the intervention will be effective and is aligned with their beliefs surrounding good patient care [12]. Second, nurses must be appropriately trained according to a comprehensive training programme. Training should preferably be spread out over time, allowing and facilitating nurses to practice to refine their skills and to discuss how to address perceived difficulties, such as patient engagement and motivation to participate in the intervention. Third, to engage nurses, the developed skills should be transferable for use with other patients and behaviours. Fourth, to enhance success of the intervention, behaviour change interventions should be structured around BCTs that were highly valued by nurses, such as goal setting, action planning, reviewing behavioural goal(s), feedback on behaviour, self-monitoring, and problem solving. In addition, these BCTs are likely to be successful in changing behaviour [40–46]. Fifth, it is important for researchers and policymakers to acknowledge that adapting complex interventions on the part of providers takes time, as provider and patient behaviour change is a lengthy process [47].

Conclusion
Delivering a behaviour change intervention is challenging as nurses have to change their traditional consultation style towards a more patient-centred consultation style. A process of acquiring and refining knowledge and skills is needed to deliver such interventions without jeopardizing treatment fidelity. Nurses were positive about delivering the intervention using a structured approach with facilitating tools and support. Comprehensive training and practising of their skills requires ongoing support to refrain from traditional habits and optimise their delivery of interventions. The nurses perceived the Activate intervention feasible in routine practice; however, incorporating the intervention into routine consultations is challenged by competing other clinical demands. This qualitative study contributes to our understanding of the complexity of changing nurses'

behaviour towards a more patient-centred consultation style. The findings can be used to enhance our understanding of the effectiveness of the Activate trial and may provide guidance for the development and evaluation of future behaviour change interventions delivered by nurses in primary care.

Abbreviations

BCT: Behaviour change technique; BCW: Behaviour Change Wheel; COM-B: Capability/opportunity/motivation – behaviour; COREQ: Consolidated criteria for reporting qualitative studies; CVD: Cardiovascular disease; MI: Motivational Interviewing

Acknowledgements

The authors would like to thank the primary care nurses who participated in the interviews.

Funding

This study was funded by the Dutch Ministry of Health, Welfare and Sports, ZonMw grant number 520001002.

Authors' contributions

HW, JT, CS, MS and SV conceived the study. YK, PS, HW carried out the interviews. YK, PS, HW, SV developed the interview guide and carried out the data coding from the transcripts. All authors designed the study and contributed to analysis and interpretation of results. CS was involved as expert on qualitative research. CS and SV provided content expertise to the analysis findings. All authors contributed to the writing of the manuscript and read and approved the final version.

Consent for publication

Not applicable

Competing interests

The authors declare that they have no competing interests.

Author details

[1]Julius Center for Health Sciences and Primary Care, University Medical Center Utrecht, HP Str. 6.131, PO 85500, 3508, GA, Utrecht, The Netherlands. [2]Department of Cardiology, Radboud University Medical Center, Nijmegen, The Netherlands. [3]Center of Excellence in Rehabilitation Medicine, Brain Center Rudolf Magnus, University Medical Center Utrecht, University Utrecht and De Hoogstraat Rehabilitation, Utrecht, the Netherlands. [4]Department of Acute Psychiatry, Psychiatric Center GGZ Central, Amersfoort, The Netherlands. [5]Cancer Center, University Medical Center Utrecht, Utrecht, The Netherlands. [6]Education Center, UMC Utrecht Academy, University Medical Center Utrecht, Utrecht University, Utrecht, The Netherlands.

References

1. Effing T, Kerstjens H, van der Valk P, Zielhuis G, van der Palen J. (cost)-effectiveness of self-treatment of exacerbations on the severity of exacerbations in patients with COPD: the COPE II study. Thorax. 2009; 64(11):956–62.
2. Chodosh J, Morton SC, Mojica W, Maglione M, Suttorp MJ, Hilton L, Rhodes S, Shekelle P. Meta-analysis: chronic disease self-management programs for older adults. Ann Intern Med. 2005;143(6):427–38.
3. Zwerink M, Brusse Keizer M, van der Valk PDLPM, Zielhuis G, Monninkhof E, van der Palen J, Frith P, Effing T. Self management for patients with chronic obstructive pulmonary disease. Cochrane Database Syst Rev. 2014;3: CD002990.
4. Barlow J, Wright C, Sheasby J, Turner A, Hainsworth J. Self-management approaches for people with chronic conditions: a review. Patient Educ Couns. 2002;48(2):177–87.
5. Newman S, Steed L, Mulligan K. Self-management interventions for chronic illness. Lancet. 2004;364(9444):1523–37.
6. Baan CA, Hutten JBF, Rijken PM. Afstemming in de zorg: Een achtergrondstudie naar de zorg voor mensen met een chronische aandoening. [Coordination of care. A study into the care for people with a chronic condition]. Bilthoven, The Netherlands: RIVM; 2003.
7. Craig P, Dieppe P, Macintyre S, Michie S, Nazareth I, Petticrew M. Developing and evaluating complex interventions: the new Medical Research Council guidance. BMJ. 2008;337:a1655.
8. Elissen A, Nolte E, Knai C, Brunn M, Chevreul K, Conklin A, Durand-Zaleski I, Erler A, Flamm M, Frolich A, Fullerton B, Jacobsen R, Saz-Parkinson Z, Sarria-Santamera A, Sonnichsen A, Vrijhoef H. Is Europe putting theory into practice? A qualitative study of the level of self-management support in chronic care management approaches. BMC Health Serv Res. 2013;13:117–6963 –13-117.
9. Wagner EH. Chronic disease management: what will it take to improve care for chronic illness? Eff Clin Pract. 1998;1(1):2–4.
10. Bodenheimer T, Lorig K, Holman H, Grumbach K. Patient self-management of chronic disease in primary care. JAMA. 2002;288(19):2469–75.
11. Taylor C, Shaw R, Dale J, French D. Enhancing delivery of health behaviour change interventions in primary care: a meta-synthesis of views and experiences of primary care nurses. Patient Educ Couns. 2011;85(2):315–22.
12. Kennedy A, Rogers A, Bowen R, Lee V, Blakeman T, Gardner C, Morris R, Protheroe J, Chew-Graham C. Implementing, embedding and integrating self-management support tools for people with long-term conditions in primary care nursing: a qualitative study. Int J Nurs Stud. 2014;51(8):1103–13.
13. Beighton C, Victor C, Normansell R, Cook D, Kerry S, Iliffe S, Ussher M, Whincup P, Fox Rushby J, Woodcock A, Harris T. "It's not just about walking....it's the practice nurse that makes it work": a qualitative exploration of the views of practice nurses delivering complex physical activity interventions in primary care. BMC Public Health. 2015;15:1236.
14. McDonald R, Rogers A, Macdonald W. Dependence and identity: nurses and chronic conditions in a primary care setting. J Health Organ Manag. 2008; 22(3):294–308.
15. Jonkman N, Groenwold RHH, Trappenburg JCA, Hoes A, Schuurmans M. Complex self-management interventions in chronic disease unravelled: a review of lessons learnt from an individual patient data meta-analysis. J Clin Epidemiol. 2017;83:48–56.
16. Craig P, Dieppe P, Macintyre S, Michie S, Nazareth I, Petticrew M. Developing and evaluating complex interventions: the new Medical Research Council guidance. Int J Nurs Stud. 2013;50(5):587–92.
17. Moore G, Audrey S, Barker M, Bond L, Bonell C, Hardeman W, Moore L, O'Cathain A, Tinati T, Wight D, Baird J. Process evaluation of complex interventions: Medical Research Council guidance. BMJ. 2015;350:h1258.
18. Conn V. Unpacking the black box: countering the problem of inadequate intervention descriptions in research reports. West J Nurs Res. 2012;34(4):427–33.
19. Michie S, Abraham C. Interventions to change health behaviours: evidence-based or evidence-inspired? Psychol Health. 2004;19(1):29–49.
20. Michie S, van Stralen MM, West R. The behaviour change wheel: a new method for characterising and designing behaviour change interventions. Implement Sci. 2011;6:42–5908 -6-42.
21. Michie S, Richardson M, Johnston M, Abraham C, Francis J, Hardeman W, Eccles MP, Cane J, Wood CE. The behavior change technique taxonomy (v1) of 93 hierarchically clustered techniques: building an international consensus for the reporting of behavior change interventions. Ann Behav Med. 2013;46(1):81–95.
22. Slootmaker SM, Chin A Paw MJM, Schuit AJ, van Mechelen W, Koppes LLJ. Concurrent validity of the PAM accelerometer relative to the MTI Actigraph using oxygen consumption as a reference. Scand J Med Sci Sports. 2009; 19(1):36–43.
23. Westland H, Bos Touwen ID, Trappenburg JCA, Schröder C, de Wit NJ, Schuurmans MJ. Unravelling effectiveness of a nurse-led behaviour change intervention to enhance physical activity in patients at risk for cardiovascular disease in primary care: study protocol for a cluster randomised controlled trial. Trials. 2017;18(1):79.
24. Braun V, Clarke V. Using thematic analysis in psychology. Qual Res Psychol. 2006;3(2):77–101.

25. Guba E, Lincoln Y. Competing Paradigms in Qualitative Research. In: Denzin NK, Lincoln YS, editors. Handbook of Qualitative Research. London: Sage; 1994. p. 105–17.

26. Creswell J. Qualitative Inquiry & Research Design: Choosing Among Five Approaches. 3rd revised edition ed. California: Sage Publications Inc.; 2012.

27. Tong A, Sainsbury P, Craig J. Consolidated criteria for reporting qualitative research (COREQ): a 32-item checklist for interviews and focus groups. Int J Qual Health Care. 2007;19(6):349–57.

28. Hardeman W, Michie S, Fanshawe T, Prevost AT, Mcloughlin K, Kinmonth A. Fidelity of delivery of a physical activity intervention: predictors and consequences. Psychol Health. 2008;23(1):11–24.

29. Mead N, Bower P. Patient-centred consultations and outcomes in primary care: a review of the literature. Patient Educ Couns. 2002;48(1):51–61.

30. Weldam SWM, Lammers J, Zwakman M, Schuurmans MJ. Nurses' perspectives of a new individualized nursing care intervention for COPD patients in primary care settings: a mixed method study. Appl Nurs Res. 2017;33:85–92.

31. Bellg A, Borrelli B, Resnick B, Hecht J, Minicucci D, Ory M, Ogedegbe G, Orwig D, Ernst D, Czajkowski S. Enhancing treatment fidelity in health behavior change studies: best practices and recommendations from the NIH behavior change consortium. Health Psychol. 2004;23(5):443–51.

32. Wells M, Williams B, Treweek S, Coyle J, Taylor J. Intervention description is not enough: evidence from an in-depth multiple case study on the untold role and impact of context in randomised controlled trials of seven complex interventions. Trials. 2012;13:95.

33. Westland H, Schröder C, de Wit J, Frings J, Trappenburg JCA, Schuurmans MJ. Self-management support in routine primary care by nurses. Br J Health Psychol. 2018;23(1):88–107.

34. Bleijenberg N, Ten Dam V, Steunenberg B, Drubbel I, Numans M, De Wit NJ, Schuurmans MJ. Exploring the expectations, needs and experiences of general practitioners and nurses towards a proactive and structured care programme for frail older patients: a mixed-methods study. J Adv Nurs. 2013;69(10):2262–73.

35. Boase S, Kim Y, Craven A, Cohn S. Involving practice nurses in primary care research: the experience of multiple and competing demands. J Adv Nurs. 2012;68(3):590–9.

36. van der Weegen S, Verwey R, Spreeuwenberg M, Tange H, van der Weijden T, de Witte L. It's LiFe! Mobile and web-based monitoring and feedback tool embedded in primary care increases physical activity: a cluster randomized controlled trial. J Med Internet Res. 2015;17(7):e184.

37. Harris T, Kerry S, Victor C, Ekelund U, Woodcock A, Iliffe S, Whincup P, Beighton C, Ussher M, Limb E, David L, Brewin D, Adams F, Rogers A, Cook D. A primary care nurse-delivered walking intervention in older adults: PACE (pedometer accelerometer consultation evaluation)-lift cluster randomised controlled trial. PLoS Med. 2015;12(2):e1001783.

38. Harris T, Kerry S, Limb E, Victor C, Iliffe S, Ussher M, Whincup P, Ekelund U, Fox Rushby J, Furness C, Anokye N, Ibison J, DeWilde S, David L, Howard E, Dale R, Smith J, Cook D. Effect of a primary care walking intervention with and without nurse support on physical activity levels in 45- to 75-year-olds: the pedometer and consultation evaluation (PACE-UP) cluster randomised clinical trial. PLoS Med. 2017;14(1):e1002210.

39. Mutrie N, Doolin O, Fitzsimons C, Grant PM, Granat M, Grealy M, Macdonald H, MacMillan F, McConnachie A, Rowe D, Shaw R, Skelton D. Increasing older adults' walking through primary care: results of a pilot randomized controlled trial. Fam Pract. 2012;29(6):633–42.

40. Bravata D, Smith Spangler C, Sundaram V, Gienger A, Lin N, Lewis R, Stave C, Olkin I, Sirard J. Using pedometers to increase physical activity and improve health: a systematic review. JAMA. 2007;298(19):2296–304.

41. Greaves C, Sheppard K, Abraham C, Hardeman W, Roden M, Evans P, Schwarz P. Systematic review of reviews of intervention components associated with increased effectiveness in dietary and physical activity interventions. BMC Public Health. 2011;11:119.

42. Hankonen N, Sutton S, Prevost AT, Simmons R, Griffin S, Kinmonth A, Hardeman W. Which behavior change techniques are associated with changes in physical activity, diet and body mass index in people with recently diagnosed diabetes? Ann Behav Med. 2015;49(1):7–17.

43. Williams SL, French DP. What are the most effective intervention techniques for changing physical activity self-efficacy and physical activity behaviour-- and are they the same? Health Educ Res. 2011;26(2):308–22.

44. Ivers N, Jamtvedt G, Flottorp S, Young J, Odgaard Jensen J, French S, O'Brien M, Johansen M, Grimshaw J, Oxman A. Audit and feedback: effects

14

Nurses' and pharmacists' learning experiences from participating in interprofessional medication reviews for elderly in primary health care

H. T. Bell[1,2]*, A. G. Granas[3], I. Enmarker[4,5], R. Omli[1,4] and A. Steinsbekk[2]

Abstract

Background: Traditionally, drug prescription and follow up have been the sole responsibility of physicians. However, interprofessional medication reviews (IMRs) have been developed to prevent drug discrepancies and patient harm especially for elderly patients with polypharmacy and multimorbidity. What participating nurses and pharmacists learn from each other during IMR is poorly studied. The aim of this study was to investigate nurses' and pharmacists' perceived learning experience after participating in IMRs in primary health care for up to two years.

Methods: A qualitative study with semi-structured focus group interviews and telephone interviews with nurses and pharmacists with experience from IMRs in nursing homes and home based services. The data was analysed thematically by using systematic text condensation.

Results: Thirteen nurses and four pharmacists were interviewed. They described some challenges concerning how to ensure participation of all three professions and how to get thorough information about the patient. As expected, both professions talked of an increased awareness with time of the benefit of working as a team and the perception of contributing to better and more individual care. The nurses' perception of the pharmacist changed from being a controller of drug management routines towards being a source of pharmacotherapy knowledge and a discussant partner of appropriate drug therapy in the elderly. The pharmacists became more aware of the nurses' crucial role of providing clinical information about the patient to enable individual advice. Increasingly the nurses learned to link the patient's symptoms of effect and side effect to the drugs prescribed.

Conclusions: Although experiencing challenges in conducting IMRs, the nurses and pharmacists had learning experiences they said improved both their own practice and the quality of drug management. There are some challenges concerning how to ensure participation of all three professions and how to get thorough information about the patient.

Keywords: Medication review, Nurse, Pharmacist, Learning, Inappropriate drug use, Primary care

* Correspondence: hege.t.bell@nord.no
[1]Department of Pharmacy, Faculty of Health Sciences, Nord University, Namsos, Norway
[2]Department of Public Health and General Practice, Norwegian University of Science and Technology, Trondheim, Norway
Full list of author information is available at the end of the article

Background

Elderly living at home and in nursing homes use many drugs [1] and are therefore at risk of experiencing adverse drug reactions and increased risk of falls [2]. Physicians have traditionally been responsible for drug prescription and follow up, but it has e.g. been shown that they renew prescriptions without assessing if the medication is still indicated [3]. In addition frequent changes in caregivers both between secondary and primary care but also within primary care, make elderly patients and patients with complex care needs more vulnerable to drug discrepancies that can lead to drug errors [4]. As a result systems for medication reconciliation and interprofessional medication reviews (IMRs) have been developed [5]. IMRs by physicians, nurses and pharmacists have been showed to reduce drug-related problems and improve quality of prescribing in hospitals and nursing homes patients [6, 7].

Primary health care workers often face additional challenges compared to those working in a hospital setting due to lack of geographical proximity of the team members [8]. Facilitators and barriers to interprofessional collaboration in primary health care has been identified as being both structural and cultural like the need of shared facilities, written procedures, shared communication tools, accessibility, trust, value and leadership [9, 10]. Collaboration between nurses and community pharmacists in primary care concerns mainly product advice and dispensing issues [11], but when nurses and pharmacists collaborate in an inpatient medical setting they can learn to appreciate each other's roles [12].

The existing research on IMR has mainly focused on the outcome of the intervention of the drug-related problems [13] or the different participants' perception of the collaboration process [14]. However, we have found no research focusing on what nurses and pharmacists perceive to learn when participating in IMRs. The aim of this study is therefore to describe what nurses and pharmacists perceive to learn from participating in interprofessional drug review teams in a primary health care setting for up to two years.

Methods

This qualitative study is part of a larger study with focus group and individual interviews performed between October 2014 and February 2016 in Norway. The Regional Committees for Medical and Health Research Ethics in Central Norway approved the study (2014/1140).

Setting, training and practice

In Norway the municipalities are responsible for social welfare and health care for all its inhabitants, including home based health and social care and nursing homes [15]. Part-time contracted general practitioners (GPs) most commonly provide the medical services in nursing

homes [16] and the home dwelling elderly with home based health and social care receive their medical service from their GP with assistance from home care nurses [17]. The nurses in home care services often work alone as nurses, supported by staff with less or no formal nursing education [18]. The majority of Norwegian pharmacists work in privately owned community pharmacies or hospital pharmacies. The municipalities have contracts with a hospital or community pharmacy to provide services to inspect drug management or to perform medication reviews [19].

Interprofessional medication reviews is not established in primary health care in Norway, but since 2013 the GP legislation states that patients prescribed four or more drugs, the GP should perform medication reviews if this is necessary from a medical point of view [20]. There is yet no such legislation for patients in nursing homes. In 2011–13 the Norwegian Patient Safety Programme "In safe hands" was implemented throughout Norway. Two of the 12 focus areas were to establish interprofessional teams on medication reviews in nursing homes and home based health and social care services [21]. The centres for Development of Institutional and Home Care Services [22] in each of Norway's 19 counties were responsible for spreading the program to municipalities in their own county, following a national guideline based on the Intergrated Medicines Management (IMM-model) [23].

The IMM-model consists of four main steps [23] and is based upon the original version from Northern Ireland [24]. In the first step, the nurses interview and go through a checklist with the patient, order blood samples and construct a drug list based on the available information. In the second step, the nurses pass this information to the pharmacist who identifies potential drug-related problems and checks if the prescribing is according to national guidelines. In the third step, the drug review is performed at a case conference where the responsible physician, nurse and the pharmacist meet and perform medication reconciliations and reviews where they discuss the best drug regime for that specific patient. The physician is responsible for the overall treatment. Finally, the nurse updates information of the drug regime agreed upon in the patient's journal. They also observe how the patient responds to any changes and give feed back to the GP when necessary [21]. The drug reviews require consent from the patient that allows health information to be shared in between the three professions involved.

The municipalities were encouraged to form interprofessional teams, consisting of at least one representative from the three professions; physician, nurse and pharmacist. In a course consisting of three structured learning meetings throughout one year the interprofessional teams of health professionals, were introduced to the methodology in the IMM-model, introduction to why IMRs are useful for the elderly patient, encouraged to initiate inter-professional cooperation and to establish interprofessional medication reviews (IMRs) [25]. The interprofessional teams were encouraged to start practicing medication rec-onciliations and IMRs after the first meeting in the course [21]. The nurses within each team were charged with de-veloping local routines for the selection of eligible pa-tients, routines for how to organize IMR-tasks on top of everyday tasks, and how to book case conferences. They were also responsible for spreading of knowledge on IMR to their colleagues. Only two physicians from the 11 par-ticipating municipalities attended the implementation course and only at the first meeting. It was therefore up to the team leaders, who were nurses, to recruit an appropri-ate physician from their municipality to their team. In some of the municipalities no physician was recruited and the IMRs were performed with only nurse and pharmacist present. In these teams the pharmacist first presented her findings to the nurse who then gave her input before she later was responsible of presenting the revised results from the discussion to the physician.

Informants and data collection

We aimed to recruit physicians, nurses and pharmacists who had participated in the patient safety program and who had experience of performing IMR. To ensure a representative sample, we wanted to have teams represent-ing different municipality size, different length of experi-ence with IMR and from both nursing homes and home based health and social care. The reports given by the dif-ferent teams after the course were used to select teams based on these criteria.

To recruit informants, the appointed team leaders in 11 municipalities in Central Norway were contacted by e-mail and then by phone. They were told that they could volunteer teams even though not all team members in each team wanted to participate. This approach only lead to the recruitment of two pharmacists participating in several teams each and therefore additional two phar-macists were recruited through the hospital pharmacies in the county.

The semi-structured focus group interviews were con-ducted with representatives from all included teams 1–2 years after initiation of the course in their county. Focus group is particularly useful for exploring people's com-mon experiences, attitudes and views in environments where people interact. The use of group interaction is an explicit part of the method [26]. The focus group inter-views were either conducted at a nursing home or at the city hall in the municipality. An interview guide with open-ended questions focused on the following themes was used; perceived learning and gained knowledge in addition to perceived facilitators and barriers to be able to perform interprofessional medication reviews in

primary health care [27] (Additional file 1). The focus group interviews lasted approximately one and a half hour, were digitally recorded and led by the first author (HTB). The telephone interviews lasted approximately 20 min performed by the first author using the same inter-view guide. Participants were provided with written and oral information about the study and informed that they could withdraw at any time. Written informed consent was obtained from the participants before the interviews were conducted.

Data analysis

The interviews were digitally recorded and transcribed ver-batim. They were analysed using the method of systematic text condensation [28], according to an iterative four-step process. In the first step, all authors read a selection of the transcripts to identify preliminary themes, which were dis-cussed. In the second step, the transcripts were searched in detail by the first author to identify meaning units, which were sorted under the preliminary themes and these were presented to the other authors. In the third step, the mean-ing units were arranged into subthemes. In all these steps the preliminary themes were adjusted. Then a narrative condensate was made of the meaning units sorted under each theme and subtheme. In the last step, an analytic text was produced based upon each theme and subtheme. The themes and the analysis were discussed among the authors several times and also in an extended research group to en-sure validity. During the whole process, the authors went back to the original transcripts to ensure that the analysis was based upon them.

Results

A total of thirteen nurses from five different nursing homes and three home-based care units and four pharmacists were interviewed. There were three focus group interviews consisting of nurses only but from both nursing homes and home based care, and two with nurses from different workplaces and a pharmacist. The remaining two pharma-cists were interviewed by telephone. Further participant characteristics are presented in Table 1.

The perceived learning from participating in structural interprofessional medication reviews in primary health care are arranged in the following five themes; Learning about each other's role, A more comprehensive documen-tation of drug management, Challenge the physician's role, Importance of detailed information about each patient and Linking patient's symptoms and medication use.

Learning about each other's role

It was new for the nurses in the nursing home and home based health and social care to learn during the interpro-fessional medication reviews (IMRs) that pharmacists could provide advice and guidance on appropriate drug

Table 1 Participant characteristics

	Nurses (n = 13)	Pharmacists (n = 4)
Working in nursing homes	8	-
Rural	5	3
Urban	3	4
Working in home-based care	5	-
Rural	2	-
Urban	3	-
≤1 year experience of performing IMR in primary health care	5	1
>1 year experience of performing IMR in primary health care	8	3
Experience from performing IMR in hospital	-	3
Experience of performing IMR with a physician present	10	4
Experience of performing IMR without a physician present	3	3

use for the elderly patients. This was contrary to their previous experience of pharmacists as someone who came on irregular visits and primarily focused on controlling their drug management routines. After taking part in IMRs, however, they now perceived the pharmacist as a supportive partner who could give them useful advice on pharmacology and pharmacotherapy. They especially appreciated the pharmacists' knowledge concerning drug monitoring data for laboratory values like haematology, proteins, hormones, vitamins and drugs such as digoxin with a small therapeutic window. The pharmacists said that after the establishment of the IMR-teams, the number of telephone and e-mail inquires from both nurses and physicians regarding drug therapy questions had increased.

The pharmacists gave us a very good impression by showing how much they could contribute regarding knowledge on drugs and drug therapy. They knew much more than we thought they did. Our previous impression was that they sold plasters and handled the drugs at the pharmacies. (Nurse, less than one year of experience with IMR)

The pharmacists did not meet with the patients themselves and therefore talked about a dependency on the patient information given by the nurses. Preparing for the IMRs could be challenging for the pharmacists when not having access to updated drug monitoring data and complementary patient documentation. They perceived the majority of the nurses to provide good information and documentation, but there were also examples of the contrary like e.g. nurses who did not know the patient well.

"A case has many sides and I only know the patient through his drug list. So it is very important for me to get the additional information from the nurses. Like when a patient has pain. When does he have pain and what type of pain?" (Pharmacist, more than 2 years experience of IMR)

A more comprehensive documentation of drug management

Taking part in the IMR, the nurses talked about how they learned to become more critical towards their own drug management routines and talked about a raised awareness on better documentation of these routines in everyday work. In addition, especially the nurses working in home based health and social care, learned the importance of medication reconciliation that ensured an updated list of drugs in use due to the high number of carer that could be involved. An updated drug list which they trusted to be correct also helped them to get a more complete and documented overview of the patient's medical situation and to later link this to the drugs in use.

When the other professions regarding drug management raised challenging questions the nurses said they learned the need for accurate, updated and detailed information in the patient journals about drugs in use and the need for a broader focus on drug management as a whole. This included having all the patient's diagnosis listed in the journal and to ensure written indications for the different drugs to be available for all health personnel involved with the patients. Participating in IMRs were therefore said to promote an understanding of comprehensive documentation of the drug management as a nurse task just as important as the other nursing tasks. It was highlighted that staff without any formal nursing education, who often are the ones to hand out the drugs and spend most time with the patients, especially appreciated this quality improvement.

"In the beginning when the indications were vague and not always written on the patient's medicine card it was difficult to evaluate the usefulness of the drugs. Especially since it was not written why they were put on those drugs." (Nurse, less than one year of experience of IMR)

Challenge the physician's role

The nurses with experience of performing IMRs together with both a physician and a pharmacist said that the pharmacist challenged the physician's role as the only drug expert. In particular this involved posing other types of questions, comments and solutions than the nurses did. This was said to stimulate the physicians to reflect upon their previous drug prescribing and in some instances forced the physicians to argue their case when there where disagreements. Both professions perceived disagreements as strength for the quality of drug therapy for the patients, because it triggered the physician to review the drug therapy choices initiated by themselves or other prescribers. Some nurses felt that the pharmacists' questions echoed comments and questions previously raised by themselves to the physicians, but where they hitherto had failed to argue their case or gave in without getting a clear answer. However, when the pharmacists asked questions during the team discussions the physicians responded better and more clearly.

"The pharmacist sees it from another angel and uses her own specialist knowledge to come up with new alternatives that the physician has not thought of – as far as I can see that must increase the quality."
(Nurse, with more than one year experience of IMR)

The nurses that had performed IMRs without having a physician present did not compliment the pharmacist in the same way and said that the physician was the one who knew what was best for the patient regardless the pharmacist's suggestions. These nurses sometimes perceived the physicians as headstrong but it was also emphasized that the physicians often had long experience in the municipality and therefore had a better insight into the totality of the patient's situation. In some of the cases the experience was also that when the nurses presented the suggestions to the physicians after the IMR with the pharmacist the physician rarely if at all took the suggestions into account.

"We presented it to the physician. And since they were only suggestions he did not go for them." (Nurse, with less than one year of experience of IMR and IMR without physician)

The pharmacists that had experienced IMR without a physician appreciated the nurse's contribution during the drug review, but found it unsatisfactory not being able to discuss and argue their case directly with the physician. Not knowing whether their suggestions were followed were also highlighted as a disadvantage since they perceived to learn less when missing out the discussions with the physician in particular. When the physician was present the pharmacists perceived that the physicians in the majority of the cases appreciated their contributions, but there were also experience of the contrary. With time the pharmacists said to understand better why their theoretical grounded suggestions not always were accepted by the physicians, mainly due the physicians' knowledge of a larger totality of the patients' situation than themselves. This was said to contribute to a wider understanding of some of the choices taken by

the primary care physician and to enable the pharmacists to view a case from another perspective than they usually did.

"We get the physicians view of the patient. A GP know the patient and his history better than I do and I might suggest a change that might have been tried out before (...) which the physician find difficult to implement (...) because the patient might refuse."
(Pharmacist, more than 2 years experience of IMR)

Importance of detailed information about each patient
In some municipalities the pharmacists experienced that the nurses struggled to find time to do their part of the preparatory work, such as interviewing the patient, order drug monitoring blood samples and filling in the patient checklist. This resulted in delayed or deficient documentation to the pharmacist. These drug reviews were perceived as unsatisfactory since the pharmacist then only could give generic advice and not tailor the suggestions for the patient in question.

"The advices we give might be good, but it might not be the best for that specific patient. For example I set up an optimal list of drugs based upon the guidelines, but then maybe the patient is not able to swallow tablets or remember to take the tablets twice a day. There is a lot of extra information I need to be able to set up an appropriate list of drugs." (Pharmacist, more than 2 years experience of IMR)

As a consequence, one pharmacist had changed the preparing routines prior the IMR and now spent the whole day at the nursing home or home based health care. Information about the patient were gathered and collected by the pharmacist using information from the patient's journals and talking to the nurses. The preparations took place in the morning and then the IMR was performed in the afternoon. This was said to give a better access to the existing documentation and also gave the pharmacists the opportunity to ask the nurses and other staff of supplementary information when needed.

None of the drug reviews were performed with the patient present. Perceiving themselves as the patient's voice at the drug review made the nurses discover that detailed knowledge of each patient was a necessity to be able to answer questions raised by the other two professions at the IMR. Contrary, the nurses felt awkward when presenting patients they did not know well or relied on second hand information. Good cooperation with nursing assistants or other care workers was perceived as important when collecting necessary information on function level and behaviour. Likewise, it was said to be important to discuss the observations of each patient in the nurse collegium since different persons perceived the patients differently. This was especially important in home based health care service as opposed to nursing homes, because the nurses spend only a short time with domiciliary patients.

It was also expressed as difficult to convey patient information, when the nurse interviewing and collecting the information about the patient might not be the same presenting at the drug review. The teams that perceived good backing for the IMR tasks in the municipality and who had managed to develop good routines throughout the collegium were also those who found collecting these data least difficult.

"I felt sometimes – oh I should have known more about this patient. I do not believe that I will be the one that continues performing drug reviews." (Nurse, less than one year experience of IMR)

Linking patient's symptoms and medication use
The pharmacists experienced that the nurses gradually showed a deeper engagement for the medication reviews, such as being more updated on the patients' conditions, symptoms and the prescribed drugs. The nurses said that during the medication reviews they had learned new things about pharmacotherapy, especially how drugs work and drug-drug interactions. Examples were knowledge about drugs with anticholinergic effect and drugs that can increase the risk of falls in their patients.

"We have learned more about combination of different drugs and anticholinergic effects. (...) Being more aware on pain relief – the need to assess the treatment more often and at an earlier stage. Previously they had Paracetamol 1 g x 3 without us assessing, but now we ask them whether they still need them. The questions pop up more frequently." (Nurse, more than one year experience of IMR)

A stronger knowledge on pharmacotherapy made the nurses more observant and capable of interpreting patients' behaviour possibly linked to the drug use – both effects and side effects. They said that they became more curious and critical, therefore asking more questions to the physicians and pharmacists. They also became more aware of the need for a more comprehensive documentation of the drug management. New awareness was said to be transferrable to other patients not yet part of IMRs such as assessing drug therapy at an earlier stage, for example in long-term pain treatment. Participation in IMR with both pharmacist and physician heighten their awareness on drug treatment as a whole and were said to contribute to the perception of more individual care.

"We have gained a greater awareness on drugs (...) You become a little more aware when you see a drug sheet. "Can this be correct?" (...) You become more critical." (Nurse, with more than one year experience of IMR)

When asked if the learning emerged from participating in the course or from performing IMR, both the professions linked the learning to active participation in IMRs. They said that at a course you were only a passive recipient, whereas during IMR you had to use your adopted knowledge actively which again led to learning. Arguing their case was particularly highlighted to contribute to learning. The nurses who had performed IMRs without a physician present spoke less of what they had learned during this period.

"I believe that IMR give something extra since you have to use what you know actively. You get forced to think through what you are doing. Why do we do this IMR, and you look at the check list and think of the patient's drugs and how the whole situation is for the patient." (Nurse, more than one year experience of IMR)

Discussion
In this study it was found that both professions reported to learn more about each other's role when performing interprofessional medication reviews (IMRs). The nurses' perception of the pharmacist changed from being a controller of drug management routines towards being a source of pharmacotherapy knowledge and a discussant partner for appropriate drug therapy in the elderly. The pharmacists became more aware of the nurses' crucial role of providing clinical information about the patient to enable individual advice. Increasingly the nurses learned to link the patient's symptoms to the prescribed drugs due to having learned more about pharmacology and pharmacotherapy and also the importance of comprehensive drug management and detailed information about each patient. With time both professions jointly spoke of an increased awareness of the benefit of working as a team and the perception of contributing to better and more individual care. Through this they learned to challenge the physicians' knowledge and prescribing decisions. IMRs were found to be unsatisfactory without the physician's input and without thorough information about the patient's condition.

Learning from each other and the experience of mutual interdependence
Others have found that pharmacists can have other roles than controlling and checking up on the other professions' drug handling [29] and that other professions' awareness of the pharmacists' clinical skills increases with time

[12, 30]. This is in line with our findings. The most prominent learning reported by the informants in this study was how they came to appreciate each other's role during the medication reviews and how this created a sense of mutual interdependence. Participating in IMR were said to lift the focus on medication management as an important nurse task and that the pharmacists' contributions during the IMRs elevated the nurses' own performance. Nurses and physicians have both stated a perceived elevation of performance and educational benefit from working together with pharmacists [12].

It has been found that effective teamwork demands role clarity and an understanding of roles and responsibilities [8, 31], where working together can create a sense of mutual interdependence when different professions learn to know each other's roles [32]. Pharmacists cooperating with other professions have been shown to facilitate a team approach that improved the patient's drug related outcomes [12, 30]. This is in line with our study. The discussions during the IMRs where all professions were present were especially perceived as beneficial and therefor indicate that doing IMRs together can contribute to both learning and the perception of mutual interdependence.

Challenges when applying IMRs in primary health care

Lack of mandate for the pharmacist's role [10], the time the pharmacist was on site and funding of the pharmacists [14] has been found as barriers for pharmacists participating in interprofessional teams in primary health care. The model of IMM provides guidelines for the role of the pharmacists in IMRs [23], but the funding is dependent on the municipalities' willingness to pay for the pharmacist and can be a limitation for the continuation of IMRs in primary care. Our findings also concur with findings in studies from Supper et al. and Bell et al. which found that limited access to the complete medical history and relevant monitoring data can be perceived as a barrier for the pharmacist [10, 33]. In our study it was particularly evident that the main barrier was if there were delayed or deficient documentation about the patient's condition given to the pharmacist prior to the IMRs.

The physician has a pivotal role in decisions making about the prescribed medicines [34]. No surprise, when the physician is not present at the IMR, the interviewees said that they learned less. Accessibility has been shown to be a premise for interprofessional collaboration particularly between physicians and allied health professionals [9]. Not having all professions present is also a deviation from the IMM-model [24]. When team members have separate bases or buildings they are less integrated with the team [8]. However, it was perceived as

challenging to gather all professions for joint meetings in primary care. The same was found in studies of interprofessional cooperation in family health teams and family medicine clinics that describe challenges according to management, leadership, time, space and governance [32, 35]. Thus, there seems to be a need for innovative solutions to overcome obstacles such as finding common time and booking meeting facilities for the case conferences, in home based care and in rural municipalities.

Another challenge experienced by our informants was how to ensure good and correct information about each patient. Shift work and part-time positions in addition to nurses spending little time with home dwelling patients, made it difficult to collect the relevant patient information. Thus it can be a challenge to gather and collect comprehensive and objective information about the patient from all personnel involved prior to the medication reviews. This raises the question whether the patients themselves, unlike today [34], should be present during IMR to make sure that the patients' perspectives are taken into account. From an ethically perspective patients should be included in decisions about their own care [36]. We have, however, not found any studies investigating such a solution in IMRs.

Medication management in primary care – more than right medicine to right patient

Since service users in primary care receive lower level of medical service intensity compared to hospital patients, the need to observe, document and report effects of the medical treatment has been reported to be an even more crucial task for the nurses [37, 38]. This includes monitoring medication administration, adherence and the effect medicines have on patients' symptoms [39]. The findings in this study indicates that this could be problematic due to the infrequent contact with the patient in home based care and not being challenged to report specifically on these issues. It is therefore reassuring that the IMR was experienced as an arena where the nurses became more aware of the importance of thorough medication handling routines and a need for written high quality instructions on all the steps in the medication management process.

Strengths and limitations

The strength of this study was that the informants had real life experience with doing interprofessional medication reviews over time and the variation in the clinical situations the IMRs were conducted. In addition, there were variation in geography and population. It was a limitation that the interviewees came from one county in Norway and none of the municipalities were a large city. However, as others have similar findings [12, 30] this does not seem to limit the transferability. The lack of the physicians as informants is another limitation. The physicians were invited on equal terms as the other two professions, but none of the physicians involved responded to the invitation. There is therefore a need for studies in the physicians' perspectives but also on the patients' perspective.

The focus groups purposefully consisted of teams that had participated in the course and performed medication reviews together. This contributed to a relaxed and freely speaking environment. Former disagreements could have limited discussions of topics they knew could cause disagreement and even hamper future collaboration. Furthermore, the fact that HTB is a pharmacist could have limited criticism of the pharmacists' role. However, the review of the transcripts indicates that the interviewees spoke also about disagreements during the interviews.

From the interviews, it seemed like the nurses learned more from the pharmacists than the other way around. This is likely to be due to the predominance of nurses among the informants, but it might also be due to the nurses getting access to a new profession's knowledge and skills, which was unlike the pharmacists whom the majority had former experience from IMR in hospitals.

Conclusion

From the nurses' and pharmacists' perspective in this study, IMRs in primary health care can be a learning arena for the participating professions. It was experienced to contribute to improving their own practice and the quality of drug management, resulting in better and more individualised care. There are some challenges especially concerning how to ensure participation of all three professions and how to get thorough information about the patient.

Abbreviations
GP: General practitioner; IMM: Integrated medicines management; IMR: Interprofessional medication review

Acknowledgements
The authors thank the health professionals who participated in the study.

Funding
The study was funded by Nord University.

Authors' contributions
HTB and RO conducted the interviews in the study. HTB, RO, AS and AGG analyzed the data and HTB, AS and AGG wrote the manuscript by providing critical appraisals. HTB, RO and IE particpated in the design of the study and all authors contributed to the content in the manuscript and read the final manuscript. All authors read and approved the final manuscript.

Competing interests
The authors declare that they have no competing interests neither financial nor non-finacial.

Consent for publication
Not Applicable.

Author details
[1]Department of Pharmacy, Faculty of Health Sciences, Nord University, Namsos, Norway. [2]Department of Public Health and General Practice, Norwegian University of Science and Technology, Trondheim, Norway. [3]School of Pharmacy, University of Oslo, Oslo, Norway. [4]Centre for Care research Mid- Norway, Steinkjer, Norway. [5]Department of Nursing, Mid University, Østersund, Sweden.

References
1. Tommelein E, Mehuys E, Petrovic M, Somers A, Colin P, Boussery K. Potentially inappropriate prescribing in community-dwelling older people across Europe: a systematic literature review. Eur J Clin Pharmacol. 2015;71(12):1415–27.
2. de Groot MH, van Campen JP, Moek MA, Tulner LR, Beijnen JH, Lamoth CJ. The effects of fall-risk-increasing drugs on postural control: a literature review. Drugs Aging. 2013;30(11):901–20.
3. Bell HT, Steinsbekk A, Granas AG. Factors influencing prescribing of fall-risk-increasing drugs to the elderly: a qualitative study. Scand J Prim Health Care. 2015;33(2):107–14.
4. Coleman EA, Smith JD, Raha D, Min SJ. Posthospital medication discrepancies: prevalence and contributing factors. Arch Intern Med. 2005;165(16):1842–7.
5. Garfinkel D, Ilhan B, Bahat G. Routine deprescribing of chronic medications to combat polypharmacy. Ther adv drug saf. 2015;6(6):212–33.
6. Chisholm-Burns MA, Kim Lee J, Spivey CA, Slack M, Herrier RN, Hall-Lipsy E, et al. US pharmacists' effect as team members on patient care: systematic review and meta-analyses. Med Care. 2010;48(10):923–33.
7. Kaur S, Mitchell G, Vitetta L, Roberts MS. Interventions that can reduce inappropriate prescribing in the elderly: a systematic review. Drugs Aging. 2009;26(12):1013–28.
8. Xyrichis A, Lowton K. What fosters or prevents interprofessional teamworking in primary and community care? a literature review. Int J Nurs Stud. 2008;45(1):140–53.
9. Costa DK, Barg FK, Asch DA, Kahn JM. Facilitators of an interprofessional approach to care in medical and mixed medical/surgical ICUs: a multicenter qualitative study. Res Nurs Health. 2014;37(4):326–35.
10. Supper I, Catala O, Lustman M, Chemla C, Bourgueil Y, Letrilliart L. Interprofessional collaboration in primary health care: a review of facilitators and barriers perceived by involved actors. J Public Health (Oxf). 2015;37(4):716–27.
11. While A, Shah R, Nathan A. Interdisciplinary working between community pharmacists and community nurses: the views of community pharmacists. J Interprof Care. 2005;19(2):164–70.
12. Makowsky MJ, Schindel TJ, Rosenthal M, Campbell K, Tsuyuki RT, Madill HM. Collaboration between pharmacists, physicians and nurse practitioners: a qualitative investigation of working relationships in the inpatient medical setting. J Interprof Care. 2009;23(2):169–84.
13. Lehnbom EC, Stewart MJ, Manias E, Westbrook JI. Impact of medication reconciliation and review on clinical outcomes. Ann Pharmacother. 2014;48(10):1298–312.
14. Bajorek B, LeMay K, Gunn K, Armour C. The potential role for a pharmacist in a multidisciplinary general practitioner super clinic. Australas med J. 2015;8(2):52–63.
15. Rosstad T, Garasen H, Steinsbekk A, Haland E, Kristoffersen L, Grimsmo A. Implementing a care pathway for elderly patients, a comparative qualitative process evaluation in primary care. BMC Health Serv Res. 2015;15:86.
16. Ruths S, Sorensen PH, Kirkevold O, Husebo BS, Kruger K, Halvorsen KH, et al. Trends in psychotropic drug prescribing in Norwegian nursing homes from 1997 to 2009: a comparison of six cohorts. Int J Geriatr Psychiatry. 2013;28(8):868–76.

17. Helsedirektoratet. Fastlegestatistikk: http://www.Helsedirektoratet.no; [cited 2017 20th of February]. Available from: https://helsedirektoratet.no/statistikk-og-analyse/fastlegestatistikk#fastlegestatistikk-2015.
18. Sneltvedt T, Bondas T. Proud to be a nurse? Recently graduated nurses' experiences in municipal health care settings. Scand J Caring Sci. 2016;30(3): 557–64.
19. Apotekforeningen. Apotek og legemidler, nøkkeltall 2015. Oslo: Apotekforeningen; 2014. [cited 2017 20th of February]. Available from: http://www.apotek.no/fakta-og-ressurser/statistikk.
20. Forskrift om fastlegeordning i kommunene (Regulation on regular GP arrangement in the municipality) 2012. Available at: https://lovdata.no/dokument/SF/forskrift/2012-08-29-842?q=fastlegeforskriften. [Accessed 20 Feb 2017].
21. Norwegian Ministry of Health and Care Services. The Norwegian Patient Safety Programme: In safe hands. 2011. [cited 2017 20th February]. Available from: http://www.pasientsikkerhetsprogrammet.no.
22. Utviklingssenter for sykehjem og hjemmetjenester. About Centre for Development of Institutional and Home Care Services http://www.utviklingssenter.no: Utviklingssenter for sykehjem og hjemmetjenester; [cited 2017 20 th of February]. Available from: http://www.utviklingssenter.no.
23. Andersen A, Wekre L, Sund J, Major A, Fredriksen G. Evaluation of implementation of clinical pharmacy services in central Norway. Eur J Hosp Pharm. 2014;21:125–8.
24. Scullin C, Scott MG, Hogg A, McElnay JC. An innovative approach to integrated medicines management. J Eval Clin Pract. 2007;13(5):781–8.
25. Andreassen Devik S. Riktig legemiddelbruk i kommunehelsetjenesten - erfaringer fra læringsnettverk i nord-trøndelag. Midt-Norge: Senter for omsorgsforskning; 2014.
26. Malterud K. Fokusgrupper som forskningsmetode for medisin og helsefag. 1st ed. Oslo: Universitetsforlaget; 2012.
27. Bell HT. Interview guide, supplementary material. 2016.
28. Malterud K. Systematic text condensation: a strategy for qualitative analysis. Scand J Public Health. 2012;40(8):795–805.
29. Halvorsen KH, Stensland P, Granas AG. A qualitative study of physicians' and nurses' experiences of multidisciplinary collaboration with pharmacists participating at case conferences. Int J Pharm Pract. 2011;19(5):350–7.
30. Pottie K, Haydt S, Farrell B, Kennie N, Sellors C, Martin C, et al. Pharmacist's identity development within multidisciplinary primary health care teams in Ontario; qualitative results from the IMPACT project. Res Social Adm Pharm. 2009;5(4):319–26.
31. Drummond N, Abbott K, Williamson T, Somji B. Interprofessional primary care in academic family medicine clinics: implications for education and training. Canadian fam physician Medecin de famille canadien. 2012;58(8):e450–8.
32. Gum L, Greenhill J, Dix K. Clinical simulation in maternity (CSiM): interprofessional learning through simulation team training. Qual Saf Health Care. 2010;19(5):e19.
33. Bell JS, Aslani P, McLachlan AJ, Whitehead P, Chen TF. Mental health case conferences in primary care: content and treatment decision making. Res Social Adm Pharm. 2007;3(1):86–103.
34. Helsedirektoratet. Veileder om legemiddelgjennomganger. Oslo: Helsedirektoratet; 2015. [cited 2016 20th of May]. Available from: https://helsedirektoratet.no/retningslinjer/veileder-om-legemiddelgjennomganger.
35. Goldman J, Meuser J, Rogers J, Lawrie L, Reeves S. Interprofessional collaboration in family health teams: an Ontario-based study. Can fam physician Medecin de famille canadien. 2010;56(10):e368–74.
36. Coulter A, Entwistle VA, Eccles A, Ryan S, Shepperd S, Perera R. Personalised care planning for adults with chronic or long-term health conditions. Cochrane Database Syst Rev. 2015;3:Cd010523.
37. Elliott M, Liu Y. The nine rights of medication administration: an overview. Br J Nurs (Mark Allen Publishing). 2010;19(5):300–5.
38. Voyer P, McCusker J, Cole MG, Monette J, Champoux N, Ciampi A, et al. Nursing documentation in long-term care settings: New empirical evidence demands changes be made. Clin Nurs Res. 2014;23(4):442–61.
39. Edwards S, Axe S. The 10'R's of safe multidisciplinary drug administration. Nurse Prescribing. 2015;13(8):398–406. 9p.

15

A prospective clinical trial of specialist renal nursing in the primary care setting to prevent progression of chronic kidney: a quality improvement report

Rachael C Walker[1,2†], Mark R Marshall[3,4*†] and Nick R Polaschek[5]

Abstract

Background: Early detection and effective management of risk factors can potentially delay progression of chronic kidney disease (CKD) to end-stage kidney disease, and decrease mortality and morbidity from cardiovascular (CV) disease. We evaluated a specialist nurse-led intervention in the primary care setting to address accepted risk factors in a study sample of adults at 'high risk of CKD progression', defined as uncontrolled type II diabetes and/or hypertension and a history of poor clinic attendance.

Methods: The study was a non-controlled quality improvement study with pre- and post- intervention comparisons to test feasibility and potential effectiveness. Patients within two primary care practices were screened and recruited to the study. Fifty-two patients were enrolled, with 36 completing 12-months follow-up. The intervention involved a series of sessions led by the nephrology Nurse Practitioner with assistance from practice nurses. These sessions included assessment, education and planned medication and lifestyle changes. The primary outcome measured was proteinuria (ACR), and the secondary outcomes estimated glomerular filtration rate (eGFR) and 5-year absolute CV risk. Several 'intermediary' secondary outcomes were also measured including: blood pressure, serum total cholesterol, glycosylated haemoglobin (HbA1c), body mass index (BMI), prevalence of active smoking, a variety of self-management domains, and medication prescription. Analysis of data was performed using linear and logistic regression as appropriate.

Results: There was a significant improvement in ACR (average decrease of −6.75 mg/mmol per month) over the course of the study. There was a small but significant decrease in eGFR and a reduction in 5 year absolute CV risk. Blood pressure, serum total cholesterol, and HbA1c all decreased significantly. Adherence to lifestyle advice improved with a significant reduction in prevalence of active smoking, although there was no significant change in BMI. Self-management significantly improved across all relevant domains.

Conclusions: The results suggest that a collaborative model of care between specialist renal nurses and primary care clinicians may improve the management of risk factors for progression of CKD and CV death. Further larger, controlled studies are warranted to definitively determine the effectiveness and costs of this intervention.

Keywords: Chronic kidney disease, Quality improvement, Primary care, Nurse practitioner, Prevention

* Correspondence: mrmarsh@woosh.co.nz
†Equal contributors
3Counties Manukau District Health Board, Auckland, New Zealand
4Faculty of Medical and Health Sciences, University of Auckland, Auckland, New Zealand
Full list of author information is available at the end of the article

Background

Chronic kidney disease (CKD) is a global public health issue. In New Zealand, end stage kidney disease (ESKD) alone accounts for 1-2% of total health care expenditure, a figure comparable to that in the United Kingdom [1,2]. The group with highest attributable risk of progressive CKD is those with diabetes mellitus, and this risk is exacerbated by hypertension, obesity and dyslipidaemia [3,4]. In addition, CKD is an independent risk factor for cardiovascular (CV) morbidity and mortality through reduced glomerular filtration rate (GFR) and proteinuria [5,6]. In New Zealand, indigenous groups (Maori and Pacific peoples) are over represented in their rates of ESKD, accounting for 44% and 29% of those commencing renal replacement therapy in New Zealand, respectively [7]. These indigenous groups also have highest prevalence of CKD and associated risk factors for progression.

It is generally accepted that early detection and effective management of CKD is the prime strategy to reduce progression to ESKD, decrease CV morbidity and mortality, and ultimately limit resource consumption [3,8-10]. However despite this knowledge, efforts to manage CKD have not proven effective and the number of patients reaching ESKD continues to increase. Within New Zealand, there are numerous reported barriers that hamper effective management of CKD in the community including socio-economic factors, poor accessibility to primary care, poor health literacy, lack of knowledge of CKD and sub-optimally controlled diabetes and blood pressure [11,12]. Alternative models of healthcare delivery are needed to address these issues.

A promising intervention is adjunctive support from nephrology Nurse Practitioners (NPs), which has been recently shown to reduce the rate of CKD progression and improve renal outcomes [13]. Although this intervention can be regarded as multifaceted, a key element in the role of NPs is coaching to improve self-management by patients. Although the researchers in the aforementioned study did not assess for change in self-management, there have been other randomized control trials (RCTs) involving specifically designed self-management interventions for CKD patients. These have shown measurable improvements in health behaviours and a reduction in the duration and number of hospital admissions [14], although a recent systematic review of literature has highlighted the small effect of self-management interventions upon level of adherence [15].

In 2010 the New Zealand Ministry of Health funded several initiatives to improve outcomes for New Zealanders with CKD through more effective management in the primary care setting. In New Zealand, secondary and tertiary services such as nephrology are provided free of charge to all patients through public hospitals funded by taxation.

By contrast, primary care (where most CKD is managed) is provided in private medical practices, where consultations are only partially publicly subsidized. In this article, we describe a quality improvement intervention involving collaboration between a regional nephrology service and local primary care clinicians to manage a group of patients with CKD at high risk of progression. The intervention utilized the resource of a nephrology NP, who in New Zealand is a highly-trained specialist nurse practicing autonomously and able to assess, diagnose and prescribe within their scope of practice [16]. The Ministry of Health funded the time of the NP working with clinicians in their primary care practice, thus enabling the service to be free to the patients.

In this study, we present an evaluation of this intervention in order to demonstrate the clinical potential of the model of care. We employed the reporting framework suggested by the Standards for Quality Improvement Reporting Excellence (SQUIRE) publication guidelines for reporting healthcare quality improvement research (http://squire-statement.org/assets/pdfs/SQUIRE_guidelines_table.pdf) [17].

Methods

Ethical issues

The study was approved by the Regional Ethics Committee (IRB00008714) of the New Zealand Ministry of Health (IORG0000895), conditional upon local ethics committee approval which was granted by the Institutional Review Board of the Hawke's Bay District Health Board after a full review of the study protocol. Patients were invited to participate in the intervention, given verbal and written information regarding the study and what their involvement would include, and informed that they were able to withdraw from participation at any stage.

Setting

The geographical setting for this study was Hawke's Bay, New Zealand, a rural district situated on the east coast of New Zealand with a population of approximately 170,000. The population of Hawke's Bay is notable for a high degree of socioeconomic deprivation, with 26% of the population in the lowest two national deciles of deprivation. The area is also notable for a high prevalence of New Zealand Maori (the indigenous ethnic group), comprising 25% of the population compared to 15% nationally.

The intervention in this study was conducted by Hawke's Bay District Health Board Nephrology Service in collaboration with two primary care practices located in the highest areas of socioeconomic deprivation in the region. Each practice served a catchment at the time of between 5000–7000 people, with clinicians that included General Practitioners (GPs) and practice nurses, registered nurses employed to work with GPs within the practice.

Patients were studied over a 12 month period, with an accrual period from 1st June 2011 to 15th September 2011.

Planning the intervention

Patients were screened and recruited through the primary care practices. Inclusion criteria required that all of the following conditions were met: 'high risk of CKD progression' (as defined below), age >18 years, diagnosis of type two diabetes mellitus, hypertension, and albuminuria defined as an albumin to creatinine ratio (ACR) >30 mg/mmol on at least three occasions separated by at least 1 week [18]. The main exclusion criterion was CKD due to renal parenchymal disease other than diabetic nephropathy. Patients at "high risk of CKD progression" were defined as those with at least 12 months of uncontrolled diabetes and/or hypertension (glycoslyated haemoglobin (HbA1c) >8% and blood pressure (BP) >140/90 mmHg [19,20]) *and* a history of poor attendance and engagement with their GP (history of unplanned non-attendance of 25% or more of scheduled appointments over the course of 12 months). Over 500 patients were

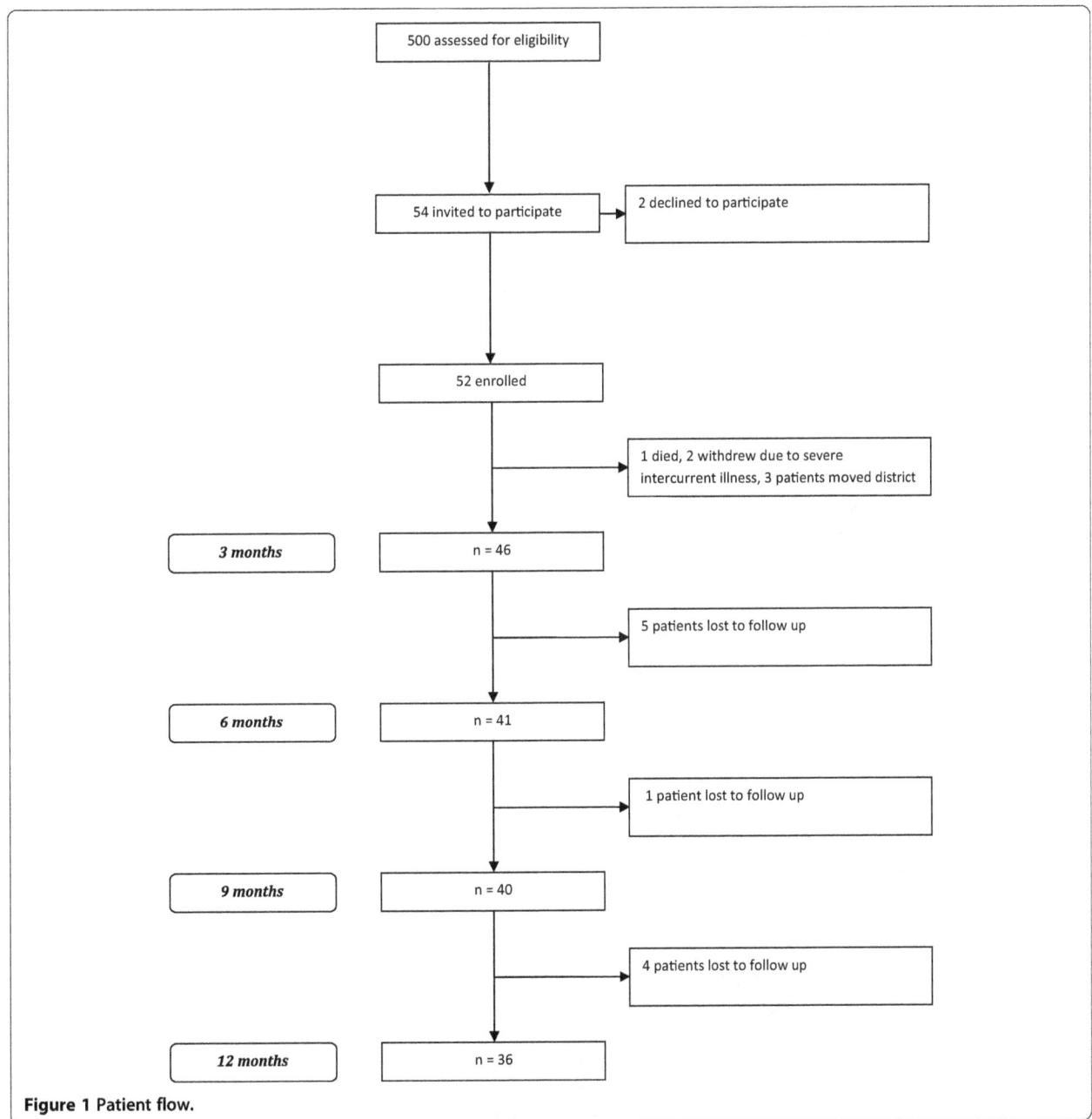

Figure 1 Patient flow.

identified from the initial screen within the practices and fifty-four high risk patients were identified by the primary care teams as also meeting the criteria for poor attendance. These fifty-four were given written information and invitation to participate by their GP or practice nurse. All were subsequently re-contacted by phone to answer any questions, and offered an initial assessment. Fifty two patients subsequently enrolled and participated in the study (Figure 1).

The intervention involved a series of sessions led by the nephrology NP with the assistance of the practice nurse. Patients were seen fortnightly for 12 weeks by the NP and the practice nurse, followed by a monitoring phase to 12 months. At baseline, a comprehensive patient history, health literacy and self-management assessment, physical assessment, and laboratory review was performed. Patient history included: medical history, family and social history and lifestyle behaviours including diet, smoking status, salt intake, exercise, and current knowledge of condition and medication. Physical assessment included office measurement of BP according to standardised protocol (JNC 7 [21]), pulse, height, weight, review of home capillary blood sugar records, and clinical cardiac assessment, conducted by the NP. Laboratory review included HbA1c, serum creatinine, estimated glomerular filtration rate (GFR), ACR and serum lipid levels.

Initial sessions involved tailored education and the development of individualised care plans based on best practice guidelines and using self-management and patient-centered theory utilizing the Flinders Chronic Care model [22]. A detailed patient education package was developed for the study and included information on diabetes and its complications, blood pressure management, lifestyle modifications, medication adherence, smoking cessation and dietary advice including low salt intake (dietary sodium intake less than 2.3 g/day). All patients were also given a booklet on self-management developed for the study where they could record all clinical results, self-care goals, individualised medication charts and other important information.

Subsequent sessions involved implementation of the individualized care plans, re-assessment of patients and management plan changes and implementations as required. A stepwise BP protocol was developed for the project with titration of antihypertensives at each fortnightly review to target a BP of 130/80 mmHg [19,20,23]. The protocol of medication escalation involved the stepwise addition of angiotensin converting enzyme inhibitors (ACEi) or angiotensin receptor blockers (ARB), thiazide diuretic, calcium channel blocker, and beta blocker or alpha blocker. Patients were provided with free transport to their study appointments, and all medications subjected to usual patient payments and subsidies without additional

cost or reimbursement. All patients in the study continued to receive usual health care (appointments as requested by patients or scheduled chronic disease management routine appointments, which are in general less than 15 minutes and 3 monthly at most) from their GP and primary health care team. Patients underwent baseline and three monthly

Table 1 Clinical characteristics of the study cohort at baseline

Variable		
Number	N	52
Practice	A	28 (54)
	B	24 (46)
Age	Years	57.5 (47–64)
Gender	Male	25 (48)
	Female	27 (52)
Ethnicity	New Zealand European	5 (10)
	Cook Island Maori/Samoan	10 (19)
	New Zealand Maori	37 (71)
Appropriate secondary specialist care		15 (29)
Total chronic medical illness burden	CIRS Score	6.92 (2.27)
2 or more diagnoses (CIRS domains)	%	33
3 or more diagnoses (CIRS domains)	%	3
4 or more diagnoses (CIRS domains)	%	0
Albumin to creatinine ratio	mg/mmol	34.9 (14.2-150.9)
5-year absolute cardiovascular risk	%	20 (15–27)
Estimated GFR	mL/min/1.73 m^2	63 (48–77)
Systolic BP	mmHg	150 (144.5-160)
Diastolic BP	mmHg	90 (80–110)
Serum total cholesterol	mmol/L	5.25 (4.1-6)
Glycosylated haemoglobin	%	8.8 (7.7-10.7)
Body mass index	kg/m^2	37 (32.5-43.5)
Active smoking		18 (35)
Self-management	Score	
Overall score (scale 0 to 104)		82 (72–91)
Knowledge of medications (scale 0 to 8)		6 (5–8)
Knowledge of condition (scale 0 to 8)		6 (4–7)
Medication adherence (scale 0 to 8)		8 (5–8)
Healthy lifestyle (scale 0 to 8)		6 (4–8)
Prescribed aspirin	%	31 (60)
Prescribed ACEi / ARBs	%	45 (87)
Prescribed HMG-CoA reductase inhibitors	%	32 (62)
Number of prescribed anti-hypertensives	n	2 (1–3)

All data are presented as n (%) or median (IQR).

Table 2 Frequency of New Zealand deprivation scores

Deprivation score	Frequency	Percent	Cumulative percent
1	1	1.9	2.0
2	1	1.9	4.0
3	1	1.9	6.0
4	1	1.9	8.0
7	1	1.9	10.0
8	3	5.8	16.0
9	13	25.0	42.0
10	29	55.8	100.0
Total	50	96.2	
Missing	2	3.8	
Total	52	100.0	

assessments of study end-points over the period of observation. All patient information and results was entered directly into the primary care health care record.

Planning the study of the intervention

We chose a validated method of measuring and describing the co-morbidities and multi-morbidity in the patient cohort. We extracted co-morbidity data from the medical history of patient records, and classified multi-morbidity using the Cumulative Illness Rating Scale (CIRS) [24]. This scale has been validated and applied in primary care settings, and has been used widely including the Australasian setting [25]. The scale rates the presence and severity of illness in 14 organ systems to provide an index of total chronic medical illness burden [26]. In this study, we assessed multimorbidity using 3 operational definitions: namely, 2 or more diagnoses (or CIRS domains), 3 or more diagnoses (or CIRS domains), and 4 or more diagnoses (or CIRS domains). We assessed the socioeconomic status of the patient cohort using the NZDep score, which combines nine variables from the census that reflect eight domains of deprivation (income, home ownership, social support, employment, academic qualifications, living space, access to a telephone, access to a car). The index provides a score for each meshblock in New Zealand, which are defined geographical areas defined by Statistics New Zealand containing a median number of approximately 87 people in 2006. The NZDep score divides New Zealand into deciles, e.g. a value of 10 indicates the meshblock is in the most deprived 10% of the New Zealand population, and a value of 1 indicates that the meshblock is in the least deprived [27].

Table 3 Change in observed outcome as a function of time

Primary outcome	Change per unit per month (linear), or change in odds ratio per month (binary categories)	(95% Confidence Interval)	P Value
ACR	−6.75	−10.98, −2.52	0.002
Secondary outcomes			
Estimated GFR	−0.34	−0.55, −0.12	0.002
5-year absolute cardiovascular risk	−0.24	−0.40, −0.09	0.002
"Intermediary" secondary outcomes - participant			
Systolic blood pressure (mmHg)	−1.65	−2.02, −1.28	<0.01
Diastolic blood pressure (mmHg)	−1.07	−1.33, −0.81	<0.001
Serum total cholesterol (mmol/L)	−0.05	−0.08, −0.02	0.002
HbA1c (%)	−0.09	−0.13, −0.06	<0.001
BMI (kg/m²)	−0.06	-.13, −0.008	0.08
Active smoking (odds ratio)	0.69	0.54, 0.88	0.003
Self-management			
Overall score (scale 0 to 104)	1.11	0.72, 1.50	<0.001
Knowledge of medications (scale 0 to 8)	0.17	0.12, 0.22	<0.001
Knowledge of condition (scale 0 to 8)	0.14	0.10, 0.18	<0.001
Medication adherence (scale 0 to 8)	0.05	0.001, 0.09	0.044
Healthy lifestyle (scale 0 to 8)	0.06	0.02, 0.11	0.005
"Intermediary" secondary outcomes - provider			
Prescribed aspirin (odds ratio)	1.61	1.23, 2.11	<0.001
Prescribed ACEi/ARB (odds ratio)	1.97	1.04, 3.72	0.037
Prescribed HMG-CoA reductase inhibitors (odds ratio)	1.26	1.08, 1.46	0.003
Number of prescribed anti-hypertensives	0.05	0.03, 0.07	<0.001

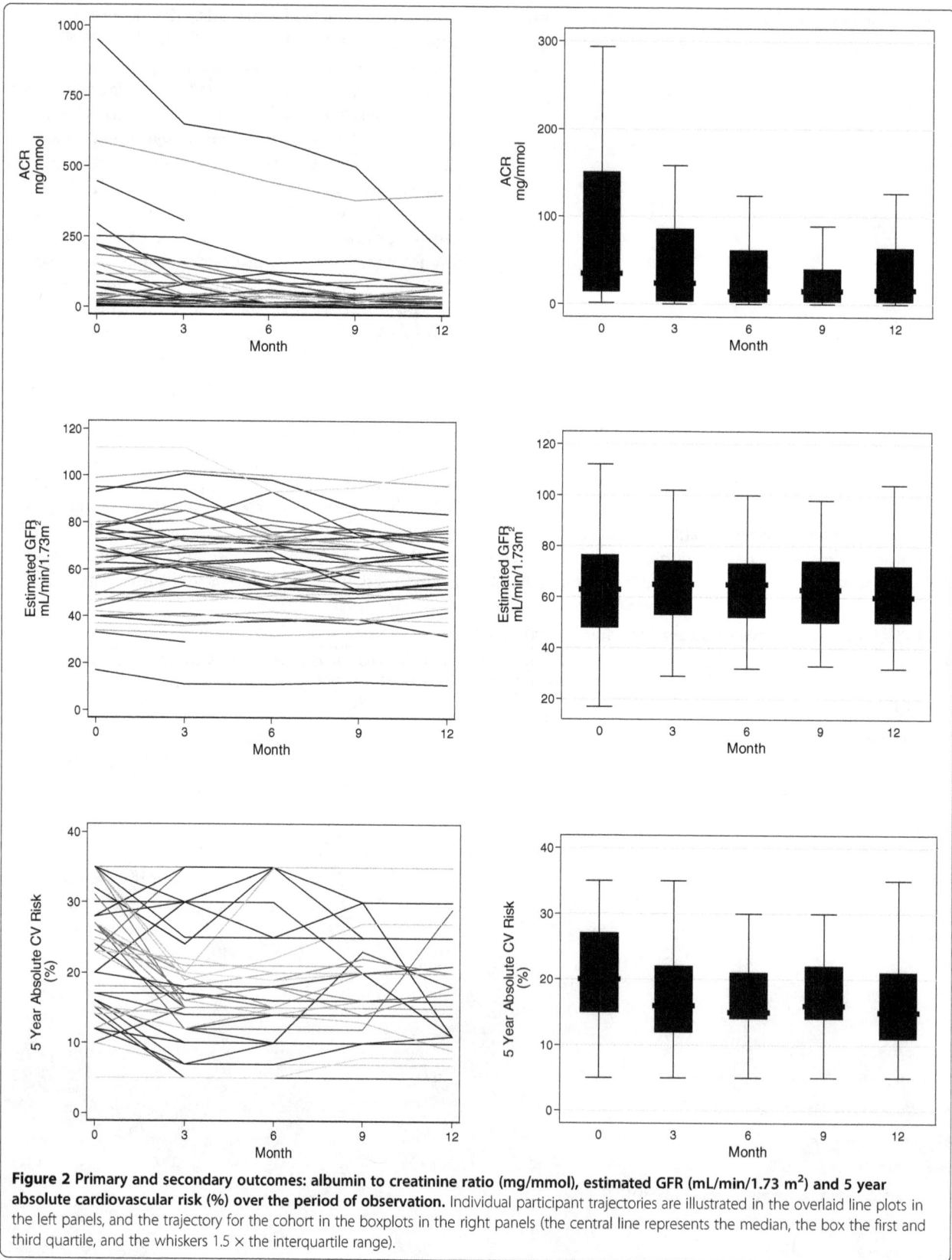

Figure 2 Primary and secondary outcomes: albumin to creatinine ratio (mg/mmol), estimated GFR (mL/min/1.73 m²) and 5 year absolute cardiovascular risk (%) over the period of observation. Individual participant trajectories are illustrated in the overlaid line plots in the left panels, and the trajectory for the cohort in the boxplots in the right panels (the central line represents the median, the box the first and third quartile, and the whiskers 1.5 × the interquartile range).

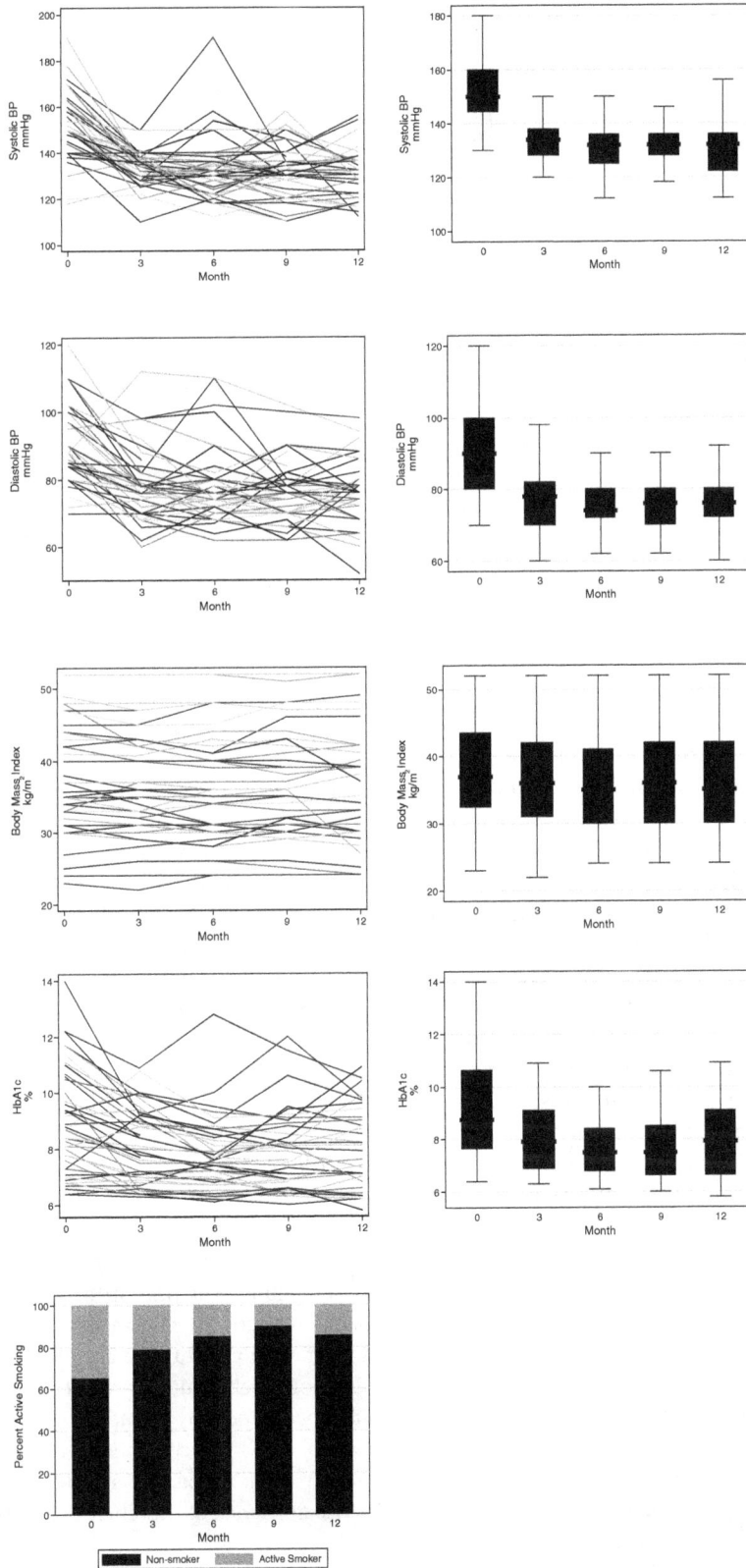

Figure 3 (See legend on next page.)

(See figure on previous page.)

Figure 3 'Intermediary' secondary outcomes related to the patient: BP (mmHg), serum total cholesterol, BMI (kg/m^2), HbA1c (%), prevalence of active smoking over the period of observation. For continuous variables, individual participant trajectories are illustrated in the overlaid line plots in the left panels, and the trajectory for the cohort in the boxplots in the right panels (the central line represents the median, the box the first and third quartile, and the whiskers 1.5 × the interquartile range). For categorical variables, bar plots indicate proportions for the entire cohort.

We assessed the outcomes of implementing the quality improvement program through the attendance of the participants to appointments, the attendance of both the NP and the practice nurse for the combined clinics, and staff satisfaction.

We measured the overall clinical impact of the quality improvement program through assessment of study outcomes over the 12 month period of the intervention. Measurements of outcomes (other than for health knowledge, medication knowledge, and self-management) were made at baseline, and endpoints consisted of measurements at 3, 6, 9 and 12 months. Measurements of health knowledge, medication knowledge, and self-management were made at baseline, and endpoints consisted of measurements at 3 and 12 months.

The primary outcome was proteinuria, assessed as the ACR on a random urine specimen taken prior to or at the combined clinic consultation. The secondary outcomes were: estimated GFR as assessed from serum creatinine and the 175 4-variable MDRD equation [28] (which to date remains the standard method rather than the CKD-EPI formula throughout New Zealand), and 5-year absolute cardiovascular risk (defined as the likelihood of a cardiovascular event over 5 years) [23].

We also assessed 'intermediary' secondary outcomes. These outcomes were either related to processes of care, or related to clinical outcomes accepted as being intermediate on casual pathways leading to either progression of CKD or to increased cardiovascular risk. Such outcomes were chosen as being the most likely mechanisms through which the study intervention might improve outcomes.

For intermediary secondary outcomes related to the participant, we assessed BP according to standardised protocol (JNC 7 [21]), serum total cholesterol, BMI, HbA1c and the prevalence of active smoking through patient clinical records. We assessed overall self-management, overall medical knowledge (knowledge of condition and medication), adherence to medication and adoption of a healthy lifestyle through a self-management reporting scale (Partners In Health Score, PIH score) [29]. The PIH score and questionnaire was developed for the Australian healthcare context, and is used to assess changes in patient self-management knowledge, skill and ability. The assessments are made from both the patient's own perspective and from the perspective of the treating clinician. The ratings span across twelve domains, or

areas of patient knowledge and health-related behaviour. The PIH scores provide a validated longitudinal record of how well patients are coping with and managing their chronic conditions [29].

For intermediary secondary outcomes related to the provider, we assessed prescribing patterns through patient clinical records.

Laboratory measurements were made in a central laboratory using standardized equipment (Abbott Aeroset®, Abbott Laboratories (N.Z.) Limited, Auckland, New Zealand). Serum creatinine assays were performed using the Jaffe method, and calibrated to isotope dilution mass spectroscopy.

Methods evaluation and analyses

The study data are in the form of a cross-sectional time-series, otherwise known as a panel, with repeated clinical observations obtained from the same patient over time. The data produce an unbalanced panel, as a result of missing observations pertaining to both truly missing data and also observations that are recorded during some months but not others. Of note, all study data from all participants were modelled, including baseline and follow-up results for those who died and dropped out, up until the time of their termination within the study.

We conducted the analysis of study data using regression models within Stata 12.1 MP software (College Station, TX, USA). For continuous data, we used linear models (xtreg procedure) and for categorical ones we used logistic models (xtlogit procedure). To account for internal correlation between repeated patient observations, a random effect model was used for each dependent variable that included all data from all time periods simultaneously, with observations over time from the same patient sharing the same random effects, assuming different random effects for different patients. To account for non-response bias, regression coefficients were estimated using the maximum likelihood method. Time was modelled as a continuous variable, and all coefficients are the modelled change in each parameter per month, with the p value referring to the significance of this change over time.

Results
Participants

Of the original 52 participants, 36 were still available for follow-up 12 months later (see Figure 1). Baseline clinical

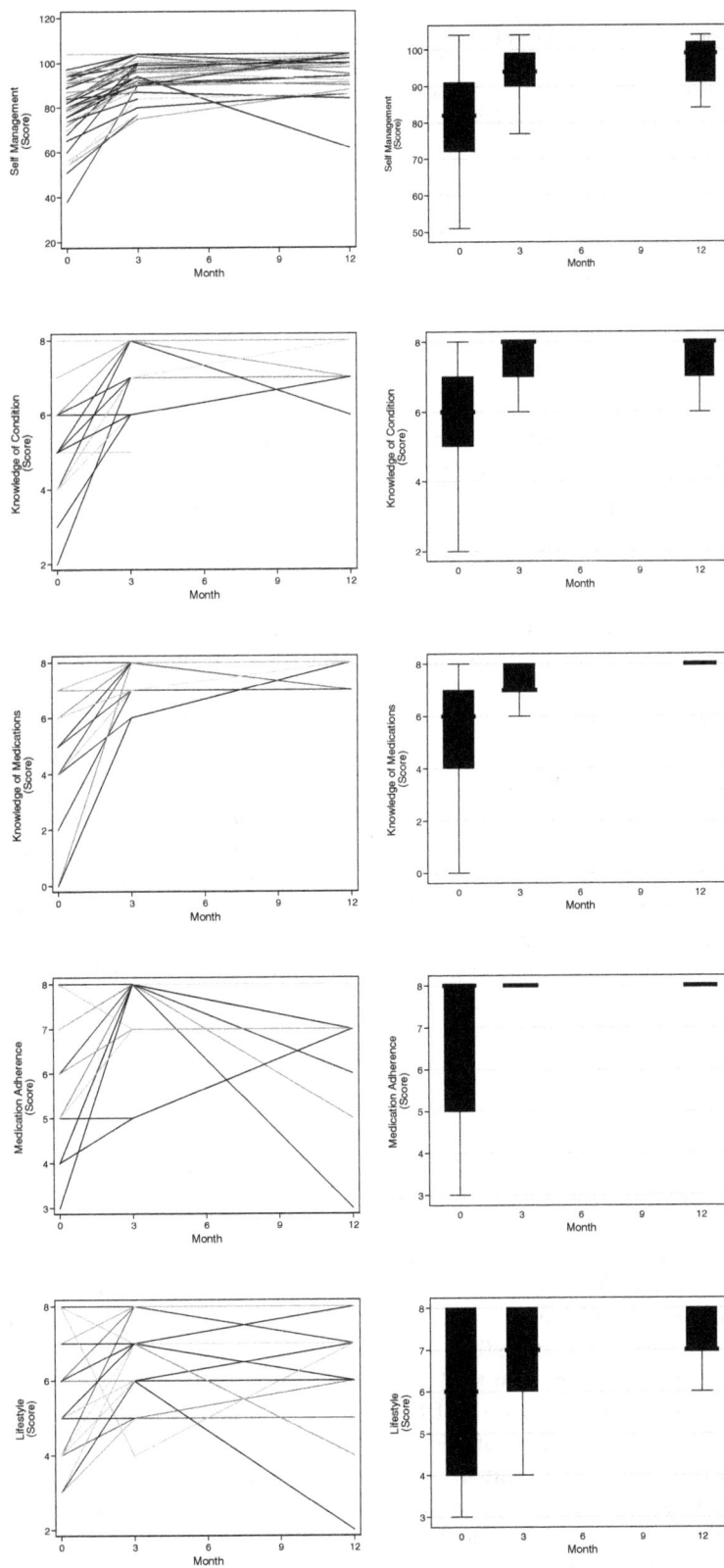

Figure 4 (See legend on next page.)

(See figure on previous page.)
Figure 4 'Intermediary' secondary outcomes related to the patient: self-management, medical knowledge (knowledge of condition and medication), adherence to medication, and adoption of a healthy lifestyle over the period of observation. Individual participant trajectories are illustrated in the overlaid line plots in the left panels, and the trajectory for the cohort in the boxplots in the right panels (the central line represents the median, the box the first and third quartile, and the whiskers 1.5 × the interquartile range).

---

characteristics of participants are provided in Table 1, and details of their total chronic medical illness burden in Additional file 1: Table S1. Socio-economic status of participants is described in Table 2, and illustrates the high level of deprivation with 84% of participants living in the 9 or 10th decile.

Course and success in implementation of intervention

Attendance of both the NP and the practice nurse was required as an integral component of the study intervention, and was 100% for the combined clinics. Staff satisfaction was surveyed as a routine part of clinical operations at the primary care practices, and was reported as high for all practice nurses and GPs involved in this initiative. All patients who were lost to follow up either died, withdrew due to severe intercurrent illness (one stroke, one myocardial infarction), or moved out of the district. 'Did not attend' rates were less than 5% for all participants remaining eligible over the entire period of observation.

Outcomes

Results of regression modelling and rank sum testing for study outcomes are provided in detail in Table 3.

There was a significant change in the primary outcome, ACR, over the course of the study, amounting to an average decrease of –6.75 mg/mmol per month over the period of observation. There were also significant changes in the secondary outcomes. There was a significance decrease in estimated GFR of –0.3 mL/min/1.73 m^2 per month, indicating that progression of CKD was still occurring within the study cohort amounting to a loss of 3–4 mL/min/1.73 m^2 per annum. There was a significant decrease in the 5 year absolute cardiovascular risk by –0.2% per month. Changes in these primary and secondary outcomes are illustrated in Figure 2.

There were significant changes in intermediary secondary outcomes related to the participant. Blood pressure decreased significantly over the course of the study, with a median baseline measurement of 150/90 and a corresponding 12 month measurement of 132/76. Serum total cholesterol and HbA1c also decreased significantly, with median baseline measurements of 5.25 mmol/L and 8.75%, respectively, and corresponding 12 month measurements of 4.6 mmol/L and 7.55%, respectively. Adherence to lifestyle advice improved, with a significant decrease of active smoking from 35%

to 10%, although there was no significant change in BMI. Self-management significantly improved across all relevant domains, with an increase in median overall self-management score from 82 to 99 over the period of observation. These changes are illustrated in Figures 3, 4 and 5.

There were significant changes in intermediary secondary outcomes related to the provider. The prescription of ACEi/ARBs, aspirin and lipid lowering medications, increased significantly to 97%, 86%, and 80% respectively. The mean number of prescribed anti-hypertensives increased significantly from 2 to 3.

Discussion

This report evaluates a primary care based intervention for CKD patients at high risk of CKD progression. The intervention utilized the nephrology NP within this setting to improve risk factors for progression of CKD. The baseline data for this group of participants indicated sub-optimal management for an extended period of time, with clinical care and outcomes that were not meeting customary targets suggested in clinical practice guidelines. Such characteristics define a common, problematic group of patients, both within New Zealand and internationally. One study from the United Kingdom typifies this experience, with only a fifth of those with diabetes and CKD having a BP of 130/80 mmHg or less, and fewer than half on angiotensin-converting-enzyme inhibitor or angiotensin-receptor blocker [30]. Similar findings have been reported from the United States [31].

This study supports the feasibility and potential effectiveness of an integrated model of care for management of CKD. During the course of the nurse-led intervention there was improved control of accepted risk factors for progression of CKD. Patient adherence to medication and lifestyle advice both improved over the duration of the intervention, indicating that high risk patients are sometimes willing to engage in lifestyle modifications when afforded adequate support and education about management of their condition, combined with empowerment through improved self-management skills.

Several other studies have shown similar success. An algorithm-based, primary care disease-management programme for patients with CKD in the United Kingdom also associated with better control of BP, lower serum cholesterol, and reduced the rate of kidney function loss supporting the notion of a community based model of

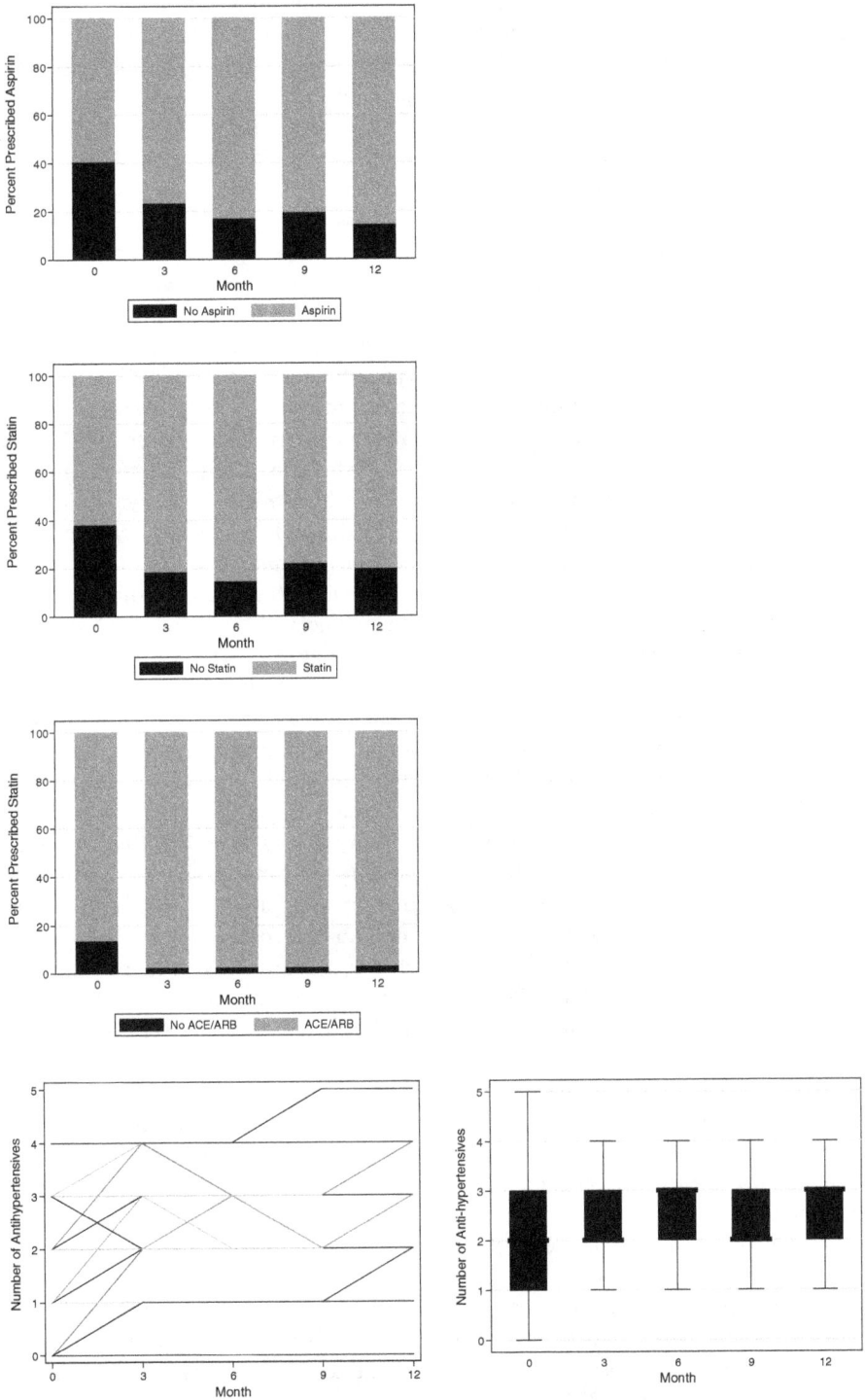

Figure 5 'Intermediary' secondary outcomes related to the provider: prescription of angiotensin converting enzyme inhibitors (ACEi) or angiotensin receptor blockers (ARB), aspirin and lipid lowering medications, and number of antihypertensive medications. For continuous variables, individual participant trajectories are illustrated in the overlaid line plots in the left panels, and the trajectory for the cohort in the boxplots in the right panels (the central line represents the median, the box the first and third quartile, and the whiskers 1.5 × the interquartile range). For categorical variables, bar plots indicate proportions for the entire cohort.

care as being both efficacious and cost-effective [32]. A community based (but not primary care based) initiative within New Zealand has also reported similar results in this population, with improvements in both renal and cardiac endpoints [33]. A RCT involving intensified NP involvement reduced the decline in kidney function and improved renal outcomes in patients with prevalent CKD over a sustained follow-up period [13].

The intervention described in this study involved collaboration between the regional secondary nephrology service and primary care practices. The nephrology NP worked primarily with practice nurses in the GP practices, with liaison with GPs as required. Interactions between these clinicians allowed for education around best practice and evidence-based management of CKD, and provided opportunities for learning through case reviews. This collaborative model also had the effect of enhancing the currently limited linkages between these primary care practices and the secondary nephrology service in the region.

There is no study in the literature that can be used to determine effect size between improved self-management and improved clinical outcomes. Other studies have assessed self-management as an outcome in itself, but only two have assessed effect on patient-centred outcomes such as HRQoL [34,35]. Ours is the first to have assessed effect on clinical outcomes. One could question the clinical significance of the small improvement in self-management that we observed in this study, although we note that as with other studies that there is sustained improvement of clinical markers over time, suggesting a sustained and long-term effect that might persist and even increase beyond the period of observation in this study [13]. The improvement in clinical outcomes observed in this study are small but significant. For instance, although the decrease in the 5 year absolute cardiovascular risk seems small at −0.2% per month, this is equivalent to a 1.2% annual decrease in the risk of a cardiovascular event for this study sample. This effect should be considered in the light of the global burden of diabetic patients with CKD, which is the primary diagnosis causing kidney disease in 20–40% of people starting treatment for ESKD [36]. The rates of progression of newly diagnosed type 2 diabetics between the stages of normoalbuminuria, microalbuminuria, macroalbuminuria and kidney failure are 2–3% per year, as evidences in the United Kingdom Prospective Diabetes Study [37]. The annual mortality rate in this population is approximately 7% [38], and at least 50% of these deaths will be cardiovascular in nature. As such, a seemingly small 1-2% annual decrease in the risk of cardiovascular morbidity and mortality has the potential to avert many life-years lost, and many health-dollars spent.

The total cost of the pilot was $160,000 over two years, this included; NP and practice nurse release time, payment for GP's and nurses to attend regular planning meetings, patient transport, blood tests, administration costs, clinical and electronic equipment and support, printing and development of resources, administration and reporting time. A large proportion of the cost was used in planning the pilot in the six months prior. Further studies should provide more detailed cost benefit analysis.

The success of the intervention suggests a goal for secondary nephrology services, in using their expertise to up-skill primary care clinicians to better manage CKD. There are several ways in which primary care practices can limit the growth of ESKD. Most importantly, practices can better screen their patient populations to identify those at different levels of risk, and work to apply evidence-based medicine to improve risk factor management amongst those with CKD. There are several major financial barriers to the scaling and implementation of programs such as the intervention in this study. The main ones relate to the impact on primary health care clinicians' work, and the corresponding impact for nephrology NPs who spend time away from their customary duties in secondary care. Self-management education should be included in all aspects of primary care and CKD management as they have proven successful in improving adherence outcomes in other chronic conditions [39,40].

As a pilot intervention, this nurse-led intervention has potential to limit growth of expensive renal replacement therapy programmes. However, it was supported on a time-limited basis by the New Zealand Ministry of Health, with funding primarily to allow deployment of a clinical resource, the nephrology NP, from secondary into primary care. The service was therefore free to the patients enrolled in the intervention, which we assume contributed to their compliance with the requirements of the programme. The feasibility of reproducing this pilot on a larger scale with an economic benefit would need to be further explored in future research. Making publicly subsidized funding of primary care contingent on clinical outcomes for practice populations may be required to incentivize adoption of different clinical activities. Financial incentive schemes employed in the United Kingdom have been shown to potentially contribute to the reduction in health inequalities in deprived areas [41].

There are several limitations of study design. Firstly, this study is a quality improvement initiative rather than a randomized controlled trial, with no comparator group or clinical data from the period prior to the intervention. As such, there is risk of bias and confounding, and no absolute certainty that the improvements were the direct results of the intervention. It is possible that they arose due to a separate and unrecognized co-intervention. It is also plausible that the improvements arose from "regression to the mean" in our study sample, which can occur when subjects are selected with outcome measures at the extremes of a given distribution. In this situation, the measures will tend to be closer to the centre of the distribution on subsequent measurements, which can often be incorrectly inferred as being an improvement in response to an intervention. The sampling frame in this study (non-adherence over the prior one-year period) reduces the risk of this occurrence, although it remains a very definite, unquantifiable limitation on the interpretation of our results. The second limitation of the study design is that it is a small-scale project, and cannot therefore be considered as proof of clinical effectiveness and cost effectiveness. Instead, the study demonstrates the feasibility of this approach and potential effectiveness. Finally, the study design did not include data collection to evaluate change in the organizational or clinical culture in primary care clinicians outside of the intervention. As such, it is not possible to evaluate whether the intervention was effective in institutionalizing a change in culture towards quality improvement in CKD care [42].

There are several limitations of study analyses that should also be acknowledged. Firstly, these were not performed in a way that allowed for causal inference, which would be the required approach to answer questions such as "did changes in proteinuria result from greater prescription of medication, or rather the improved compliance of said medication?". Such analyses may be possible using various structural modelling approaches, and will be considered further in the future. Secondly, analyses assume linear relationships over time, a prosaic approach to improve comprehensibility of the statistical models. The analyses cannot, however, address any non-linear relationships that might have occurred over the period of observation. For instance, the changes in many study variables show a pronounced early improvement, with some "rebound" at a later time. Notwithstanding, the models in this study do provide an indication of the overall effect of the intervention over the course of the study, and strongly suggest that the benefits observed over 3 months were sustained to a significant degree during the remainder of the 12 months follow-up. Future studies are planned to identify co-morbidities within the source population of our study sample, to compare multi-morbidity between the groups.

Conclusions

This study demonstrates that a model of specialist nephrology NP led clinics with primary care clinicians is feasible and may improve risk factors for progression of CKD and cardiovascular death. The cost of implementing such

as program a wider basis would be considerable, although costs maybe offset in the long-term if the future burden of ESKD is reduced. Notwithstanding, a collaborative approach to primary and secondary care may be an effective way to manage high risk patients with CKD in the primary care setting. The results of this study call for definitive studies to definitively determine the effectiveness and costs of this intervention in a controlled study on a wider scale.

Competing interests
Mark R Marshall is an employee of Baxter Healthcare Limited, as the Director of Medical Affairs Asia-Pacific (Renal). The other authors declare that they have no competing interests.

Authors' contributions
RW carried out the design and implementation of the study, collected data and drafted the manuscript. MM performed the statistical analysis and drafted the manuscript. NP helped to draft the manuscript. All authors read and approved the final manuscript.

Acknowledgements
The authors would like to acknowledge the Ministry of Health for the financial assistance and for initiating the study as part of the national CKD pilots. We thank both primary care practices, both management and clinicians, for supporting this study, as well as the patients who participated in the study. We are grateful to the nephrology and diabetes services for their leadership, guidance and support.

Author details
[1]Hawkes Bay District Health Board, Hastings, New Zealand. [2]Sydney School of Public Health, Sydney Medical School, University of Sydney, Sydney, Australia. [3]Counties Manukau District Health Board, Auckland, New Zealand. [4]Faculty of Medical and Health Sciences, University of Auckland, Auckland, New Zealand. [5]Sector Capability and Implementation, Ministry of Health, Wellington, New Zealand.

References
1. Ashton T, Marshall MR: The organization and financing of dialysis and kidney transplantation services in New Zealand. *Int J Health Care Finance Econ* 2007, **7**(4):233–252.
2. Kerr M, Bray B, Medcalf J, O'Donoghue DJ, Matthews B: Estimating the financial cost of chronic kidney disease to the NHS in England. *Nephrol Dial Transplant* 2012, **27**(Suppl 3):iii73–iii80.
3. Wheeler DC, Becker GJ: Summary of KDIGO guideline: what do we really know about management of blood pressure in patients with chronic kidney disease? *Kidney Int* 2013, **83**(3):377–383.
4. Hahr AJ, Molitch ME: Diabetes, cardiovascular risk and nephropathy. *Cardiol Clin* 2010, **28**(3):467–475.
5. Gerstein HC, Mann JF, Yi Q, Zinman B, Dinneen SF, Hoogwerf B, Hallé JP, Young J, Rashkow A, Joyce C: Albuminuria and risk of cardiovascular events, death, and heart failure in diabetic and nondiabetic individuals. *JAMA* 2001, **286**(4):421–426.
6. Go AS, Chertow GM, Fan D, McCulloch CE, Hsu C-y: Chronic kidney disease and the risks of death, cardiovascular events, and hospitalization. *N Engl J Med* 2004, **351**(13):1296–1305.
7. Grace B, Hurst K, McDonald SP: **Stock and flow.** In *ANZDATA Registry Report 2010.* Edited by Hurst K, McDonald SP. Adelaide, South Australia: ANZDATA Registry; 2012.

8. Black C, Sharma P, Scotland G, McCullough K, McGurn D, Robertson L, Fluck N, MacLeod A, McNamee P, Prescott G, Smith C: **Early referral strategies for management of people with markers of renal disease: a systematic review of the evidence of clinical effectiveness, cost-effectiveness and economic analysis.** *Health Technol Assess* 2010, **14**(21):1–184.

9. Collins AJ, Vassalotti JA, Wang C, Li S, Gilbertson DT, Liu J, Foley RN, Chen SC, Arneson TJ: **Who should be targeted for CKD screening? Impact of diabetes, hypertension, and cardiovascular disease.** *Am J Kidney Dis* 2009, **53**(3 Suppl 3):S71–S77.

10. Crowe E, Halpin D, Stevens P: **Guidelines: early identification and management of chronic kidney disease: summary of NICE guidance.** *BMJ* 2008, **337**(7673):812–815.

11. Robinson T, Simmons D, Scott D, Howard E, Pickering K, Cutfield R, Baker J, Patel A, Wellingham J, Morton S: **Ethnic differences in Type 2 diabetes care and outcomes in Auckland: a multiethnic community in New Zealand.** *N Z Med J* 2006, **119**(1235):U1997.

12. Tomlin A, Tilyard M, Dawson A, Dovey S: **Health status of New Zealand European, Maori, and Pacific patients with diabetes at 242 New Zealand general practices.** *N Z Med J* 2006, **119**(1235):U2004.

13. Peeters MJ, van Zuilen AD, van den Brand JA, Bots ML, van Buren M, Ten Dam MA, Kaasjager KA, Ligtenberg G, Sijpkens YW, Sluiter HE, van de Ven PJ, Vervoort G, Vleming LJ, Blankestijn PJ, Wetzels JF: **Nurse practitioner care improves renal outcome in patients with CKD.** *J Am Soc Nephrol* 2014, **25**(2):390–398.

14. Chen SH, Tsai YF, Sun CY, Wu IW, Lee CC, Wu MS: **The impact of self-management support on the progression of chronic kidney disease–a prospective randomized controlled trial.** *Nephrol Dial Transplant* 2011, **26**(11):3560–3566.

15. Bonner A, Havas K, Douglas C, Thepha T, Bennett P, Clark R: **Self-Management Programmes in Stages 1–4 Chronic Kidney Disease: A Literature Review.** *J Ren Care* 2014, **40**(3):194–204.

16. Jacobs SH, Boddy JM: **The genesis of advanced nursing practice in New Zealand: policy, politics and education.** *Nurs Prax N Z* 2008, **24**(1):11–22.

17. Davidoff F, Batalden P, Stevens D, Ogrinc G, Mooney S: **Publication guidelines for quality improvement in health care: evolution of the SQUIRE project.** *Qual Saf Health Care* 2008, **17**(Suppl 1):i3–i9.

18. Caring for Australians with Renal I: **The CARI guidelines: Urine protein as diagnostic test: testing for proteinuria.** *Nephrol* 2004, **9**(Suppl 3):S3–S7.

19. Chadban S, Howell M, Twigg S, Thomas M, Jerums G, Cass A, Campbell D, Nicholls K, Tong A, Mangos G, Stack A, MacIsaac RJ, Girgis S, Colagiuri R, Colagiuri S, Craig J: **The CARI guidelines: Prevention and management of chronic kidney disease in type 2 diabetes.** *Nephrol* 2010, **15**(Suppl 1):S162–S194.

20. Harris D, Thomas M, Johnson D, Nicholls K, Gillin A, Caring for Australasians with Renal I: **The CARI guidelines: Prevention of progression of kidney disease.** *Nephrol* 2006, **11**(Suppl 1):S2–S197.

21. Chobanian AV, Bakris GL, Black HR, Cushman WC, Green LA, Izzo JL Jr, Jones DW, Materson BJ, Oparil S, Wright JT Jr, Roccella EJ: **The seventh report of the joint national committee on prevention, detection, evaluation, and treatment of high blood pressure: the JNC 7 report.** *JAMA* 2003, **289**(19):2560–2572.

22. Harris MF, Williams AM, Dennis SM, Zwar NA, Davies GP: **Chronic disease self-management: implementation with and within Australian general practice.** *Med J Aust* 2008, **189**(10):17.

23. New Zealand Guidelines Group: *New Zealand Cardiovascular Guidelines Handbook: A summary resource for primary care practitioners.* 2nd edition. Wellington: (New Zealand): Ministry of Health; 2009.

24. Fortin M, Stewart M, Poitras ME, Almirall J, Maddocks H: **A systematic review of prevalence studies on multimorbidity: toward a more uniform methodology.** *Ann Fam Med* 2012, **10**(2):142–151.

25. Britt HC, Harrison CM, Miller GC, Knox SA: **Prevalence and patterns of multimorbidity in Australia.** *Med J Aust* 2008, **189**(2):72–77.

26. Hudon C, Fortin M, Soubhi H: **Abbreviated guidelines for scoring the Cumulative Illness Rating Scale (CIRS) in family practice.** *J Clin Epidemiol* 2007, **60**(2):212.

27. Salmond CE, Crampton P: **Development of New Zealand's deprivation index (NZDep) and its uptake as a national policy tool.** *Can J Public Health* 2012, **103**(8 Suppl 2):S7–S11.

28. Levey AS, Coresh J, Greene T, Stevens LA, Zhang Y, Hendriksen S, Kusek JW, Van Lente F: **Using standardized serum creatinine values in the modification of diet in renal disease study equation for estimating glomerular filtration rate.** *Ann Intern Med* 2006, **145**(4):247–254.

29. Battersby MW, Ask A, Reece MM, Markwick MJ, Collins JP: **The Partners in Health scale: The development and psychometric properties of a generic assessment scale for chronic condition self-management.** *Aust J Prim Health* 2003, **9**(3):41–52.

30. Stevens PE, O'Donoghue DJ, de Lusignan S, Van Vlymen J, Klebe B, Middleton R, Hague N, New J, Farmer CK: **Chronic kidney disease management in the United Kingdom: NEOERICA project results.** *Kidney Int* 2007, **72**(1):92–99.

31. Israni A, Korzelius C, Townsend R, Mesler D: **Management of chronic kidney disease in an academic primary care clinic.** *Am J Nephrol* 2003, **23**(1):47–54.

32. Richards N, Harris K, Whitfield M, O'Donoghue D, Lewis R, Mansell M, Thomas S, Townend J, Eames M, Marcelli D: **Primary care-based disease management of chronic kidney disease (CKD), based on estimated glomerular filtration rate (eGFR) reporting, improves patient outcomes.** *Nephrol Dial Transplant* 2008, **23**(2):549–555.

33. Hotu C, Bagg W, Collins J, Harwood L, Whalley G, Doughty R, Gamble G, Braatvedt G, Investigators D: **A community-based model of care improves blood pressure control and delays progression of proteinuria, left ventricular hypertrophy and diastolic dysfunction in Maori and Pacific patients with type 2 diabetes and chronic kidney disease: a randomized controlled trial.** *Nephrol Dial Transplant* 2010, **25**(10):3260–3266.

34. Campbell KL, Ash S, Bauer JD: **The impact of nutrition intervention on quality of life in pre-dialysis chronic kidney disease patients.** *Clin Nutr* 2008, **27**(4):537–544.

35. Yen M, Huang JJ, Teng HL: **Education for patients with chronic kidney disease in Taiwan: a prospective repeated measures study.** *J Clin Nurs* 2008, **17**(21):2927–2934.

36. U.S. Renal Data System: *USRDS 2013 Annual Data Report: Atlas of Chronic Kidney Disease and End-Stage Renal Disease in the United States.* Bethesda, MD: National Institutes of Health, National Institute of Diabetes and Digestive and Kidney Diseases; 2013.

37. Atkins RC, Zimmet P: **Diabetic kidney disease: act now or pay later.** *Nephrol Dial Transplant* 2010, **25**(2):331–333.

38. Barkoudah E, Skali H, Uno H, Solomon SD, Pfeffer MA: **Mortality rates in trials of subjects with type 2 diabetes.** *J Am Heart Assoc* 2012, **1**(1):8–15.

39. Janson SL, Fahy JV, Covington JK, Paul SM, Gold WM, Boushey HA: **Effects of individual self-management education on clinical, biological, and adherence outcomes in asthma.** *Am J Med* 2003, **115**(8):620–626.

40. Lin EH, Katon W, Von Korff M, Rutter C, Simon GE, Oliver M, Ciechanowski P, Ludman EJ, Bush T, Young B: **Relationship of depression and diabetes self-care, medication adherence, and preventive care.** *Diabetes Care* 2004, **27**(9):2154–2160.

41. Muntner P, Judd SE, Krousel-Wood M, McClellan WM, Safford MM: **Low medication adherence and hypertension control among adults with CKD: data from the REGARDS (Reasons for Geographic and Racial Differences in Stroke) Study.** *Am J Kidney Dis* 2010, **56**(3):447–457.

42. Hughes RG (Ed): *Tools and Strategies for Quality Improvement and Patient Safety.* Rockville, US: Agency for Healthcare Research and Quality; 2008.

16

The views of general practitioners and practice nurses towards the barriers and facilitators of proactive, internet-based chlamydia screening for reaching young heterosexual men

Karen Lorimer[1*], Susan Martin[2] and Lisa M McDaid[2]

Abstract

Background: Chlamydia trachomatis is a common bacterial sexually transmitted infection (STI), which disproportionately affects young people under 25 years. Commonly, more women are offered screening than men. This study obtained the views of general practitioners and practice nurses towards Internet-based screening and assessed levels of support for the development of proactive screening targeting young heterosexual men via the Internet.

Methods: Semi-structured telephone interviews with 10 general practitioners and 8 practice nurses, across Central Scotland. Topics covered: experience of screening heterosexual men for chlamydia, views on the use of the Internet as a way to reach young men for chlamydia screening, beliefs about the potential barriers and facilitators to Internet-based screening. Transcripts from audio recordings were analysed with Framework Analysis, using QSR NVivo10.

Results: Experiences of chlamydia screening were almost exclusively with women, driven by the nature of consultations and ease of raising sexual health issues with female patients; few practice nurses reported seeing men during consultations. All participants spoke in favour of Internet-based screening for young men. Participants reported ease of access and convenience as potential facilitators of an Internet-based approach but anonymity and confidentiality could be potential barriers and facilitators to the success of an Internet approach to screening. Concerns over practical issues as well as those pertaining to gender and socio-cultural issues were raised.

Conclusions: Awareness of key barriers and facilitators, such as confidentiality, practicality and socio-cultural influences, will inform the development of an Internet-based approach to screening. However, this approach may have its limits in terms of being able to tackle wider social and cultural barriers, along with shifts in young people's and health professionals' attitudes towards screening. Nevertheless, employing innovative efforts as part of a multi-faceted approach is required to ensure effective interventions reach the policy agenda.

Background

Chlamydia, the most common bacterial sexually transmitted infection (STI) in the UK [1], disproportionately affects young people under 25 years. Prevalence in the general population is mostly similar for women and men [2]. Screening for chlamydia among the target population at risk of infection can lead to early detection, reduction in transmission and to a reduction in associated morbidities [3]. Thus, early identification and treatment of infections remains paramount. There are two screening approaches: proactive, or systematic, which use population registers to invite members for a test, and; opportunistic, which involves health professionals offering tests to patients attending health care or other defined settings for unrelated reasons [4]. Various countries have taken an opportunistic approach to control the population prevalence of chlamydia including England, which has a National Chlamydia Screening Programme (NCSP). A randomised

* Correspondence: karen.lorimer@gcu.ac.uk
[1]Institute for Applied Health Research, Glasgow Caledonian University, School of Health and Life Sciences, Cowcaddens Road, Glasgow G4 0BA, Scotland
Full list of author information is available at the end of the article

controlled trial of opportunistic screening is underway in Australia, with results from the ACCEPt trial due in 2014 [5]. Norway is exploring and planning a proactive approach [6], and a recent trial conducted in three regions of the Netherlands (the Chlamydia Screening Implementation programme) [7], evaluated the effectiveness of systematic, yearly chlamydia screening. The Dutch trial found no impact on chlamydia positivity rates or on estimated population prevalence [7].

Whilst treating infections remains paramount, opportunistic approaches have largely failed to demonstrate sufficient coverage among the target population [8], have tended not to achieve sustained screening engagement over time or show effectiveness in reducing population prevalence [9]. It is also an approach which has thus far largely failed to include men to the same extent as women: the NCSP in England reached only 16% of young people aged 15–24 years (24% of women and only 8% of men) in 2007/08 [3], although some areas have since seen higher coverage. In Scotland, in 2010, 27% of all tests performed were on men [10]. Screening men is primary prevention for women and could help normalise screening and reduce the psychosocial stigma for women associated with submitting one sex to surveillance, testing and treatment [11]. However, barriers to a proactive approach include: the largely asymptomatic nature of the infection which provides no physical cue with which to seek healthcare; and the poor willingness among young people to access 'stigmatising' genitourinary medicine (GUM) or other clinical settings [12]. There is a continued need to evaluate different approaches to screening, paying attention to the involvement of young adult men.

Online social media, such as social networking sites (e.g., Facebook), blogs and chat rooms have become integral parts of adolescents' and young adults' lives. Interactive computer-based interventions for sexual health promotion were assessed in a systematic review and found to be effective tools for learning about sexual health, and showed positive effects on self-efficacy, intention and sexual behaviour [13]. Computer-based technology has also been effective in increasing condom use for HIV prevention [14]. Media such as the Internet offers exciting potential for sexual health interventions, as they can be a low cost and flexible way to reach young people and could provide the easy, convenient and confidential approach to screening that young people report they want [12]. Young people hold favourable views towards the use of technology for STI screening [15-17], want straightforward information [15], authenticity of voice on websites [18] and to be treated like adults [17]. Postal testing kits, obtained via the Internet are acceptable [19], but direct mailing of kits appear to perform better than test-request kits [20]. Internet-based approaches are also showing better screening uptake than clinic-based

approaches among men [21]. The use of the Internet for chlamydia screening has the potential to ease pressure from time-limited staff, such as general practitioners (GPs) and practice nurses (PNs), and in contexts where there is the absence of a national programme or where there may be limited availability of screening outwith specialist sexual health services, the Internet could fill a gap to act as an adjunct to clinical services. Whilst there remain challenges in building a sufficiently robust evidence-base on which to devise screening policy [9], further research questions continue to be posed, including whether sustaining a certain level of uptake with repeat systematic screening could lead to a reduction in chlamydia prevalence [7].

The intent of this study was to gather evidence to inform the subsequent design of an Internet-based approach to chlamydia screening targeting young men (aged 16–24 years). Understanding the views of GPs and PNs to the potential use of registers to contact men for chlamydia screening is vital to the future design of a randomised controlled trial (RCT) involving patient lists. Further, it is vital to understand the acceptability amongst primary care professionals regarding potential increased workloads from a new approach which may drive patients towards primary health care [22], particularly in a context where there is no existing screening programme or consistent culture of screening for chlamydia. Thus, to aid the development of our intervention, we explored the barriers and facilitators to implementing an Internet chlamydia screening approach, including the acceptability of such an approach amongst young men and health professionals. Elsewhere we report men's views from fifteen focus groups (n = 60) [17]; here we detail the views of the GPs and PNs.

Methods
Design and setting
Participants were selected purposefully, to include GPs and PNs working at practices across areas of low to high deprivation across two regions across central Scotland (known as the 'central belt' of Scotland, with Glasgow in the west through to the capital, Edinburgh, in the east). These regions contain cities with the two largest sexual health clinics as well as other hub services, falling under two major NHS Board areas; as such, we sought the views of staff working within these two key areas. We also sought practices with varying percentages of young men (aged 15–24 years) registered with the practice. This was to obtain views from professionals who *may* have different perspectives due to practice-based issues (e.g., serving a largely elderly population may not incline staff towards sexual and reproductive health services, including chlamydia screening). We set out to conduct short (around 30 minutes), focused semi-structured

telephone interviews in order to generate explanations of the specific phenomena under consideration. We aimed to recruit twenty GPs and PNs (10 of each). To reach GPs and PNs, we sent 241 letters outlining the study to practices across the two chosen regions. In the letter we stated: '*We would appreciate your consideration of this invitation and will follow-up this letter with a telephone call*'. We then began to contact a purposive sample of these (seeking to try to include practices located within high and low deprivation areas as well as those with high and low percentages of young men registered) to try to include a plurality of voices and experiences; we continued this process until we had conducted eighteen interviews and had reached data saturation, whereby the same comments were being offered to questions with no new data emerging. At saturation we ceased contacting practices so most practices were not contacted with a follow-up telephone call. As such, we do not have a full response rate for the 241 letters sent.

To identify practices, we assigned general practices with a deprivation score by using data provided online by Information Statistics Division (ISD) Scotland (http://www.isdscotland.org/Health-Topics/General-Practice/Workforce-and-Practice-Populations/Practices-and-Their-Populations/) and referring to the Scottish Index of Multiple Deprivation (SIMD) quintiles, where 1 is the most deprived and 5 is the least deprived) to link the practice postcode data with SIMD quintile for that small area. The Scottish Government website provides an interactive map to identify the SIMD rank of small areas [23]. The 2012 SIMD combines 38 indicators across 7 domains, namely: income, employment, health, education, skills and training, housing, geographic access and crime; the overall index is a weighted sum of the seven domain scores. We were also able, using ISD data, to identify the percentage of men aged 15–24 years registered at the practice – although we note that the variation was limited, with 6% of practices having fewer than 10% of young men aged 15–24 registered at the practice and a handful having

more than 45%, with the average being 13%. We therefore attempted to recruit the few practices with more extreme percentages. We offered remuneration for participants' time (£30 for GPs and £20 for PNs).

Data collection
Telephone interviews were designed to be brief, and lasted between 15 and 35 minutes, with most being around 30 minutes. The semi-structured topic guide was drawn from key areas to emerge from the focus groups with young men [17], including screening experiences, views towards the Internet-based approach and their identification of barriers and facilitators, as well as from literature on this topic [5,22,24] suggesting practitioner workload and training issues were affecting screening offers. The final topic guide focused on: experience of screening women and men (to give context to views); use of technologies within the practice around screening (for example, text results); views towards the use of the Internet as a way to reach young men for chlamydia screening; and views towards any barriers and facilitators to an Internet-based screening approach. Practice nurses were asked additional question about willingness to undertake partner notification to explore whether a future Internet approach could rely on general practice to deal with the follow-up of positives. The proposed approach as explained to GPs and PNs is illustrated in Figure 1.

Data analysis
The telephone interviews were conducted by the first author (KL) and audio recorded, then transcribed intelligent verbatim and checked for accuracy. QSR Nvivo10 was used to facilitate analysis. Transcripts were read repeatedly by SM and a thematic coding framework was developed on a collaborative, iterative basis within the team (including SM, KL, LM), with discrepancies in early interpretation being fully discussed within the team and an agreement reached; the Framework Approach was employed, where data are coded, indexed and

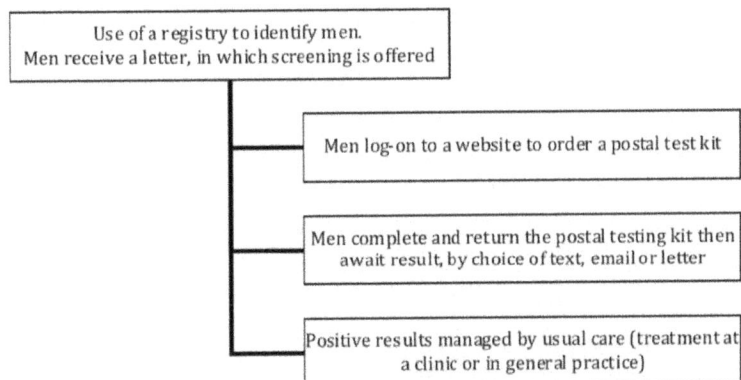

Figure 1 Process of internet-based proactive screening provided to the general practitioners and practice nurses.

charted systematically, then organised using a matrix or framework [25]. There are five key stages of Framework: familiarisation, identifying a thematic framework, indexing, charting, mapping and interpretation. Framework Analysis begins deductively from the study aims and objectives (generating prepositions), but is also inductive (using patterns and associations derived from observations) [26]. SM indexed the data using the coding framework, with a third checked by KL, before data were 'charted' into the framework matrix. The charting and interpretation stage was conducted by SM with continued dialogue and checking of the data with KL. Constant comparison was carried out to check for deviant cases as well as similarities, in an iterative process; we explored whether there were any differences in experience and views by deprivation and percentage of young men registered to the practice attributes, as well as by the gender of the GP (but not for PN as we were only able to interview female PNs) and between the GPs and PNs. There were few differences in views between GPs and PNs based on the deprivation score and percentages of men registered at the practice, but we outline them where there are.

Ethics

Ethical approval was obtained from West of Scotland Research Ethics Committee 1 (Ref: 11/AL/0398). Consent was obtained by participants being read the consent form over the telephone and verbally agreeing to each point. Participants were asked for this to be audio-recorded, so that a recorded record of the consent was obtained. A copy of the form was posted to the participants for reference. All participants agreed to the consent process and their interview being audio-recorded.

Illustrative quotes are used throughout indicating the participants' category: GP for general practitioner; PN for Practice Nurse; and the gender, practice SIMD code

and percentage of young men registered at the practice (e.g., PN1, Female, SIMD 1, 14.3%).

Results

Participant and practice demographics

We conducted telephone interviews with 10 GPs and 8 PNs between February and May 2012. Table 1 shows the spread of practices from SIMD quintiles (1 being most deprived and 5 being least deprived) and the percentages of young men aged 15–24 years registered with the practice. Whilst we recruited GPs and PNs from practices across SIMD categories, and we were able to recruit even numbers of male and female GPs to the study, we were unsuccessful in recruiting any male PNs, despite purposefully seeking them though searching the websites of practices and attempting 'snowballing' techniques. Across the eighteen practices the percentage of young men registered with the practice were broadly similar, with the exception of a few, which had either a very low percentage (e.g., 6.5%) or in one case a very high percentage (42.9%) (see Table 1); however, given many practices have similar percentages, this inclusion is not surprising.

Experiences of screening women and men for chlamydia

General practitioners, and particularly the PNs, described their experiences of chlamydia screening as being almost exclusively with women, which reflects the national testing figures for Scotland showing that 73% of tests were conducted with women [10]. Participants perceived there to be a higher attendance at general practice by women compared to men, driven by contraception consultations, cervical smear tests (Pap tests) or breast screening, and this was cited regularly by both the GPs and PNs as underlying their perceived greater opportunity for, and thus experience of, opportunistic screening of women. Perceptions of low attendance by young men were cited by both GPs and PNs as a major reason for their lower experience of

Table 1 Participant and practice demographics

	Gender	Practice SIMD quintile	Location (Glasgow/Edinburgh)	% 15–24 year old males registered		Gender	Practice SIMD quintile	Location (Glasgow/Edinburgh)	% 15–24 year old males registered
GP1	Female	1	Glasgow	12.9	PN1	Female	1	Glasgow	14.3
GP2	Male	5	Edinburgh CHP	9.6	PN2	Female	5	Glasgow	6.5
GP3	Female	5	Edinburgh CHP	42.9	PN3	Female	3	Glasgow	12.2
GP4	Male	5	Edinburgh CHP	10.2	PN4	Female	2	Glasgow	10.1
GP5	Female	1	Glasgow	18.4	PN5	Female	2	Glasgow	10.5
GP6	Female	1	Glasgow	13.7	PN6	Female	5	Edinburgh CHP	12.8
GP7	Male	1	Glasgow	14.0	PN7	Female	5	Edinburgh CHP	13.9
GP8	Female	5	Edinburgh CHP	16.1	PN8	Female	2	Glasgow	12.0
GP9	Male	4	Edinburgh CHP	10.9					
GP10	Male	2	Edinburgh CHP	11.2					

screening male patients for chlamydia. Practice Nurses, far more than the GPs, reported very few occasions of interacting with young men, even during times when screening was being encouraged by the Health Boards.

My experience of screening young men has probably been part of the opt-in enhanced service, that ran over, I think, a two-year period, and has now ceased. During that time, we were opportunistically asking people if they wanted to be screened, and that was people aged from 15 to 24, as I recall. During that time, I didn't approach any young men, because I don't think it's an age group that I actually see very often, in my particular field. (PN3, Female, SIMD3, 12.2%)

The few occasions mentioned tended to be for specific clinic attendance, such as an asthma clinic, but such clinics were not consistently available across the practices represented by the participants as they depended on patient need across practices. GPs, who saw more men than the PNs, gave their views on why they did not screen as many men as women:

I suppose [pause] - I guess one of the reasons for the differences that we see more young female patients then we see young men, we have more interaction with them, they come in for their contraceptive pill and they generally consult more frequently. We don't see that in many 20 year old men in and about the place so that would probably explain the difference in my testing rates between the two groups. (GP4, Male, SIMD5, 10.2%)

However, when participants were asked to describe the percentage of their practice list that were young men under 25 years, and to reflect on the frequency of the visits these young men may make over a 12 month period, it often prompted GPs to reassess their perceptions of men's low attendance, whilst PNs continued to assert that they had few opportunities to interact with young men.

I: ok. In terms of the proportion of young people on the list, would you say it's kind of high or low?

R: Yes, we've got a lot of young people. [pause]. Hmm, yeah, I mean I suppose yeah they are here. (GP2, Male, SIMD5, 9.6%)

I: OK, so you have about 1 in 10 on your list are young men.

R: As much as that? But I would say personally I can't remember the last time I gave a guy a bottle, probably about six months ago, a urine test for chlamydia.

I: Mm-hmm, mm-hmm. Do you see many young men at all?

*R: No, no.
(PN5, Female, SIMD2, 10.5%)*

Experiences of screening for chlamydia were strongly linked to the nature of the patient-led consultation, with many believing it easier to raise issues of sexual health with patients when attending for related issues. There was a common belief from both GPs and PNs that women are exposed more, or are used to, health-related messages pertaining to sexual and reproductive health as well as being more used to routine screening (e.g., cervical screening).

I think women are easier to talk to about things like that, especially younger women, and especially you've got them in for things like smears and stuff, you know, and sometimes when they come in for things like that they tend to open up a bit more about other things, especially to a woman who again they can maybe relate to being a bit like their mum, if you see what I mean! [laugh] (PN6, Female, SIMD5, 12.8%)

Many GPs described their reluctance to initiate conversations around sexual health with men. Descriptions of such encounters by GPs were often characterised as 'difficult', 'awkward' and 'challenging'. As a consequence, any tests they conducted with men were largely driven by the men self-reporting symptoms, which would then lead to STI conversations and investigation.

It can be a bit awkward. It's sort of how you gauge it. (GP6, Female, SIMD1, 13.7%)

Fewer nurses offered such comments, perhaps reflecting their infrequent contact with young men. Such embarrassment and discomfort was not always a key factor in failing to raise the issue of screening with men, particularly for those based at practices in areas of higher deprivation, who were not confident that chlamydia was a high priority for their patients.

... most of the young men I see are not coming in for sore knees, they're coming in for methadone prescriptions and often quite complicated consultations...(GP10, Male, SIMD2, 11.2%).

Both GPs and PNs spoke of being uneasy with 'unsolicited health care intervention' and with making health promotion 'leaps'.

I'd go out of my way to avoid randomly bringing up new things because we've got enough staff to deal with

it and I'm always running 15 or 20 minutes late anyway. The fewer new unsolicited healthcare intervention the better [laughs] and we've got all the QOF [Quality Outcomes Framework] stuff to do. We're already bugging people enough...
(GP4, Male, SIMD5, 10.2%)

However, when probed, participants admitted they asked unsolicited questions about smoking or alcohol, including to patients seeking advice for sports-related injuries.

These 'leaps' were justified by GPs because they were part of the practices' contractual issues and related to financial incentives. The fewer PNs who spoke about these issues were related to the infrequency with which they interacted with men in their practice, but, like GPs, they still spoke more generally of ever present time pressures within the practice environment.

I think it's just that there's so much else going on in general practice at the moment that, you know, sort of screening the young male population just isn't on the agenda. (GP8, Female, SIMD5, 16.1%)

I: What do you think might be the barriers of such an approach?

R: The cost. [pause] And the QOF, I mean that's increased our workload year on year since I started doing this job so one more little thing. (PN6, Female, SIMD5, 12.8%)

Participants spoke of chlamydia screening being higher in their practice when payments were offered but witnessing, and participating in, a subsequent reduced concern once there was no longer a financial incentive for the practice.

We used to do it [screening] a bit more when it was run by the Health Board...we would get a payment for every test done, so probably its dropped a bit since that was withdrawn. (PN2, Female, SIMD5, 6.5%)

Although this PN worked at an affluent and low percentage practice, in terms of men registered, there seemed to be a real focus on payment and time-concerns, and little attention paid to the low percentages of young men registered. Such a focus was mirrored in the views of a PN from an affluent and higher percentage practice. She reflected on this payment period and suggested that in her practice there were so few positive infections identified that the £10 payment per screen was *'quite a lot of money to be spent on health, to reassure somebody'* (PN3, Female, SIMD3, 12.2%). Thus, their views coalesced around similar issues: payments and time.

Views towards proactive, Internet-based screening

No GP or PN dismissed this approach outright as unworkable or unrealistic. All spoke in favour of it, in general terms, but offered a variety of views towards the ways it could be successful and reach the targeted populations for a high uptake, and the perceived challenges to its success. Views ranged from it being "wholly appropriate" and "entirely the way to reach" young men through to the still supportive, but tentative, "potentially quite a clever idea" and "worthwhile exploring". The unanimous support for the use of the Internet for screening was commonly borne of the belief that technologies fall within the domain of 'youth', and are thus entirely appropriate for this population.

I presume that like technology is maybe the right way forward with this. Because that's, you never see a young person that does not have a mobile phone. (PN8, Female, SIMD2, 12.0%)

Two GPs spoke of the reduction of hours for GPs if a nation-wide service with funding was introduced, leading to a favourable view towards an Internet-based approach.

...certainly if it [screening] was done at health board level, well I think all GPs would be happy with it (laughs) because it would be...yeah, out of their hands. (GP8, Female, SIMD5, 16.1%)

Barriers and facilitators
Design and recruitment facilitators

The facilitators of an Internet-based approach to screening young people for chlamydia identified by participants focused on ease of access and convenience, as well as the importance of anonymity and confidentiality.

The easier it is for them, the better, probably. The more convenient it is for them, the better. (GP3, Female, SIMD5, 42.9%)

Almost every participant spoke of the anonymous or confidential nature of an Internet-based screening approach as being vital if it is to appeal to young people. For PNs in particular, this was borne out of their reflections of the potential for no anonymity in GP attendance, in particular the potential to 'bump into' someone.

I think they're [young people] always concerned about the anonymity of things and GP practice, you go the doctors and you bump into your next door neighbour or your mother's friend... (PN8, Female, SIMD2, 12.0%)

Confidentiality issues were raised by around half of all participants in relation to the type of data that would be accessed from registers for this approach; it was acceptable for age and date of birth data to be accessed but not detailed medical records. Most made the point that registers are being used for screening programmes, such as for cervical and bowel cancer. Four GPs and two PNs pondered whether some people may get annoyed at receiving an unsolicited screening letter, which might have a knock-on effect to practices.

Six GPs and two PNs mentioned practical issues that would need to be considered for an Internet screening approach so as not to become barriers, including who sends screening invitation letters and the accuracy of address information for young people. One GP believed there would need to be a *'very small step between the screening invitation and actually being able to do the test'* (GP9, Male, SIMD4, 10.9%).

Most participants spoke with ease about targeting particular populations for health education or screening offers, often referring to examples within their own practice such as previous efforts to screen for chlamydia or to reach out to young smokers on their practice list. The approach of targeting particular sub-populations, based on age, was not questioned. Although one GP did question whether men may face scrutiny by partners relating to infidelity if there was a lack of understanding that all young men were being offered screening.

...if the young man lives with a partner, and if the partner sees 'chlamydia screening', she needs to be told that it's purely screening, and not that her partner's been cheating around, and someone has asked for the partner to be tested, in case he's got an infection because of his infidelity. (GP7, Male, SIMD1, 14.0%).

This underscores the importance of ensuring these processes are thought through carefully if they are not to become barriers to screening.

Socio-cultural barriers
Participants were often keen to stress that an Internet screening approach could be successful if young people considered testing as a normal thing to do. Half of all participants believed that normalisation of testing could be assisted by a nation-wide marketing campaign to kick start it, but also the need for such a campaign to continue so as to help keep momentum by keeping the service in young people's minds.

...we didn't have a screening process for cervical cancer when I was younger. So the first time I had one here I was like, oh why am I getting this? But now it's...I expect it every three years and it's not something

that fazes me when it comes through the door. So again I think it's... it would then become a bit more engrained that this is part of your health like having your blood pressure checked and things like that. (PN7, Female, SIMD5, 13.9%)

For some, such a widespread awareness of the screening taking place for all age-eligible young people may lead to relationships not becoming jeopardised by the screening letter arriving in the post.

Participants also stressed perceived barriers pertaining to gender-related issues, including perceptions among young people that chlamydia is a 'woman's disease', associated with infertility and promiscuous women. Consequently, these participants believed that such young people fear the stigma of attending for a STI test where they can be seen and identified as promiscuous. No participant spoke about men in this way, but some did mention the embarrassment men may feel asking for a STI test. Support for the Internet approach therefore rested on the anonymity of the approach and non-clinic attendance. Young men were described as reluctant in general to discuss issues relating to their sexual health, although some went on to widen their thoughts on this to the issue of youth's low perception of risk for STIs.

...the ostrich sort of thing - let's not think about it. it'll not happen, sort of thing (PN8, Female, SIMD2, 12.0%).

Participants also described women as more likely to be at ease with screening offers, given their experiences of cervical screening, but also with other regular medical intrusions in their lives due to contraception appointments. Reproductive health conversations were perceived to occur more often with women, and as such respondents questioned whether an approach that included men without an accompanying educational element might not ultimately reach men.

if you've got somebody who's already got their awareness raised, and who's thinking, "I probably ought to get this screening done, but I'm too embarrassed to go and talk to a GP about it." If you've got somebody in that situation then, obviously, I think doing it on the Internet would be good. (GP10, Male, SIMD2, 11.2%).

Discussion
This study obtained the views of GPs and PNs in Scotland towards Internet-based screening and assessed levels of support for the development of proactive screening targeting young heterosexual men via the Internet. The limitations include the small sample size and no male practice nurse being included in our sample, to allow

for exploration of gender differences within PNs. Data were gathered from short but focused telephone interviews, which limit the richness of the available descriptions. We also recognise that, as is common across qualitative research, these views may not be representative of all GPs and PNs across Scotland, particularly those working at rural practices. Nevertheless, themes reflect those identified by GPs and PNs in other contexts [22], and provide valuable insights into the views of this group of health professionals concerning the acceptability and feasibility of this proposed intervention, should it become an approach to become implemented in a context with no current screening programme. The non-clinical background of the interviewer, made apparent to participants, acted to draw a fuller explanation from participants, who did not assume in-depth knowledge about primary care processes and policies, for example.

Our findings reveal the screening experiences of both GPs and PNs were largely with women, tied to beliefs that women simply consult more than men and that it is easier to raise sexual health issues within the type of consultations women are seeking, such as contraception or cervical screening. Screening men was low on the agenda, despite financial payment previously incentivising screening. Participants reported awkwardness and embarrassment in raising chlamydia screening with men, particularly if unrelated to the consultation; however, other unrelated health matters were often raised, tied to contracts, payment and workload. These findings are consistent with research conducted in England (where there is a National Chlamydia Screening Programme), particularly in relation to the barriers of raising sexual health with patients [22], and the role of financial incentives [24]. In the Scottish context, where there has never been a screening programme for chlamydia, the period of financial incentives failed to raise awareness of screening men, and certainly screening men was not maintained in any way after payment ceased. For men with no symptoms, they are unlikely to be offered an opportunistic test in this context. Removing the burden of screening from primary health settings by introducing an Internet-based approach could negate the need to return to the unsolved issue of training and payments by focusing the screening directly towards young men themselves.

Our findings reveal a high level of acceptability for an Internet-based screening approach, predicated partly on concerns for increased workload. A variety of views were offered concerning the ways it could be successful and reach the populations for a high uptake, as well as towards the perceived challenges to its success. The ease of access and convenience of this approach were identified by GPs and PNs as being facilitators. Anonymity and confidentiality, important issues raised by young people in

other work [12,27,28], were also mentioned by participants as facilitators to an internet-based screening approach, as long as they were emphasised and assured to men. Barriers identified included the possible perception among men that they were being targeted on the basis of promiscuity or due to other perceived negative traits. Indeed, the issues raised by these health professionals were largely mirrored in the young men's views towards Internet-based screening as a way to reach them: men wanted to be reassured that the approach would be easy, convenient and also confidential and were apprehensive about feeling targeted with screening [17].

The combined data from our study with GPs and PNs as well as with young men [17] have identified barriers and facilitators that would either help or hinder an Internet screening approach. We have identified support for the approach from these health professionals if screening is offered in a particular way, including being backed by a campaign to raise awareness. The young men provided a list of key 'ingredients' that would encourage their engagement with Internet-based screening, including: use a serious not a jokey tone; convey information simply; have an authentic voice by avoiding adults masquerading as youth, and; avoid fear narratives [17]. Identifying design-related and other barriers facilitators, from the target group as well as the health professionals who could support it, has been an important first step towards developing an Internet screening intervention, and follows the guidance on developing complex interventions [29]. Key findings to influence the intervention development include serious consideration to: guaranteeing confidentiality throughout, to ensure this does not end up a barrier to screening but instead acts as a facilitator; the introduction of an accompanying media campaign to raise awareness; engagement with health professionals who may have workload concerns and low perceptions of the priority of chlamydia screening (since it is no longer part of payments or key issues to raise with patients in the Scottish context); and further education and training for health professionals to counter awkwardness in discussing sexual health issues with men in unrelated consultations. These professionals also broadly supported the use of central registers to identify potential intervention participants (similar to cervical screening), which suggests this would not pose a major barrier to the implementation of our intervention. However, our data also suggest that any future involvement by health professionals may need to involve a financial incentive, which appears to have, to some extent, worked in the past to drive up screening among women. The intervention as envisaged does not include GPs and PNs at the level of testing, but could impact on workload if positive patients seek follow-up at their general practice; therefore, how any financial payment could work requires significant further consideration.

It is important to recognise that there are broader, key challenges in moving forward with further work on the use of the Internet for chlamydia screening, which pertain to the overall effectiveness of chlamydia screening as well as wider social and cultural factors associated with young people's sexual behaviours. Concerns have been raised about the ability of screening to reach sufficient numbers of young people to reduce chlamydia prevalence and also for screening to interrupt subsequent sequelae, such as pelvic inflammatory disease [30]. The Dutch trial of a systematic approach to screening using the Internet, showed insufficient levels of uptake sustained over the three year screening period to reduce chlamydia prevalence [7]. Thus, reaching the target group, engaging them in screening and doing so repeatedly over time remains a key challenge. This is where the evidence of wider social and cultural barriers associated with young people's sexual behaviours identifies issues that could continue to impede screening reach. These health professionals were cognisant of these barriers, even amongst themselves, which is now seen across multiple studies: a systematic review of qualitative literature on factors shaping young people's behaviours found seven key themes across 268 studies, including social expectations impeding communication about sex [31].

Conclusions

Our findings suggest that health professionals within primary care support an Internet-based screening approach and would support the use of registers to facilitate a proactive approach to reaching young men. They support the need to reach young men and recognise their own inability to engage men in screening, due to time pressures, lack of financial incentive and discomfort with raising screening with men. We also now require more than just increasing access to testing and communicating the ease of testing if greater screening coverage among key groups is to be achieved. An Internet approach to screening may not be able to tackle all of these issues, if it is only focused on the delivery of a service; therefore, the limits of this as a screening approach must be acknowledged. Internet-based approaches are acceptable to young people and professionals [15-17], and are reaching men and those from low socio-economic areas [21]. However, this approach requires accompanying efforts to tackle wider social and cultural barriers. What is required is to perhaps employ such approaches within a multi-faceted approach and ensuring effective interventions reach the policy agenda [32]. This would involve, for example, clinic-based testing and screening, a media and/or social marketing campaign to raise awareness, Internet-based screening, and self-testing via postal kits made freely available in shops, education and other settings. Within this, it remains clear that health professionals in primary care

setting, such as those included in our work, may require further education and training within such a multi-faceted approach.

Competing interests
The authors declare that they have no competing interests.

Authors' contributions
KL and LM designed the study. KL collected the data; SM conducted the detailed coding and analysis, with input from KL and LM. KL wrote a first draft of the manuscript, collated comments from LM, SM and Prof Paul Flowers, thereafter re-drafting the manuscript. All authors approved the final manuscript.

Acknowledgements
We are thankful to the general practitioners and practice nurses who very kindly gave us their time and views. We are thankful to our Advisory Group: Prof Paul Flowers (Glasgow Caledonian University); Dr Julia Bailey and Prof Graham Hart (UCL); Colin Anderson (NHS Lanarkshire). This study was funded by the Chief Scientist Office at the Scottish Government (CZG/2/515). Lisa McDaid and Susan Martin are funded by the UK Medical Research Council as part of the Sexual Health programme (MC_U130031238/MC_UU_12017/2) at the MRC/CSO Social and Public Health Sciences Unit, University of Glasgow, although Susan was employed by GCU during the coding and analysis period. Ethics approval was granted by West of Scotland Research Ethics Committee 1 (Ref: 11/AL/0398).

Author details
[1]Institute for Applied Health Research, Glasgow Caledonian University, School of Health and Life Sciences, Cowcaddens Road, Glasgow G4 0BA, Scotland. [2]MRC/CSO Social and Public Health Sciences Unit, University of Glasgow, 200 Renfield Street, Glasgow G2 3QB, Scotland.

References
1. The UK Collaborative Group for HIV and STI Surveillance: **Testing Times. HIV and other Sexually Transmitted Infections in the United Kingdom.** London: Health Protection Agency, Centre for Infections; 2007.
2. Dielissen PW, Teunissen DA, Lagro-Janssen TL: **Chlamydia prevalence in the general population: is there a sex difference? a systematic review.** *BMC Infect Dis* 2013, **13**(1):534.
3. National Chlamydia Screening Programme (NSCP) in England: *The Bigger Picture Annual Report*; 2009.
4. Network SIG: *Management of Genital Chlamydia trachomatis infection.* Edinburgh: Royal College of Physicians; 2009.
5. Lorch R, Hocking J, Temple-Smith M, Law M, Yeung A, Wood A, Vaisey A, Donovan B, Fairley CK, Kaldor J: **The chlamydia knowledge, awareness and testing practices of Australian general practitioners and practice nurses: survey findings from the Australian Chlamydia Control Effectiveness Pilot (ACCEPt).** *BMC Fam Pract* 2013, **14**(1):169.
6. Low N, Cassell JA, Spencer B, Bender N, Martin Hilber A, van Bergen J, Andersen B, Herrmann B, Dubois-Arber F, Hamers FF, van de Laar M, Stephenson JM: **Chlamydia control activities in Europe: cross-sectional survey.** *Eur J Public Health* 2012, **22**(4):556–561.
7. van den Broek I, van Bergen J, Brouwers E, Fennema J, Götz H, Hoebe CJPA, Koekenbier R, Kretzschmar M, Over EAB, Schmid BV, Pars L, van Ravesteijn S, van der Sande M, de Wit GA, Low N, Op de Coul ELM: **Effectiveness of yearly, register based screening for chlamydia in the Netherlands: controlled trial with randomised stepped wedge implementation.** *BMJ* 2012, **345**:e4316.
8. Salisbury C, Macleod J, Egger M, McCarthy A, Patel R, Holloway A, Ibrahim F, Sterne JAC, Horner P, Low N: **Opportunistic and systematic screening for chlamydia: a study of consultations by young adults in general practice.** *Br J Gen Pract* 2006, **56**(523):99–103.
9. Low N: **Screening programmes for chlamydial infection: when will we ever learn?** *BMJ* 2007, **334**(7596):725–728.
10. NHS National Services Scotland: **Chlamydia Key Clinical Indicator.** 2010. Available at http://www.isdscotland.org/Health-Topics/Sexual-Health/

Publications/2011-09-27/2011-09-27-Chlamydia-KCI-Report.pdf?88894289732 (24 June 2014, date last accessed).

11. Duncan B, Hart G: **Sexuality and health: the hidden costs of screening for Chlamydia trachomatis.** *BMJ* 1999, **318**(7188):931–933.

12. Lorimer K, Reid ME, Hart GJ: **"It has to speak to people's everyday life":** qualitative study of men and women's willingness to participate in a non-medical approach to Chlamydia trachomatis screening. *Sex Transm Infect* 2009, **85**(3):201–205.

13. Bailey JV, Murray E, Rait G, Mercer CH, Morris RW, Peacock R, Cassell J, Nazareth I: **Interactive computer-based interventions for sexual health promotion [Systematic Review].** *Cochrane Database Syst Rev* 2010, **9**:6.

14. Noar SM, Black HG, Pierce LB: **Efficacy of computer technology-based HIV prevention interventions: A meta-analysis.** *AIDS* 2009, **23**(1):107–115.

15. McCarthy O, Carswell K, Murray E, Free C, Stevenson F, Bailey JV: **What Young People Want From a Sexual Health Website: Design and Development of Sexunzipped.** *J Med Int Res* 2012, **14**(5):e127.

16. Shoveller JA, Knight R, Davis W, Gilbert M, Ogilvie G: **Online Sexual Health Services: Examining Youth's Perspectives.** *Can J Public Health* 2012, **103**(1):14–18.

17. Lorimer K, McDaid L: **Young Men's Views Toward the Barriers and Facilitators of Internet-Based Chlamydia Trachomatis Screening: Qualitative Study.** *J Med Int Res* 2013, **15**(12):e265.

18. Davis WM, Shoveller JA, Oliffe JL, Gilbert M: **Young people's perspectives on the use of reverse discourse in web-based sexual-health interventions.** *Culture, Health Sexual* 2012, **14**(9):1065–1079.

19. Greenland KE, Op de Coul ELM, van Bergen JEAM, Brouwers EEHG, Fennema HJSA, Götz HM, Hoebe CJPA, Koekenbier RH, Pars LL, van Ravesteijn SM: **Acceptability of the Internet-Based Chlamydia Screening Implementation in the Netherlands and Insights Into Nonresponse.** *Sex Transm Dis* 2011, **38**(6):467.

20. Scholes D, Heidrich FE, Yarbro P, Lindenbaum JE, Marrazzo JM: **Population-based outreach for Chlamydia screening in men: Results from a randomized trial.** *Sex Transm Dis* 2007, **34**(11):837–839.

21. Woodhall S, Sile B, Talebi A, Nardone A, Baraitser P: **Internet testing for Chlamydia trachomatis in England, 2006 to 2010.** *BMC Public Health* 2012, **12**(1):1095.

22. McNulty CAM, Freeman E, Howell-Jones R, Hogan A, Randall S, Ford-Young W, Beckwith P, Oliver I: **Overcoming the barriers to chlamydia screening in general practice–a qualitative study.** *Fam Pract* 2010, **27**(3):291–302.

23. The Scottish Government, Scottish Index of Multiple Deprivation: [http://www.scotland.gov.uk/Topics/Statistics/SIMD]

24. Ma R, Clark A: **Chlamydia screening in general practice: views of professionals on the key elements of a successful programme.** *J Family Plan Reprod Health Care* 2005, **31**(4):302–306.

25. Ritchie J, Lewis J: *Qualitative research practice: A guide for social science students and researchers.* Sage Publications Ltd; 2003.

26. Pope C, Ziebland S, Mays N: **Analysing qualitative data.** *BMJ* 2000, **320**(7227):114–116.

27. Baraitser P, Pearce V, Holmes J, Horne N, Boynton PM: **Chlamydia testing in community pharmacies: evaluation of a feasibility pilot in south east London.** *Qual Safety Health Care* 2007, **16**(4):303–307.

28. Buston K, Wight D: **Self-reported sexually transmitted infection testing behaviour amongst incarcerated young male offenders: findings from a qualitative study.** *J Fam Plann Reprod Health Care* 2010, **36**(1):7–11.

29. Craig P, Dieppe P, Macintyre S, Michie S, Nazareth I, Petticrew M: **Developing and evaluating complex interventions: the new Medical Research Council guidance.** *BMJ* 2008, **337**:979–983.

30. Low N, Bender N, Nartey L, Shang A, Stephenson JM: **Effectiveness of chlamydia screening: systematic review.** *Int J Epidemiol* 2009, **38**(2):435–448.

31. Marston C, King E: **Factors that shape young people's sexual behaviour: a systematic review.** *Lancet* 2006, **368**(9547):1581–1586.

32. Low N, Broutet N, Adu-Sarkodie Y, Barton P, Hossain M, Hawkes S: **Global control of sexually transmitted infections.** *Lancet* 2006, **368**(9551):2001–2016.

17

The evolution of nursing in Australian general practice: a comparative analysis of workforce surveys

Elizabeth J Halcomb[1*], Yenna Salamonson[2], Patricia M Davidson[3], Rajneesh Kaur[4] and Samantha AM Young[5]

Abstract

Background: Nursing in Australian general practice has grown rapidly over the last decade in response to government initiatives to strengthen primary care. There are limited data about how this expansion has impacted on the nursing role, scope of practice and workforce characteristics. This study aimed to describe the current demographic and employment characteristics of Australian nurses working in general practice and explore trends in their role over time.

Methods: In the nascence of the expansion of the role of nurses in Australian general practice (2003–2004) a national survey was undertaken to describe nurse demographics, clinical roles and competencies. This survey was repeated in 2009–2010 and comparative analysis of the datasets undertaken to explore workforce changes over time.

Results: Two hundred eighty four nurses employed in general practice completed the first survey (2003/04) and 235 completed the second survey (2009/10). Significantly more participants in Study 2 were undertaking follow-up of pathology results, physical assessment and disease specific health education. There was also a statistically significant increase in the participants who felt that further education/training would augment their confidence in all clinical tasks (p < 0.001). Whilst the impact of legal implications as a barrier to the nurses' role in general practice decreased between the two time points, more participants perceived lack of space, job descriptions, confidence to negotiate with general practitioners and personal desire to enhance their role as barriers. Access to education and training as a facilitator to nursing role expansion increased between the two studies. The level of optimism of participants for the future of the nurses' role in general practice was slightly decreased over time.

Conclusions: This study has identified that some of the structural barriers to nursing in Australian general practice have been addressed over time. However, it also identifies continuing barriers that impact practice nurse role development. Understanding and addressing these issues is vital to optimise the effectiveness of the primary care nursing workforce.

Keywords: Practice nurse, Nursing workforce, Survey, Office nurse, General practice, Primary care, Australia

* Correspondence: ehalcomb@uow.edu.au
[1]School of Nursing & Midwifery, University of Wollongong, Sydney, Australia
Full list of author information is available at the end of the article

Background

A practice nurse (PN), is a registered or an enrolled nurse who provides nursing services within a general practice setting. Practice nurses can be either registered nurses (RN), who are baccalaureate prepared, or enrolled nurses (EN), who have undertaken diploma level training [1,2]. These differences in educational preparation impact on the regulated scope of the nurses clinical practice. The general practice nurse is not as well recognised as an independent nursing specialty in Australia [3], as it is in the United Kingdom (UK) and New Zealand (NZ) [4,5]. The general practice nurse in the UK has evolved from a task-oriented position to a key player within an integrated, multidisciplinary primary care team [6]. A major distinction between the current state of nursing in general practice within the UK and NZ and the current Australian role is the presence of career frameworks, comprised of salary structures and levels of nursing practice which articulate roles based on the nurses experience, education and scope of practice [7]. In Australia, there remains no defined career pathway [7] and PN roles have been demonstrated to often be linked to funding schemes that provide reimbursement for specific activities [8,9].

The nursing role in Australian general practice has undergone significant expansion over the past decade. Changes in health policy, funding models and nurse education are transforming the landscape of Australian primary care [10,11]. Policy makers are seeking to build sustainable primary care services to reduce the burden of chronic and complex disease. Financial incentives are being offered to provide evidence based care for specific disease groups, many of which are nurse-led. Nurse education providers are increasingly seeking to prepare graduates to work in primary care and to provide postgraduate courses with a primary care focus [12]. This transformative agenda is being driven by the increasing burden of non-communicable diseases, a need for improved coordinated management of chronic and complex conditions and the increasing evidence for the value of preventative care [13]. Monitoring and responding to both push and pull factors in the health workforce is important in ensuring a dynamic and responsive primary care workforce.

In 2003, 40% of Australian general practices employed a nurse and it was estimated that there was 2349 nurses employed in Australian general practice [14]. In response to policy change this number grew rapidly, and in 2008, it was estimated that there were approximately one nurse per 2.3 general practitioners [3,14], a ratio similar to that of NZ [3]. By 2009, 56.9% of Australian general practices were reported to employ one or more of the 8914 estimated nurses now working in Australian general practice [15]. Such rapid workforce growth has significant implications for both nurses, the workforce as

a health care team and the system within which they practice.

Several investigations have sought to examine the Australian PN workforce at various points in its evolution. In the early period, Patterson [16] undertook a case study of the role of nurses employed within a single region of general practices. This study described differences in perception of the nature of the nursing role in general practice between general practitioners and nurses. Through this work, Patterson [16] identified a lack of understanding of the boundaries of the nurses scope of practice. Several years later the Royal Australian College of General Practitioners and the Royal College of Nursing, Australia sought to investigate the roles of nurses working in general practice across Australia [17,18]. Whilst this study identified a diversity of roles within Australian general PNs, they found four common elements, namely; clinical care; clinical organization; practice administration and integration of the practice with external organizations [17,18]. This work also identified a number of factors that impacted on the current and future practice nurse role, including lack of education pathways, clarification of nurse roles, systems issues, legal, funding and workforce issues [18]. Whilst these factors were identified, the nature of the impact which they had on the nurses' role was unclear.

More recently, Joyce & Piterman [3,19,20] have examined the nurses role in Australian general practice. This work involved a cross-sectional national survey which explored nurse demographics, work environments and duties [19] and nurse-patient encounters in Australian general practice [3,20]. This work identified a gap in knowledge around nurses' roles in patient care and a need for better monitoring of the practice nurse workforce [19]. This literature provides important insights into the various stages of the evolution of practice nursing in Australia. However, in order to truly appreciate how the workforce has evolved it is important to trace the trends in workforce characteristics, roles and the work environment over time. In this paper, we compare and contrast the findings of two Australian investigations of the practice nurse workforce to examine the evolution in demographic, work roles and employment characteristics of practice nurses over the past ten years.

Methods
Design

A national cross-sectional survey of nurses employed in general practice was conducted during both 2003–04 and 2009–10 using a structured survey tool as a part of two larger mixed methods investigations of the clinical roles of these nurses [8,21]. This paper provides a comparative analysis of the data from these two surveys to explore the trends in workforce development over time.

Sample/participants

As there is no central or local register that identifies practice nurses, both surveys used a multifaceted approach to participant recruitment. Nurses working in general practice were recruited to complete the survey from delegates attending the Australia General Practice Nursing Conference, via advertisements disseminated through the Divisions of General Practice, Australian Practice Nurses Association and State/Territory industrial nursing organisations or via direct email from Divisional practice nurse program staff. Potential participants who contacted the research team were either sent a copy of the information sheet and survey form directly from the research team or via Divisions of General Practice or Australian Practice Nurses Association. Links to the survey form and advertisements about the research were also placed on relevant professional websites and in relevant professional publications. Email reminders were sent to all potential participants who provided contact details to the research team and to the Divisional Staff who facilitated survey distribution. Despite the limitations of such convenience sampling, the lack of employment data precluded the use of more representative sampling techniques.

The first survey involved 284 nurses employed in general practice across six Australian states. These data have been previously reported [8,21]. The second survey involved 235 nurses employed in general practice across six Australian states.

Survey tool

For the first study, a survey tool was developed following a review of the literature and key informant consultation. This tool was pilot tested with 14 respondents before widespread distribution. This method has been previously reported [8]. The survey was comprised of three sections; (i) demographic, employment and workplace characteristics, (ii) barriers and facilitators to role expansion, and (iii) the clinical role. The third section provided a list of clinical tasks and asked participants to identify tasks that they currently undertook in their practice, tasks that they felt were appropriate for a nurse in general practice and tasks for which they felt they required additional education/training. These tasks were selected to represent the kinds of activities that a nurse might contribute to in terms of their role in the assessment, ongoing management and self-management support of individuals with chronic disease.

The second survey comprised of items repeated from the first survey and some additional items related specifically to chronic disease management. This paper reports the data from the items which were collected in both surveys.

Ethical considerations

The Human Research Ethics Committee of the University of Western Sydney granted approval for the conduct of both surveys (Approval No. HEC 03/166 & H6774) before the commencement of data collection. Return of the completed survey form was considered indication of the participants consent to participate.

Data analysis

All data analyses were executed using the SPSS Version 21.0 software. Descriptive statistics were summarised using frequencies and percentages for categorical variables, frequencies, mean, standard deviations and ranges for continuous variables. Inferential statistical analyses were also undertaken. Distributions of continuous variables were first checked for normality using Smirnov-Kolmogorov test. The Mann–Whitney U test was used to assess for group differences of continuous variables that were not normally distributed (independent t-test for normally distributed continuous variables), and Pearson chi-square test for group differences in categorical variables. The $p < 0.05$ value was set as the cut-off for statistical significance.

Validity and reliability

The content validity of the tool was established in the first survey by a panel of clinical nurses and research experts. A further panel of experts reviewed the second survey instrument prior to survey administration.

Results

Participant demographics

Table 1 summarises the sociodemographic and practice related variables of the two data collections. Whilst similar recruitment methods were employed in both surveys, a slightly smaller sample size was achieved in study 2 (284 versus 235) despite a growth in the overall population of nurses working in general practice. This should be considered in the interpretation of these data. Participants in study 2 were slightly, but not significantly, older than those in study 1 (mean age 47.52 yrs versus 45.83 yrs; $p=0.022$). Whilst only one male nurse responded to the first study, study 2 included 8 male respondents ($p=0.007$). The number of enrolled nurse participants more than doubled from study 1 to study 2 (6.3% versus 14.0%). Additionally, participants in Study 2 were more likely to hold an advanced certificate or tertiary qualification (54.3% versus 35.5; $p<0.001$).

Both datasets included responses from the 6 Australian States, however, there were more respondents from South Australia (22.3% versus 5.4%) and significantly less from NSW (36.8% versus 44.4%) and Victoria (7.3% versus 20.1%) in study 2 compared to study 1 ($p<0.001$). Despite this geographical variation there was no significant difference

Table 1 Socio-demographic characteristics of participants in two studies

Characteristic	Study 1 (2003/04) n = 284	Study 2 (2009/10) n = 235	p
Age (mean SD), years	45.83 (7.30)	47.52 (9.26)	0.022[a]
Sex (Female)%	99.6	96.5	0.007[c]
Hours per week as PN (mean SD) hours	26.22 (9.80)	26.84 (14.39)	0.89[b]
Nursing Classification %			
Non-nursing	2.1	2.1	0.02[c]
Enrolled nurse	6.3	14	
Registered nurse	85.6	77	
Clinical nurse specialist/Clinical nurse consultant/Nurse manager	6.0	6.8	
Nursing qualification %			
Hospital trained	64.5	45.7	<0.001[c]
Advanced certificate or tertiary education	35.5	54.3	
Years of practice as a qualified nurse (mean SD)	20.58 (8.28)	21.58 (9.97)	0.219[a]
Duration worked as PN (mean SD) years	7.51 (6.86)	6.40 (6.38)	0.068[b]
Locality of practice %			
Inner city/urban	38.1	44.2	0.096[c]
Rural/Regional	40.6	33.8	
Rural/Remote	19.8	22.1	
Postcode by practice %			
NSW	44.4	36.8	<0.001[c]
Victoria	20.1	7.3	
Queensland	17.2	15.9	
South Australia	5.4	22.3	
Western Australia	9.7	15.5	
Tasmania	3.2	2.3	
Own room/treatment area %	94.7	91.2	0.121[c]
Current policy/procedure manual (Yes) %	73.0	77.6	0.241[c]

Note: [a]Independent samples t test/[b]Mann–Whitney U test (non-normal distribution of scores)/[c] Pearson χ^2 test.

in the locality of practice between the two datasets (p=0.096), with a mix of rural, inner city and remote practice nurses participating in both surveys.

Overall no significant differences were found between hours worked per week as PN, years of practice as qualified nurse and years worked as a practice nurse in both studies. This finding is interesting given the passing of time between the studies. If nurses were retained in the workforce it would be expected that the years worked as a practice nurse would increase between the two studies. This finding adds further weight to the anecdotal evidence of significant turnover within the practice nurse

workforce and issues of retention of nurses. These data also demonstrate that the predominance of part-time workers within the workforce that has maintained steady across the two time periods.

Nurse roles in general practice

Participants were provided a list of clinical activities and a matrix to identify which activities they felt were appropriate tasks for nurses within general practice, which tasks they currently undertook within their practice and which tasks they felt that they needed additional education or training in order to be confident. There was a small but non-significant rise in the number of participants in the two surveys who felt that the clinical activities identified were appropriate tasks for practice nurses (Table 2). Data from the initial study demonstrated that roles of nurses employed in general practice focussed on core clinical skills that attracted remuneration for the Practice, such as wound dressings, immunisation. In contrast, Table 2 demonstrates the broader services now being delivered by practice nurses. A statistically significant increase was observed in the number of participating nurses undertaking follow-up of pathology results (p=0.001), physical assessment (p<0.001), and providing disease specific health education (p<0.001).

The only clinical activity that was reportedly significantly less frequently undertaken was counselling for mental health issues (p=0.002). Significantly fewer participants in study 2 felt that this was an appropriate task for nurses within general practice (p<0.001). This finding may be related to the recent introduction of specialist mental health nursing services to Australian primary care. Additionally, as can be seen from Figure 1, this was the clinical activity which participants rated themselves as being least confident. However, level of confidence on a 10-point Likert scale did not completely explain whether or not participants undertook an activity. Whilst over half of participants (n=152; 54.9% and n=153; 65.1%) reported feeling that undertaking case management was within their role, the mean level of confidence in undertaking this task was only 6.27.

When asked whether further education/training would increase their confidence in undertaking each activity, a statistically significant increase was noted for each clinical activity between the two datasets (Table 3). These data confirmed the areas in which nurses within general practice had identified as those in which they were last confident to practice.

Barriers to role development

As can be seen from Figure 2, the barriers to the expansion of the nurses' role in general practice have changed in many ways between the two studies. Three barriers, in particular, were seen as much less of a barrier to role

Table 2 Clinical activities undertaken

Clinical activity	Do you think this is an appropriate activity for a practice nurse?					Do you undertake this activity in your clinical practice?				
	Study 1		Study 2		p	Study 1		Study 2		p
	n	%	n	%		n	%	n	%	
Vital signs measurement	265	95.7%	219	93.2%	0.219	256	91.8%	208	88.5%	0.216
Follow up of pathology results	172	62.1%	174	74.0%	0.004	132	47.3%	147	62.6%	0.001*
ECG testing	257	92.8%	217	92.3%	0.850	241	86.4%	188	80.0%	0.052
Physical Assessment	213	76.9%	184	78.3%	0.705	127	45.5%	148	63.0%	<0.001*
Counselling for mental health issues	162	58.5%	96	40.9%	<0.001*	87	31.2%	45	19.1%	0.002*
Disease-specific health education	210	75.8%	197	83.8%	0.025	120	43.0%	158	67.2%	<0.001*
Assessment of social support	205	74.0%	181	77.0%	0.430	125	44.8%	126	53.6%	0.046
Assessment of medication regimes	133	48.0%	116	49.4%	0.761	74	26.5%	67	28.5%	0.615
Case-management/Co-ordination	152	54.9%	153	65.1%	0.019	79	28.3%	90	38.3%	0.016

*statistically significant.

expansion in study 2 than they had been in study 1. Firstly, whilst slightly more than half the participants in study 1 (51.6%) reported legal implications as a barrier, only a quarter of participants in study 2 (25.1%; p<0.001) felt that this still negatively impacted role development for nurses within general practice. Secondly, patient's perceptions of nurses' role expansion improved significantly. Compared to study 1 (16.1%) half the number of nurses' in study 2 considered patient's perceptions of their role as a barrier to their role development (8.5%; p=0.01).

Additionally, the impact of general practitioners (GPs) attitude on the role of nurses within general practice development has changed significantly. Whilst 28.7% of

participants in study 1 saw this as a barrier, only 20% reported this as an impediment in study 2 (28.7%; p=0.02). However, a number of barriers related to the GP were consistent across the two surveys. These included; GPs not understanding the nurses' scope of practice, lack of teamwork between GPs and nurses', unwillingness of some GPs to delegate tasks to the nurse, and variation in practice between GPs.

Conversely, three barriers were identified by more respondents in study 1 than in study 2, namely lack of job description, low confidence to negotiate with general practitioners, and a lack of the nurses' personal desire to enhance their role. None of these differences were statistically significant (Figure 2).

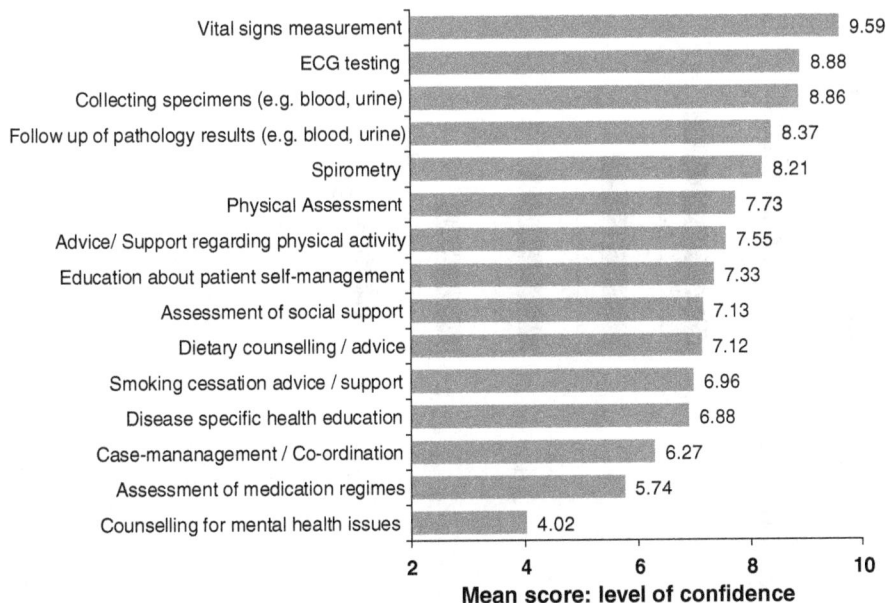

Figure 1 Mean confidence with clinical activities.

Table 3 Need for further education/training

Clinical activity	Would further education/training increase your confidence in undertaking this activity?				
	Study 1		Study 2		p
	n	%	n	%	
Vital signs measurement	10	3.6%	47	32.9%	<0.001*
Follow up of pathology results	68	24.4%	91	38.7%	<0.001*
ECG testing	37	13.4%	73	31.1%	<0.001*
Physical Assessment	83	30.1%	117	49.8%	<0.001*
Counselling for mental health issues	122	43.7%	147	62.6%	<0.001*
Disease-specific health education	125	45.3%	142	60.4%	0.001*
Assessment of social support	83	30.1%	119	50.6%	<0.001*
Assessment of medication regimes	104	37.7%	141	60.0%	<0.001*
Case-management/Co-ordination	96	34.8%	127	54.0%	<0.001*

*statistically significant.

Facilitators of role development

Between the two periods three key changes in the facilitators to role development were apparent. Despite the GPs attitudes being seen as less of a barrier to nurses' role development, collaboration with the GP was reported less as a facilitator of the nurses' role in study 2 compared with study 1 (S1 87.6% versus S2 77%; p=0.002). Similarly, positive consumer feedback (S1 54.6% versus S2 43.8%; p=0.015) and employment conditions (S1 29.1% versus S2 23.4%; p=0.146) were reported as a facilitator of role development by fewer participants in study 2 compared with study 1 (Figure 3).

The only facilitator that saw a significant increase between the two datasets was access to education and training. Significantly more participants in study 2 considered access to education and training as a facilitator in their role development compared to study 1 (S1 65.6% versus S2 79.6%; p<0.001).

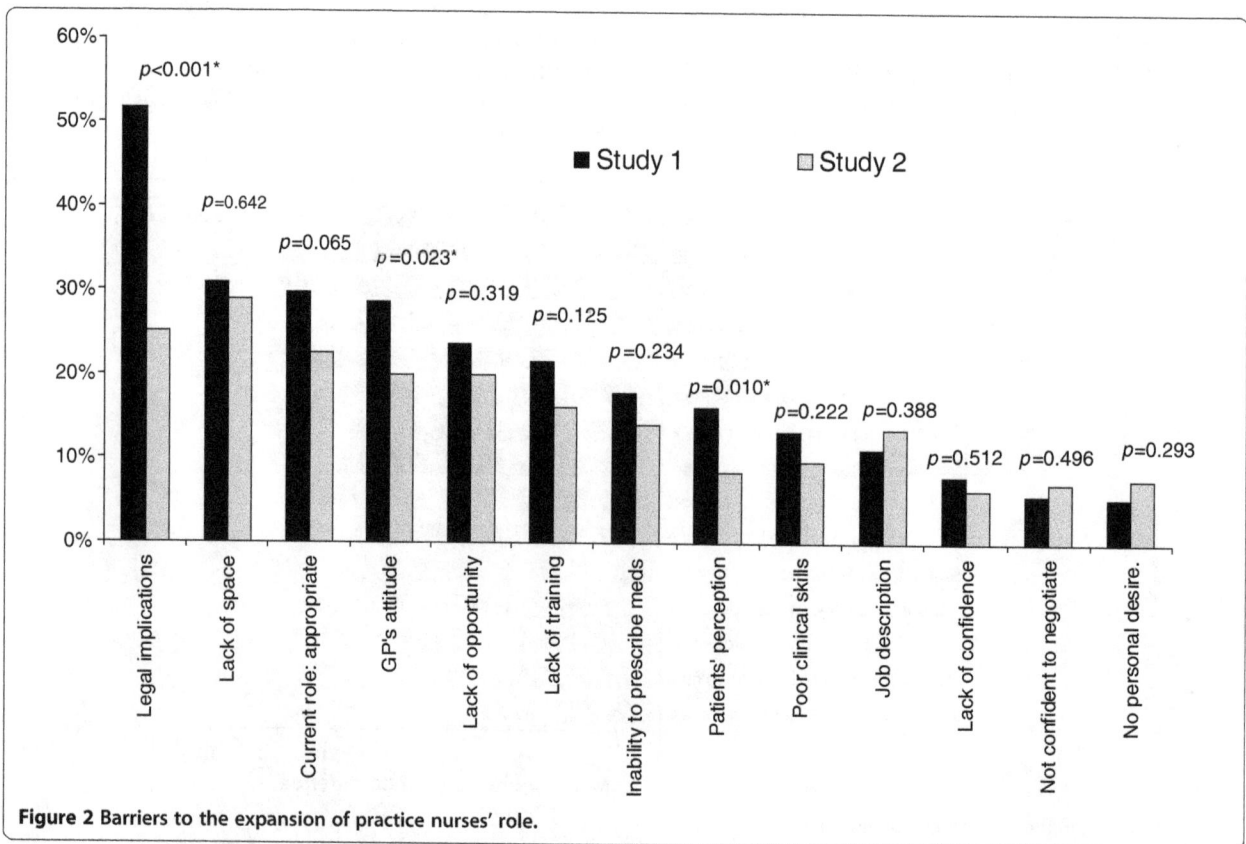

Figure 2 Barriers to the expansion of practice nurses' role.

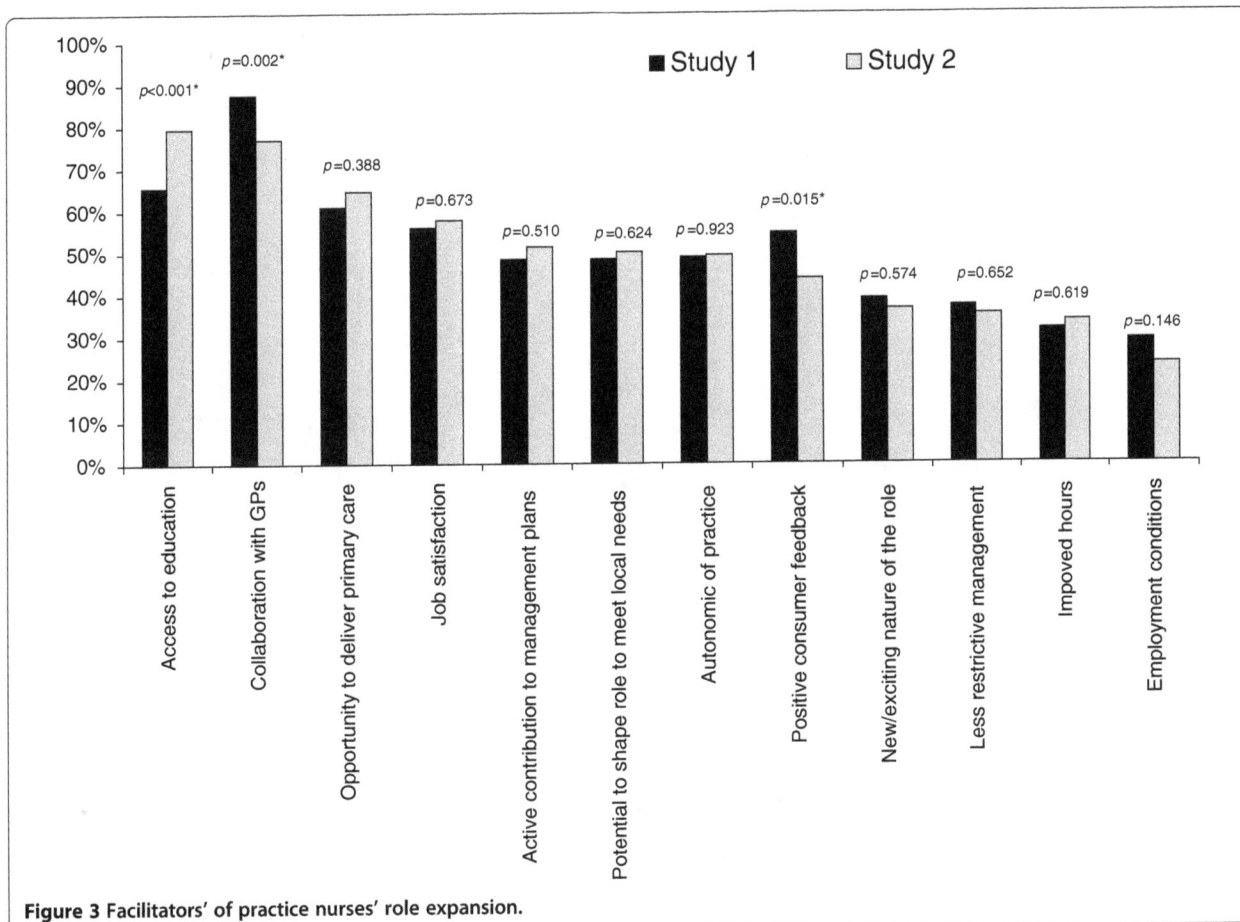

Figure 3 Facilitators' of practice nurses' role expansion.

Levels of optimism

Participants were asked to rate on a five point Likert scale their level of optimism regarding the development of the practice nurse role in Australia. Nurses in both studies continue to have high level of optimism regarding their role expansion (S1 n=237, 87.0%; S2 n=180, 83.7%). The mean score for level of optimism was 4.22 in Study 1 compared to 4.07 in Study 2. However, whilst in Study 1 2.6% (n=7) participants were somewhat pessimistic, in Study 2 5.1% (n=11) participants were somewhat pessimistic and a further 2.3% (n=5) participants extremely pessimistic (Figure 4).

Discussion

These data provide some salient observations regarding the changing nature of nursing in Australian general practice. Such observations have clear implications for peak bodies and policy makers, as well as for clinicians and consumers. The complexity of the clinical tasks undertaken in general practice is increasing and may be attributable to the increasing numbers of nurses employed and the significant investments in nurse training and development to date [22]. The expansion of advanced and diversified clinical activities is encouraging.

However, some key activities continue to demonstrate low confidence amongst nurses within general practice and a need for further education and training. Additionally, in spite of this increase in the complexity of PN role, there was no change in the perception of professional autonomy. The slight increase in pessimism around the role of nurses within general practice and the emerging evidence of poor retention of nurses, may be indicative of a level of frustration around the slow progress in achieving true role development and the continued lack of career pathway for this specialty [22,23]. Despite much attention to such issues in the literature, minimal progress has been made in terms of developing career pathways in the Australian setting. In their Australian study, Parker et al. [23] identified that 85% of practice nurse participants did not have a career pathway in their organisation. Participants also reported a strong feeling that they were regarded as less important than their acute care colleagues [23]. Given the increasing emphasis on providing care within general practice to address the growing burden of chronic disease, there is an urgent need for peak bodies and policy makers to address the workforce issues to promote the retention of skilled, motivated nurses.

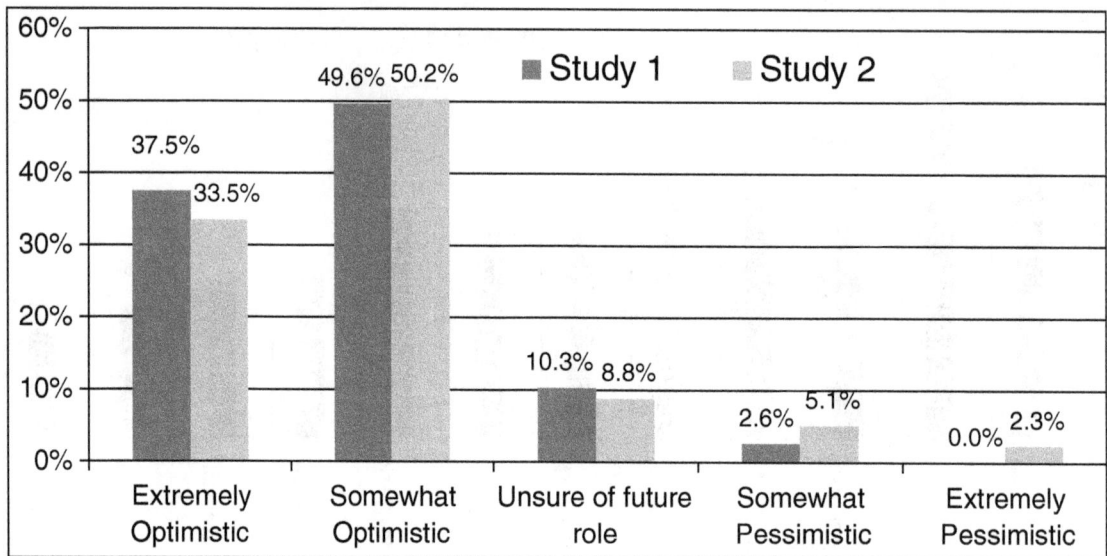

Figure 4 Levels of practice nurse optimism regarding role.

It was not clear from this study how many participants had undergone specific formal education programs focussed on general practice nursing. It is recognised that there are limited opportunities for specific formal higher education programs for nurses within general practice [24]. The continuing professional development needs of Australian nurses working in general practice are currently more likely to be met by short courses and workshops [22,24]. Data from this study highlighted the need for focussed education and training to support the nurses' role.

The limited uptake in postgraduate programs is an impediment to role development as ad hoc training sessions do not provide the structured learning and professional development necessary for advanced roles. In their review of the impact of Masters level education on patient care, Cotterill-Walker [25] identified that graduates demonstrate increased confidence and self-esteem; enhanced communication; personal and professional growth; knowledge and application of theory to practise; and analytical thinking and decision making following completion of their programs. Similarly, Drennan [26] identified that Masters graduates demonstrated significant gains in leadership and management skills as a result of completing their higher degree. Despite the existence of some postgraduate programs for practice nurses in Australia, the uptake of these programs has been variable. Barriers such as cost, lack of familiarity with university education, time commitment and lack of perceived value by practice management have been identified as impediments to PNs undertaking postgraduate programs [22]. As part of developing a career framework, attention needs to be paid to developing a formal education pathway to enhance the clinical and professional skills of nurses in the general practice setting.

Patients' perceptions of the role of nurses within general practice were seen by the nurses to be much less of a barrier in the second survey. This is supported by findings from both Australia and New Zealand which identify that consumers are largely satisfied with practice nurse services and comfortable with the nurse role in general practice [27-29]. A barrier across both surveys was the perceived lack of collaboration with GPs. This is significant in general practice given the frequent employee/employer relationship between PNs and GPs. It highlights the need for strategies to be implemented to promote the kind of multidisciplinary teamwork that has been demonstrated to improve health outcomes. The concerns expressed by participants in this study about GPs understanding the nurses' scope of practice, unwillingness to delegate tasks, variation in practice between GPs and unwillingness to delegate are echoed by the experience of McCarthy et al. [24] in Ireland. McCarthy et al. [24] demonstrated that despite some congruence of opinion between GPs and PNs, there remained a degree of divergent opinion regarding the nursing roles, with GPs underestimating the PN scope of practice. Similarly, in their study of culturally and linguistically diverse solo Australian GPs, Halcomb et al. [30] reported that GPs did not feel confident about the roles of nurses and their scope of practice. A factor complicating this issue in the Australian setting is the employment of both EN and RNs in general practice. The different educational preparation and subsequent scopes of practice of EN and RNs adds complexity, particularly for GPs in understanding the nursing role. Whilst there have been attempts to improve teamwork between GPs and nurses, implementing a truly multidisciplinary model of care in Australian general practice requires organisational changes [24,31]. The growing burden of chronic and complex disease facing primary care, and the high level evidence to support the efficacy of multidisciplinary models of care, underscores the importance of actively striving towards such models of care.

This study has a number of limitations. Firstly, the sampling frame and method of this survey challenge the representativeness of this sample. With no means of identifying the population of nurses employed in general practice in either time period it is not possible to calculate a response denominator. Additionally, the sample size is small considering the growing nursing workforce in Australian general practice. However, the sampling techniques used in this study are similar to those used in other Australian investigations and the sample size comparable to others reported in the literature [18,24]. Like any survey, the data collected in these investigations was self-reported and therefore may be subject to recall bias. However, these data provide an important snapshot of trends over time in the Australian general practice nursing workforce. They also underscore the need for data collection methods to monitor issues in human resources for health not just in the general practice setting but globally [32].

Australian general practice is in a dynamic state of growth and faces both challenges and opportunities. As changes occur within this environment these have flow on effects to both the nursing workforce and its role in providing clinical care. There is an increased strategic emphasis on the importance of primary care and primary health care organisations. These data suggest the importance of workforce factors in driving general practice reforms. As in many areas of nursing, retention is a critical concern and this is linked to satisfaction in the workplace. Increasing the emphasis on the specialisation of nursing in primary care will continue to be an important strategic initiative. In order to achieve this, an increased professional profile, including in undergraduate and post graduate nursing courses will be critical. Promoting models of interdisciplinary practice and role definition and refinement may also be of use.

Conclusion

This study has provided a snapshot across two critical time periods in Australian general practice and provides useful information for nursing workforce planning and models of care. It has identified some of the structural organisational barriers to the nurses role in general practice. The results demonstrate that although strategies to develop workforce capacity have made some inroads to supporting the general practice nurse workforce to grow their role, further attention to workforce development is required. There is a clear need to build structured career pathways with embedded formal practice nurse education

programs to facilitate transition of the practice nurse from novice to clinical expert.

These data also emphasise the importance of promoting teamwork and collaborative practice in Australian primary care. They highlight the need to promote interprofessional collaboration and teamwork between GPs and nurses, as well as open discussions between clinicians about how they can best contribute to health care within their professional scope of practice.

Competing interests
The authors declare that they have no competing interests.

Author contributions
Study Design (EH, YS, PD), Data Collection and Analyses (EH, YS, PD, RK, SY), Manuscript Preparation (EH, YS, PD, RK, SY). All authors read and approved the final manuscript.

Acknowledgements
This study would not have been possible without the enthusiastic assistance of the general practice nurses who responded to the survey. We also wish to thank the Australian Practice Nurses Association, Royal Australian College of Nursing and Divisions of General Practice, in particular Western Sydney, St George, Mid-North Coast, Wide Bay, North Shore & ACT Divisions, for their assistance with survey distribution.

Funding
EH was a doctoral candidate supported by an Australian Postgraduate Award from the Australian Department of Education and Training and a Top-Up grant from the University of Western Sydney at the time of the initial survey. A Research Seed Grant from the University of Western Sydney funded the conduct of the initial survey. The second survey was funded by a Research Grant from the University of Western Sydney.

Author details
[1]School of Nursing & Midwifery, University of Wollongong, Sydney, Australia. [2]School of Nursing & Midwifery, University of Western Sydney, Sydney, Australia. [3]Johns Hopkins University School of Nursing, Baltimore, USA. [4]University of New South Wales, Sydney, Australia. [5]University of Newcastle, Sydney, Australia.

References
1. Nursing and Midwifery Boards of Australia: *National competency standards for the registered nurse.* Melbourne, Victoria: Nursing and Midwifery Board of Australia; 2006.
2. Australian Nursing Federation: *Competency standards for nurses in general practice.* Melbourne, Australia: Australian Nursing Federation; 2005.
3. Joyce CM, Piterman L: **The work of nurses in Australian general practice: a national survey.** *Int J Nurs Stud* 2011, **48**(1):70–80.
4. Royal College of Nursing: *Agenda for Change and nurses employed outside the NHS.* London, England: RCN Direct; 2004.
5. Prior P, Wilkinson J, Neville S: **Practice nurse use of evidence in clinical practice: a descriptive study.** *Nurs Prax N Z* 2010, **26**(2):14–25.
6. Redsell SA, Cheater FM: **Nurses' roles in primary care: developments and future prospects.** *Qual Prim Care* 2008, **16**(2):69–71.
7. Parker RM, Keleher HM, Francis K, Abdulwadud O: **Practice nursing in Australia: a review of education and career pathways.** *BMC Nursing* 2009, **8:**6p.
8. Halcomb EJ, Davidson PM, Salamonson Y, Ollerton R: **Nurses in Australian general practice: Implications for chronic disease management.** *J Clin Nurs* 2008, **17**(5A):6–15.
9. Halcomb EJ, Davidson PM, Brown N: **Uptake of Medicare chronic disease items in Australia by practice nurses and Aboriginal health workers.** *Collegian* 2010, **17**(2):57–61.
10. Halcomb E, Moujalli S, Griffiths R, Davidson P: **Effectiveness of general practice nurse interventions in cardiac risk factor reduction among adults.** *Int J Evid Based Healthc* 2007, **5**(3):269–295.

11. Senior E: **How general practice nurses view their expanding role.** *Aust J Adv Nurs* 2008, **26**(1):8–15.
12. Halcomb EJ, Peters K, McInnes S: **Practice nurses experiences of mentoring undergraduate nursing students in Australian general practice.** *Nurse Educ Today* 2012, **32**(5):524–528.
13. Knight AW, Ford D, Audehm R, Colagiuri S, Best J: **The Australian Primary Care Collaboratives Program: improving diabetes care.** *BMJ Qual Saf* 2012, **21**(11):956–963.
14. Australian Divisions of General Practice Ltd.: **National practice nurse workforce survey 2003.** http://amlalliance.com.au/__data/assets/pdf_file/0007/46735/2003-National-Practice-Nurse-Workforce-Survey.pdf.
15. Australian General Practice Network: **National practice nurse workforce survey 2009.** http://amlalliance.com.au/__data/assets/pdf_file/0005/46733/2009-National-Practice-Nurse-Workforce-Survey.pdf.
16. Patterson EA, Del Mar C, Najman J: **Medical receptionists in general practice: who needs a nurse?** *Int J Nurs Pract* 2000, **6**:229–236.
17. Pascoe T, Foley E, Hutchinson R, Watts I, Whitecross L, Snowdon T: **The changing face of nurses in Australian general practice.** *Aust J Adv Nurs* 2005, **23**(1):44–50.
18. Watts I, Foley E, Hutchinson R, Pascoe T, Whitecross L, Snowdon T: *General practice nursing in Australia.* Canberra, ACT: Royal Australian College of General Practitioners and Royal College of Nursing, Australia; 2004.
19. Joyce CM, Piterman L: **Farewell to the handmaiden? Profile of nurses in Australian general practice in 2007.** *Aust J Adv Nurs* 2009, **27**(1):48–58.
20. Joyce CM, Piterman L: **Nurse-patient encounters in general practice: patterns in general practitioner involvement and use of nurse-specific Medicare items.** *Aust J Prim Health* 2010, **16**(3):224–230.
21. Halcomb EJ, Davidson PM, Griffiths R, Daly J: **Cardiovascular disease management: time to advance the practice nurse role?** *Aust Health Rev* 2008, **32**(1):44–55.
22. Halcomb EJ, Davidson PM: *Practice Nurse Continuing Professional Development Program Evaluation.* Australia: The Australian Government Department of Health and Ageing and the Australian Practice Nurses Association; 2009.
23. Parker R, Keleher H, Forrest L: **The work, education and career pathways of nurses in Australian general practice.** *Aust J Prim Health* 2011, **17**(3):227–232.
24. McCarthy G, Cornally N, Moran J, Courtney M: **Practice nurses and general practitioners: perspectives on the role and future development of practice nursing in Ireland.** *J Clin Nurs* 2012, **21**:2286–2295.
25. Cotterill-Walker SM: **Where is the evidence that master's level nursing education makes a difference to patient care? A literature review.** *Nurse Educ Today* 2012, **32**(1):57–64.
26. Drennan J: **Masters in nursing degrees: an evaluation of management and leadership outcomes using a retrospective pre-test design.** *J Nurs Manag* 2012, **20**(1):102–112.
27. Halcomb EJ, Caldwell B, Davidson PM, Salamonson Y: **Development and psychometric validation of the General Practice Nurse Satisfaction Scale.** *J Nurs Scholarsh* 2011, **43**(3):318–327.
28. Halcomb EJ, Peters K, Davies D: **A qualitative evaluation of New Zealand consumers perceptions of general practice nurses.** *BMC Fam Pract* 2013, **14**(26). http://www.biomedcentral.com/1471-2296/14/26.
29. Halcomb E, Davies D, Salamonson Y: **Consumer satisfaction with practice nursing: a cross-sectional survey in New Zealand general practice.** *Aust J Prim Health.* in press.
30. Halcomb EJ, Salamonson Y, Cooper MK, Clausen JL, Lombardo L: **Culturally and linguistically diverse general practitioners' utilisation of practice nurse.** *Collegian* 2013, **20**(3):137–144.
31. Black DA, Taggart J, Jayasinghe UW, Proudfoot J, Crookes P, Beilby J, Powell-Davies G, Wilson LA, Harris MF: **The Teamwork Study: enhancing the role of non-GP staff in chronic disease management in general practice.** *Aust J Prim Health* 2013, **19**(3):184–189.
32. Zurn P, Dal Poz MR, Stilwell B, Adams O: **Imbalance in the health workforce.** *Hum Resour Health* 2004, **2**(1):13.

Permissions

All chapters in this book were first published in FP, by BioMed Central; hereby published with permission under the Creative Commons Attribution License or equivalent. Every chapter published in this book has been scrutinized by our experts. Their significance has been extensively debated. The topics covered herein carry significant findings which will fuel the growth of the discipline. They may even be implemented as practical applications or may be referred to as a beginning point for another development.

The contributors of this book come from diverse backgrounds, making this book a truly international effort. This book will bring forth new frontiers with its revolutionizing research information and detailed analysis of the nascent developments around the world.

We would like to thank all the contributing authors for lending their expertise to make the book truly unique. They have played a crucial role in the development of this book. Without their invaluable contributions this book wouldn't have been possible. They have made vital efforts to compile up to date information on the varied aspects of this subject to make this book a valuable addition to the collection of many professionals and students.

This book was conceptualized with the vision of imparting up-to-date information and advanced data in this field. To ensure the same, a matchless editorial board was set up. Every individual on the board went through rigorous rounds of assessment to prove their worth. After which they invested a large part of their time researching and compiling the most relevant data for our readers.

The editorial board has been involved in producing this book since its inception. They have spent rigorous hours researching and exploring the diverse topics which have resulted in the successful publishing of this book. They have passed on their knowledge of decades through this book. To expedite this challenging task, the publisher supported the team at every step. A small team of assistant editors was also appointed to further simplify the editing procedure and attain best results for the readers.

Apart from the editorial board, the designing team has also invested a significant amount of their time in understanding the subject and creating the most relevant covers. They scrutinized every image to scout for the most suitable representation of the subject and create an appropriate cover for the book.

The publishing team has been an ardent support to the editorial, designing and production team. Their endless efforts to recruit the best for this project, has resulted in the accomplishment of this book. They are a veteran in the field of academics and their pool of knowledge is as vast as their experience in printing. Their expertise and guidance has proved useful at every step. Their uncompromising quality standards have made this book an exceptional effort. Their encouragement from time to time has been an inspiration for everyone.

The publisher and the editorial board hope that this book will prove to be a valuable piece of knowledge for researchers, students, practitioners and scholars across the globe.

List of Contributors

Jodi Gray, Hossein Haji Ali Afzali and Jonathan Karnon
Discipline of Public Health, The University of Adelaide, Adelaide, South Australia

Justin Beilby
Faculty of Health Sciences, The University of Adelaide, Adelaide, South Australia

Christine Holton
Discipline of General Practice, The University of Adelaide, Adelaide, South Australia

David Banham
Office for Research Development, Health System Performance Division, SA Health, Adelaide, South Australia

Sonja ME van Dillen and Gerrit J Hiddink
Strategic Communication, Section Communication, Philosophy and Technology, Centre for Integrative Development (CPT-CID), Wageningen University, 6700 EW Wageningen, the Netherlands

Rebecca Lorch and Rebecca Guy
The Kirby Institute, University of New South Wales, Sydney, NSW, Australia

Jane Hocking, Alaina Vaisey, Anna Wood and Dyani Lewis
Melbourne School of Population and Global Health, University of Melbourne, Melbourne, VIC, Australia

Meredith Temple-Smith
Department of General Practice, University of Melbourne, Melbourne, VIC, Australia

Annemieke P. Bikker, Bridie Fitzpatrick and Stewart W. Mercer
General Practice and Primary Care, Institute of Health and Wellbeing, University of Glasgow, 1 Horselethill Road, Glasgow G12 9LX, UK

Douglas Murphy
School of Medicine, University of Dundee, Mackenzie Building, Kirsty Semple Way, Dundee DD2 4BF, UK

Verena Schadewaldt
Faculty of Health Sciences, School of Nursing Midwifery and Paramedicine, Australian Catholic University, Melbourne, Australia

Elizabeth McInnes
Nursing Research Institute, St Vincent's Health Australia/Australian Catholic University, Sydney, Australia

Janet E. Hiller
School of Health Sciences, Faculty of Health, Arts and Design, Swinburne University of Technology, Melbourne, Australia
School of Public Health, University of Adelaide, Adelaide, Australia

Anne Gardner
Faculty of Health Sciences, School of Nursing, Midwifery and Paramedicine, Australian Catholic University, Canberra, Australia
James Cook University, Townsville, Australia

Susan E. van Dijk, Judith E. Bosmans, Marcel C. Adriaanse and Maurits W. van Tulder
Department of Health Sciences and the EMGO Institute for Health and Care Research, Vrije Universiteit, Amsterdam, De Boelelaan 1085, 1081 HV Amsterdam, The Netherlands

Alide D. Pols
Department of Health Sciences and the EMGO Institute for Health and Care Research, Vrije Universiteit, Amsterdam, De Boelelaan 1085, 1081 HV Amsterdam, The Netherlands
Department of General Practice & Elderly Care Medicine and EMGO Institute for Health and Care Research, VU University Medical Centre, Amsterdam, The Netherlands

Debbie Overkamp
Department of General Practice & Elderly Care Medicine and EMGO Institute for Health and Care Research, VU University Medical Centre, Amsterdam, The Netherlands

Harm W. J. van Marwijk
Department of General Practice & Elderly Care
Medicine and EMGO Institute for Health and
Care Research, VU University Medical Centre,
Amsterdam, The Netherlands
CLAHRC Greater Manchester and NIHR School
for Primary Care Research, the University of
Manchester, Manchester, UK

Karen Schipper
Department of Medical Humanities, EMGO+
Institute, VU Medical Centre (VUmc), Amsterdam,
The Netherlands

Mieke Van Der Biezen
Radboud Institute for Health Sciences, Scientific
Center for Quality of Healthcare, Radboud
University Medical Center, The Netherlands

Michel Wensing
Radboud Institute for Health Sciences, Scientific
Center for Quality of Healthcare, Radboud
University Medical Center, The Netherlands
Department of General Practice and Health Services
Research, Heidelberg University, INF Marsilius
Arkaden, Heidelberg, Germany

Miranda Laurant
Radboud Institute for Health Sciences, Scientific
Center for Quality of Healthcare, Radboud
University Medical Center, The Netherlands
Faculty of Health and Social Studies, HAN
University of Applied Sciences, The Netherlands

Eddy Adang
Department for Health Evidence, Radboud Institute
for Health Sciences, Radboud University Medical
Center, The Netherlands

Regi Van Der Burgt
Foundation for Development of Quality Care in
General Practice, Tilburgseweg-West 100, 5652 NP
Eindhoven, The Netherlands

Mandy M N Stijnen
Department of Family Medicine, School for Public
Health and Primary Care (CAPHRI), Faculty of
Health, Medicine and Life Sciences, Maastricht
University, 6200 MD Maastricht, The Netherlands

Inge G P Duimel-Peeters
Department of Family Medicine, School for Public
Health and Primary Care (CAPHRI), Faculty of
Health, Medicine and Life Sciences, Maastricht
University, 6200 MD Maastricht, The Netherlands

Department of Patient and Care, Maastricht
University Medical Centre, 6202 MD Maastricht,
The Netherlands.

Maria W J Jansen
Public Health Service South-Limburg, 6160 HA
Geleen, The Netherlands Department of Health
Services Research, School for Public Health and
Primary Care (CAPHRI), Faculty of Health,
Medicine and Life Sciences, Maastricht University,
6200 MD Maastricht, The Netherlands

Hubertus J M Vrijhoef
Tilburg School of Social and Behavioral Sciences,
Scientific Centre for Care and Welfare (TRANZO),
Tilburg University, 5000 LE Tilburg, The Netherlands
SawSwee Hock School of Public Health, National
University of Singapore, MD3, 16 Medical Drive,
Singapore 117597, Republic of Singapore

Vivian Midtbø
National Centre for Emergency Primary Health
Care, Uni Research Health, NO 5020 Bergen,
Norway

Guttorm Raknes
National Centre for Emergency Primary Health
Care, Uni Research Health, NO 5020 Bergen,
Norway
Regional Medicines Information & Pharmacovigilance
Centre (RELIS), University Hospital of North Norway,
NO 9038 Tromsø, Norway
Raknes Research, Myrdalskogen 243, NO 5117
Ulset, Norway

Steinar Hunskaar
National Centre for Emergency Primary Health
Care, Uni Research Health, NO 5020 Bergen,
Norway
Department of Global Public Health and Primary
Care, University of Bergen, NO 5018 Bergen,
Norway

**Kirsten J. Coppell, Kiri Sharp and Joanna K.
Norton**
Edgar Diabetes and Obesity Research, Department
of Medicine, Dunedin School of Medicine, University
of Otago, Dunedin 9054, New Zealand

Sally L. Abel
Kaupapa Consulting Ltd, Napier 4110, New Zealand

Trish Freer, Terrie Spedding and Lillian Ward
Health Hawke's Bay – Te Oranga Hawke's Bay,
Hastings 4158, New Zealand

Andrew Gray
Department of Preventive and Social Medicine, Dunedin School of Medicine, University of Otago, Dunedin 9054, New Zealand

Lisa C. Whitehead
School of Nursing and Midwifery, Edith Cowan University, 270 Joondalup Drive, Joondalup 6027, Australia

Nicholas Magill and Sabine Landau
Department of Biostatistics and Health Informatics, Institute of Psychiatry, Psychology and Neuroscience, King's College London, 16 De Crespigny Park, London SE5 8AF, UK

Helen Graves, Nicole de Zoysa and Kirsty Winkley
Department of Psychological Medicine, Institute of Psychiatry, Psychology and Neuroscience, King's College London, London, UK

Khalida Ismail
Department of Psychological Medicine, Institute of Psychiatry, Psychology and Neuroscience, King's College London, London, UK
Institute of Diabetes, Endocrinology and Obesity, King's Health Partners, London, UK

Stephanie Amiel and Emma Shuttlewood
Diabetes and Nutritional Sciences Division, School of Medicine, King's College London, London, UK

Maurits W. van Tulder and Marcel C. Adriaanse
Department of Health Sciences, Amsterdam Public Health Research Institute, Faculty of Science, Vrije Universiteit Amsterdam, Amsterdam, the Netherlands

Alide D. Pols
Department of Health Sciences, Amsterdam Public Health Research Institute, Faculty of Science, Vrije Universiteit Amsterdam, Amsterdam, the Netherlands
Amsterdam Public Health Research Institute, Department of General Practice & Elderly Care Medicine, Amsterdam UMC, Vrije Universiteit Amsterdam, Amsterdam, the Netherlands

Debbie Overkamp
Amsterdam Public Health Research Institute, Department of General Practice & Elderly Care Medicine, Amsterdam UMC, Vrije Universiteit Amsterdam, Amsterdam, the Netherlands

Harm W. J. van Marwijk
Amsterdam Public Health Research Institute, Department of General Practice & Elderly Care Medicine, Amsterdam UMC, Vrije Universiteit Amsterdam, Amsterdam, the Netherlands
Division of Primary Care and Public Health, Brighton and Sussex Medical School, Mayfield House, University of Brighton, Brighton, UK

Karen Schipper
Amsterdam Public Health Research Institute, Department of Medical Humanities, Amsterdam UMC, Vrije Universiteit Amsterdam, Amsterdam, the Netherlands

Heleen Westland and Jaap C. A. Trappenburg
Julius Center for Health Sciences and Primary Care, University Medica Center Utrecht, HP Str. 6.131, 3508, GA, Utrecht, The Netherlands

Yvonne Koop
Department of Cardiology, Radboud University Medical Center, Nijmegen The Netherlands

Carin D. Schröder
Center of Excellence in Rehabilitation Medicine, Brain Center Rudolf Magnus, University Medical Center Utrecht, University Utrecht and De Hoogstraat Rehabilitation, Utrecht, the Netherlands

P. Slabbers
Department of Acute Psychiatry, Psychiatric Center GGZ Central, Amersfoort, The Netherlands

Sigrid C. J. M. Vervoort
Cancer Center, University Medical Center Utrecht, Utrecht, The Netherlands

Marieke J. Schuurmans
Education Center, UMC Utrecht Academy, University Medical Center Utrecht, Utrecht University, Utrecht, The Netherlands

H. T. Bell
Department of Pharmacy, Faculty of Health Sciences, Nord University, Namsos, Norway
Department of Public Health and General Practice, Norwegian University of Science and Technology, Trondheim, Norway

R. Omli
Department of Pharmacy, Faculty of Health Sciences, Nord University, Namsos, Norway
Centre for Care research Mid- Norway, Steinkjer, Norway

A. Steinsbekk
Department of Public Health and General Practice, Norwegian University of Science and Technology, Trondheim, Norway

A. G. Granas
School of Pharmacy, University of Oslo, Oslo, Norway

I. Enmarker
Centre for Care research Mid- Norway, Steinkjer, Norway
Department of Nursing, Mid University, Østersund, Sweden

Rachael C Walker
Hawkes Bay District Health Board, Hastings, New Zealand
Sydney School of Public Health, Sydney Medical School, University of Sydney, Sydney, Australia

Mark R Marshall
Counties Manukau District Health Board, Auckland, New Zealand
Faculty of Medical and Health Sciences, University of Auckland, Auckland, New Zealand

Nick R Polaschek
Sector Capability and Implementation, Ministry of Health, Wellington, New Zealand

Karen Lorimer
Institute for Applied Health Research, Glasgow Caledonian University, School of Health and Life Sciences, Cowcaddens Road, Glasgow G4 0BA, Scotland

Susan Martin and Lisa M McDaid
MRC/CSO Social and Public Health Sciences Unit, University of Glasgow, 200 Renfield Street, Glasgow G2 3QB, Scotland

Elizabeth J Halcomb
School of Nursing & Midwifery, University of Wollongong, Sydney, Australia

Yenna Salamonson
School of Nursing & Midwifery, University of Western Sydney, Sydney, Australia

Patricia M Davidson
Johns Hopkins University School of Nursing, Baltimore, USA

Rajneesh Kaur
University of New South Wales, Sydney, Australia

Samantha AM Young
University of Newcastle, Sydney, Australia

Index

www.ingramcontent.com/pod-product-compliance
Lightning Source LLC
Chambersburg PA
CBHW082017190326
41458CB00010B/3213